Macleod's
Clinical
Diagnosis

Macleod's

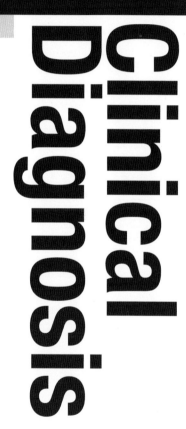

3rd Edition

Euan A Sandilands

MBChB BSc(Hons) MD FRCPE PGCertMedEd

Consultant Physician
Clinical Toxicology & Acute Medicine
Royal Infirmary of Edinburgh
Honorary Clinical Senior Lecturer
University of Edinburgh
Edinburgh, Scotland

Emma E Morrison

MBChB(Hons) PhD BSc(Hons) MRCP

Consultant Physician
Clinical Toxicology
Acute Medicine & Medicines Management
Royal Infirmary of Edinburgh
Edinburgh, Scotland

A Toby Merriman

MBChB BSc(Hons) MRCP

Specialist Registrar
Acute Medicine
Royal Infirmary of Edinburgh
Edinburgh, Scotland

ELSEVIER

First edition 2013
Second edition 2018
Third edition 2025

ISBN: 978-0-443-12503-4
     978-0-443-12504-1

Printed in China by 1010 Printing International Ltd

Last digit is the print number: 9 8 7 6 5 4 3 2 1

Content Strategist: Jeremy Bowes
Content Project Manager: Shravan Kumar
Design: Miles Hitchen
Marketing Manager: Deborah Watkins

Working together to grow libraries in developing countries

www.elsevier.com • www.bookaid.org

Contents

Preface

This is the third edition of *Macleod's Clinical Diagnosis*. Traditionally, medical education has focused on the core clinical skills of history taking and clinical examination, with platitudes such as '90% of diagnoses are made from the history' and 'clinical examination is the cornerstone of assessment' being commonplace. While these skills are critical for every clinician, it is important to understand how they fit into a contemporary clinical environment.

Our aim is to show you how to practically use your core clinical skills to maximum advantage in the modern clinical world of novel imaging techniques and point-of-care testing. Each chapter takes the reader through the diagnostic pathway, highlighting the importance of the core clinical skills in formulating a working and differential diagnosis. We then demonstrate how these core skills not only complement but can direct the use of diagnostic techniques to refine the differential.

This edition is brought to you by a new editorial team. For this updated edition, we have focused on common acute medical presentations that you are likely to come across in any acute medical unit. New chapters on poisoning and acute kidney injury have been included, while all other chapters have been updated to reflect current clinical practice. We would like specifically to acknowledge the valued contribution made by Mr Stafford Samsone, Ophthalmology Registrar, to Chapter 16. Overall, we are confident that these changes to this edition have allowed us to produce a revitalised textbook, and we hope you find it a useful and valuable resource.

Euan A Sandilands
Emma E Morrison
A Toby Merriman

Abbreviations

Abbreviations that do not appear in this list are spelled out in the main text.

AAA	abdominal aortic aneurysm	**bpm**	beats per minute
ABCDE	airway, breathing, circulation, disability, exposure	**BPPV**	benign paroxysmal positional vertigo
		BS	breath sound
ABG	arterial blood gas	**BSA**	body surface area
ABPI	ankle-brachial pressure index	**CAD**	coronary artery disease
ACE	angiotensin-converting enzyme	**CAP**	community-acquired pneumonia
ACPA	anti-citrullinated protein antibody	**CBG**	capillary blood glucose
ACS	acute coronary syndrome	**CCF**	congestive cardiac failure
ACTH	adrenocorticotrophic hormone	**CCU**	critical care unit
ADH	antidiuretic hormone	**CDT**	*C difficile* toxin
AF	atrial fibrillation	**CK**	creatine kinase
AGEP	acute generalized exanthematous pustulosis	**CKD**	chronic kidney disease
		CLO	*campylobacter*-like organism
AIDS	acquired immunodeficiency syndrome	**CMV**	cytomegalovirus
AIN	acute interstitial nephritis	**CNS**	central nervous system
AKI	acute kidney injury	**CO**	carbon monoxide
ALP	alkaline phosphatase	**COHb**	carboxyhaemoglobin
ALT	alanine aminotransferase	**COPD**	chronic obstructive pulmonary disease
AMA	antimitochondrial antibody	**CPET**	cardiopulmonary exercise test
ANA	antinuclear antibody	**CRP**	C-reactive protein
ANCA	antineutrophil cytoplasmic antibody	**CRS**	cardiorenal syndrome
APKD	adult polycystic kidney disease	**CRT**	capillary refill time
APTT	activated partial thromboplastin time	**CSF**	cerebrospinal fluid
ARDS	acute respiratory distress syndrome	**CSU**	catheter specimen of urine
AS	ankylosing spondylitis	**CT**	computed tomogram/tomography
ASMA	anti-smooth muscle antibody	**CTKUB**	computed tomography of kidneys, ureters and bladder
ASO	anti-streptolysin O		
AST	aspartate aminotransferase	**CTPA**	computed tomographic pulmonary angiography
AT	atrial tachycardia		
ATN	acute tubular necrosis	**CVP**	central venous pressure
AV	atrioventricular	**CVST**	cerebral venous sinus thrombosis
AVNRT	atrioventricular nodal reentry tachycardia	**CXR**	chest X-ray
AVRT	atrioventricular reentry tachycardia	**DAT**	direct antiglobulin test
AXR	abdominal X-ray	**DC**	direct current
BG	blood glucose	**DEXA**	dual-energy X-ray absorptiometry
BMI	body mass index	**DIC**	disseminated intravascular coagulation
BNP	brain-type natriuretic peptide (test)	**DIP**	distal interphalangeal
BP	blood pressure	**DKA**	diabetes-related ketoacidosis
BPH	benign prostatic hyperplasia	**DMARD**	disease-modifying anti-rheumatic drug

DOAC	direct oral anticoagulation		**JVP**	jugular venous pulse
DRESS	drug reaction with eosinophilia and systemic symptoms (syndrome)		**LBBB**	left bundle branch block
DVT	deep vein thrombosis		**LDH**	lactate dehydrogenase
EBV	Epstein–Barr virus		**LFT**	liver function test
ECF	extracellular fluid		**LIF**	left iliac fossa
ECG	electrocardiogram/electrocardiography		**LKM**	liver kidney microsomal (antibodies)
EEG	electroencephalogram/electroencephalography		**LLQ**	left lower quadrant
			LMN	lower motor neuron
ENA	extractable nuclear antigen		**LP**	lumbar puncture
ENT	ear, nose and throat		**LUQ**	left upper quadrant
ERCP	endoscopic retrograde cholangiopancreatography		**LV**	left ventricular
			LVH	left ventricular hypertrophy
ESR	erythrocyte sedimentation rate		**MAP**	mean arterial pressure
FBC	full blood count		**MI**	myocardial infarction
FEV1	forced expiratory volume		**MND**	motor neuron disease
FiO$_2$	fraction of inspired oxygen		**MRA**	magnetic resonance angiography
FND	functional neurological disorder		**MRCP**	magnetic resonance cholangiopancreatography
GBM	glomerular basement membrane (renal)		**MRI**	magnetic resonance imaging
GBS	Glasgow-Blatchford score		**MS**	multiple sclerosis
GCA	giant cell arteritis		**MSU**	midstream urine (specimen)
GCS	Glasgow Coma Scale (score)		**NCSE**	nonconvulsive status ellipticus
GDS	Geriatric Depression Scale		**NG**	nasogastric
GFR	glomerular filtration rate		**NSAID**	non-steroidal anti-inflammatory drug
GGT	gamma-glutamyl transferase		**NSTEMI**	non-ST-elevation myocardial infarction
GI	gastrointestinal		**N&V**	nausea and vomiting
GORD	gastro-oesophageal reflux disease		**OA**	osteoarthritis
GP	general practitioner		**OHS**	obesity hypoventilation syndrome
GPP	generalized pustular psoriasis		**PaCO$_2$**	partial pressure of carbon dioxide in arterial blood
GRACE	Global Registry of Acute Coronary Event (score)		**PaO$_2$**	partial pressure of oxygen in arterial blood
GTN	glyceryl trinitrate		**PACS**	partial anterior circulation stroke
GU	genitourinary		**PCR**	polymerase chain reaction
HAP	hospital-acquired pneumonia		**PE**	pulmonary embolism
Hb	haemoglobin		**PEFR**	peak expiratory flow rate
hCG	human chorionic gonadotrophin		**PET**	positron emission tomography
HDU	high-dependency unit		**PFTs**	pulmonary function tests
HHS	hyperosmolar hyperglycaemic state		**PID**	pelvic inflammatory disease
HIV	human immunodeficiency virus		**PIP**	proximal interphalangeal
HLA	human leukocyte antigen		**PND**	paroxysmal nocturnal dyspnoea
HR	heart rate		**PoCS**	posterior circulation stroke
IBD	inflammatory bowel disease		**PPI**	proton pump inhibitor
IBS	irritable bowel syndrome		**PR**	per rectum
ICP	intracranial pressure		**PRN**	pro re nata; whenever required
ICU	intensive care unit		**PSA**	prostate-specific antigen
ID	infectious disease		**PT**	prothrombin time
IIH	idiopathic intracranial hypertension		**PTH**	parathyroid hormone
ILD	interstitial lung disease		**PV**	per vaginam
IM	intramuscular(ly)		**PVST**	paroxysmal supraventricular tachycardia
INR	international normalized ratio		**qSOFA**	quick Sepsis Related Organ Failure Assessment
IV	intravenous(ly)			
IVU	intravenous urogram/urography			

QTc	corrected QT interval	**STEMI**	ST-elevation myocardial infarction
RBBB	right bundle branch block	**SVT**	supraventricular tachycardia
RF	rheumatoid factor	**TACS**	total anterior circulation stroke
RIF	right iliac fossa	**TB**	tuberculosis
RLQ	right lower quadrant	**TBSA**	total body surface area
RPGN	rapidly progressive glomerulonephritis	**TFT**	thyroid function test
RR	respiratory rate	**TIA**	transient ischaemic attack
RRT	renal replacement therapy	**TLC**	total lung capacity
RTI	respiratory tract infection	**TLOC**	transient loss of consciousness
RUQ	right upper quadrant	**TNF**	tumour necrosis factor
RV	residual volume	**TRAB**	thyroid receptor antibody
SA	sinoatrial	**TSH**	thyroid stimulating hormone
SAAG	serum-ascites albumin gradient	**TWI**	T wave inversion
SAH	subarachnoid haemorrhage	**UC**	ulcerative colitis
SaO$_2$	oxygen saturation of arterial blood	**U+E**	urea and electrolytes
SBP	spontaneous bacterial peritonitis	**UGIE**	upper gastrointestinal endoscopy
SC	subcutaneous(ly)	**UI**	urinary incontinence
SCAR	severe cutaneous adverse reaction	**UMN**	upper motor neuron
SIRS	systemic inflammatory response syndrome	**USS**	ultrasound scan
		UTI	urinary tract infection
SJS	Stevens-Johnson syndrome	**VA**	visual acuity
SLE	systemic lupus erythematosus	**VBG**	venous blood gas
SMA	smooth muscle antibody	**VQ scan**	ventilation/perfusion scan
SpO$_2$	peripheral (capillary) oxygen saturation	**VT**	ventricular tachycardia
SSRI	selective serotonin re-uptake inhibitor	**WBC**	white blood count

UKMLA Acute Medical Presentations and Where to Find Them

Patient presentation	Chapter	Revised?
Abdominal distension	7	
Abdominal mass	7	
Accidental poisoning	28	
Acute abdominal pain	7	
Acute change in or loss of vision	16	
Acute joint pain/swelling	18	
Acute rash	27	
Acute renal failure	29	
Altered sensation, numbness and tingling	14	
Anuria	29	
Ascites	7, 12	
Back pain	19	
Blackouts and faints	24	
Bleeding from the lower GI tract	8	
Bleeding from the upper GI tract	8	
Breathlessness	4	
Change in bowel habit	7, 8, 9	
Change in stool colour	8, 12	
Chest pain	3	
Chronic abdominal pain	7	
Chronic joint pain/stiffness	18	
Chronic rash	27	
Chronic renal failure	29	
Confusion	21	
Cough	4	
Decreased appetite	25	
Decreased/loss of consciousness	24	
Diarrhoea	9	
Diplopia	13, 14, 16	

Patient presentation	Chapter	Revised?
Skin ulcers	27	
Swallowing problems	10	
Symptoms of raised intracranial pressure (headache, vomiting, hypercalcaemia)	13	
Tinnitus	17	
Unsteadiness	17	
Vertigo	17	
Vomiting	11	
Weight loss	25	
Wheeze	4	

PART 1

The Diagnostic Process

The diagnostic process

1

The ability to diagnose accurately is fundamental to clinical practice. Only with a correct diagnosis is it possible to institute treatment, assess its effectiveness, give an informed prognosis and make follow-up arrangements. The exact method by which a diagnosis is reached will vary between clinicians. The best diagnosticians invariably use several complementary skills which have been honed through years of experience. This book aims to demonstrate how to make a diagnosis in the majority of commonly encountered clinical presentations.

Identification of an abnormality is often only the first step in the diagnostic process and additional assessments are required to characterize a condition in greater detail or search for an underlying cause. A *differential diagnosis* is a list of potential diagnoses, placed in order of likelihood, which may be causing the presentation. When assessing a patient, clinicians formulate a differential diagnosis as a stepping-stone to the final diagnosis. This list may be lengthy at the outset of the assessment but will progressively shorten as they accumulate information about the patient's condition through history-taking, examination and investigations. When one diagnosis begins to stand out from the rest as the most likely cause of the patient's presentation, it is often referred to as the *working diagnosis*. Investigations are then directed towards confirming (or refuting) this condition and thereby arriving at a *final diagnosis*. This entire process may happen very rapidly for acute presentations or may occur over a prolonged period (e.g., weeks) across several different contacts with healthcare professionals. Some conditions (e.g., irritable bowel syndrome) lack a definitive confirmatory test, and in this situation the diagnosis relies upon recognizing characteristic clinical features and ruling out alternative diagnoses. Such disorders are often referred to as *diagnoses of exclusion*.

Pattern recognition and probability analysis

Different diagnostic approaches are recognized in the literature, each with associated advantages and disadvantages. Experienced clinicians often rely on techniques such as pattern recognition and probability analysis. Pattern recognition can be a powerful technique, but it requires a clinician to have experienced a similar presentation previously, so it is less suited to the newcomer. Despite this, the most common diagnostic method utilized by medical students and junior doctors is a variant of this approach. In this case, their 'database' of patterns corresponds to the descriptions of signs and symptoms provided in textbooks rather than real-life examples. This has several limitations in that textbooks tend to present an idealized account of the way in which illnesses present, emphasizing classical signs and symptoms that may be absent in clinical practice. Furthermore, descriptions of physical signs from textbooks or lectures (e.g., pill-rolling tremor or festinating gait) are also poor substitutes for experiencing them first-hand in the clinical environment.

Probability analysis considers that diagnostic tests are inherently imperfect, so diagnoses are often regarded as statements of probability rather than hard facts. In practice, a disease is 'ruled in' when the probability of it being present is deemed to be sufficiently high, and 'ruled out' when the probability is sufficiently low. The degree of certainty depends on factors such as the consequences of missing the particular diagnosis, the side effects of treatment, and the risks of further testing. The diagnostic approach to subarachnoid haemorrhage (SAH) illustrates this. For a middle-aged patient who presents, fully conscious, with a history of sudden (within a few seconds) onset of 'the worst headache ever', the chances of a diagnosis of SAH are approximately 10%–12%. The presence of some clinical findings (e.g., photophobia, neck stiffness, cranial nerve palsies, subhyaloid haemorrhage) will increase these chances markedly, but these features may take time to develop. Even if the clinical examination is unequivocally normal, the chances of SAH are 8%–10%. Currently, there is no simple bedside test for SAH, and the initial investigation is normally a noncontrast CT scan. A positive scan will prompt appropriate treatment, possibly involving neurosurgical or neuroradiological intervention. A negative scan does not, however, exclude an SAH. The accuracy of CT scanning in detecting SAH depends on the experience of the reporting individual, the nature of the scanner (principally, its resolution), and the time interval between the onset of symptoms and the scan (accuracy falls with time). A scan performed within 6 hours by most modern scanners and interpreted by a skilled radiologist has a diagnostic accuracy of between 95% and 100%. This level of accuracy is seen as satisfactory to exclude an SAH. Therefore the patient is not put through the risk of a further diagnostic procedure. However, if the CT scan is done more than 6 hours after the onset of the headache, accuracy drops to between 85% and 90%. Given the morbidity and mortality of unrecognized and untreated SAH, this level of diagnostic accuracy is inadequate. For this reason, patients with a negative CT scan 6 hours after the onset of headache undergo a lumbar puncture. The cerebrospinal fluid (CSF) obtained must be examined by spectrophotometry in the laboratory for xanthochromia. Xanthochromia (produced from haemoglobin breakdown within the CSF) takes some time to develop, and the sensitivity of this test peaks at about 12 hours after symptom onset. The combination of a negative CT scan performed within 12 hours of symptom onset and normal CSF findings at 12 hours reduces the chances of the patient's symptoms being caused by an SAH to well below 1%—a level of probability acceptable to most clinicians and, if appropriately explained, to their patients.

Medically unexplained symptoms

Sometimes it is difficult to correlate a patient's symptoms with a specific disease. This does not mean that the symptoms are factitious or that they are malingering, merely that we are unable to identify a physical cause for the symptoms. A proportion have symptoms that cannot be readily explained by a specific diagnosis. Nevertheless, the symptoms are very real to the patient, and one of the major challenges, intellectually and practically, is to recognize which patients have organic disease.

Clusters of symptoms in recognizable patterns, in the absence of physical and investigational abnormalities, are called *functional disorders* (e.g., chronic fatigue syndrome, irritable bowel syndrome, chronic pain syndrome). Although it is important to investigate appropriately when there is any concern about underlying organic pathology, it is equally important to avoid excessive and inappropriate investigations if they are not indicated, especially when there are no specific 'red flags' in the history, they are not in a recognized at-risk group, and there are no abnormalities on clinical examination and simple bedside tests.

Treatment before diagnosis

In some situations, accurate diagnosis depends upon the patient's response to treatment. In certain scenarios, this may be life saving as well as diagnostic. Clinical examples where immediate treatment is required and acts as both a diagnostic tool and therapeutic intervention include the treatment of hypoglycaemia in a patient with altered consciousness or the administration of naloxone in a patient with a reduced level of consciousness and respiratory function resulting from opiate toxicity.

A diagnostic guide

Until clinicians gain sufficient knowledge and experience that the diagnostic process becomes second nature, we advocate a system of individual 'diagnostic guides' for the major presenting clinical problems. With experience, you will start to use your own unique methods but, at the outset, following an established framework may help to prevent potentially damaging errors.

Each chapter in Part 2 is a diagnostic guide or 'road map' for a common clinical presentation. The purpose of the guides is not to tell you which questions to ask and which examination steps to perform, but instead to explain how to use the information you have extracted from the history, examination and initial tests to work towards a final diagnosis.

To do this, we focus on the most valuable pieces of diagnostic data—those symptom characteristics, signs, and test results with the greatest potential to narrow the differential diagnosis or to rule in/rule out suspected conditions.

The guides follow a logical and consistent approach designed to reflect contemporary medical practice. They provide a secure framework to work within but are *not* rigid protocols and allow ample scope for clinical judgement.

The highest priority is always given to immediately life-threatening problems. In some cases, this means focusing on aims of assessment other than diagnosis (e.g., gauging illness severity or determining resuscitation requirements). The next aim is, wherever necessary, to exclude major pathology; for each of the most serious potential disorders, the guides will identify patients who require further investigation to rule in or rule out the diagnosis. Thereafter, we prioritize diagnostic information with the highest yield whilst avoiding data that do not significantly alter probabilities or help to target investigation. In situations where the information obtained from the routine workup is unlikely to yield a clear working diagnosis, we may opt to provide a strategy for further investigation to help narrow the differential diagnosis.

How to use the diagnostic guides

The first step is to determine which guide, if any, is the most appropriate for the patient in front of you. Ensure that you have clarified the true nature of the problem; a patient who presents with a fall may have had a blackout, whilst a patient who has had a 'funny turn' may have experienced limb weakness. In general, you should match the guide to the patient's predominant complaint.

After you have decided which guide to use, the format is simple to follow:

- Each begins with the *differential diagnosis*: a rundown of important diagnoses to consider for the particular presenting problem.

- We then present an *overview of assessment*: this is essentially a flowchart that lays out the route to diagnosis. It is vital that you understand the format of the overview, so an example is provided in Fig. 1.1 and is explained below.

- Each overview is accompanied by a *step-by-step assessment*. This is a textual companion to the overview that explains and expands on each individual step.

- Some chapters also contain details on further assessment of common disorders or abnormalities that may have been identified during the initial assessment.

The components of each overview of assessment, as seen in Fig. 1.1, are described below:

- Blue boxes are stages of action—they contain the steps of assessment that you need to undertake. This will always include methods of clinical assessment ('airway, breathing, circulation, disability, exposure [ABCDE]' or 'full clinical assessment') plus the essential basic tests (e.g., ECG, CXR) and any necessary additional examination steps. Note: The diagnostic process that follows assumes that you have performed these steps and extracted the relevant clinical information.

- Yellow boxes are stages of diagnostic reasoning—they do not show 'what to do now' but rather 'what to think about now'. Each numbered step in the diagnostic process is accompanied by a detailed explanation in the step-by-step assessment section (see above).

- Red boxes represent important elements of the assessment that are independent of the diagnostic process (e.g., evaluation of illness severity or resuscitation requirements).

- Green boxes represent the potential endpoints of the diagnostic process. As with the yellow boxes, explanatory text is provided in the accompanying step-by-step assessment. In some cases, further investigation may be required to confirm the diagnosis, refine it, assess severity or guide optimal management; if so, the necessary steps will be outlined in the text.

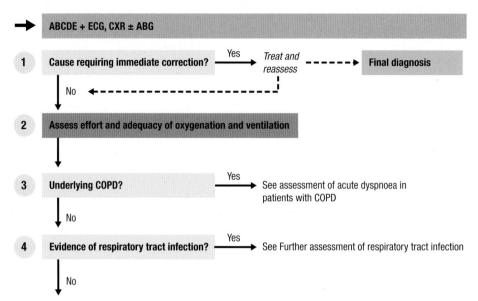

Fig. 1.1 **A guide to using the 'overview of assessment'**

PART 2

Assessment of Common Presenting Problems by System

Cardiorespiratory System

2 Shock

The term 'shock' describes a life-threatening clinical syndrome characterized by acute circulatory failure and inadequate oxygen delivery to vital organs. This results in failure of aerobic metabolism, leading to end organ dysfunction. It is recognized by features of tissue hypoperfusion (Box 2.1). Hypotension is often considered a cardinal sign; however, BP may be maintained until the advanced stages of shock, particularly in young, fit individuals.

Shock can be categorized according to the underlying physiological process involved:
1. Hypovolaemic shock: reduced circulatory volume resulting from acute fluid loss
2. Cardiogenic shock: inability of the heart to pump sufficient blood to meet the body's demands ('pump failure')
3. Distributive shock: a state of relative hypovolaemia secondary to abnormal distribution of circulating volume
4. Obstructive shock: inadequate cardiac output resulting from mechanical obstruction

These different processes can be difficult to distinguish, as components of the circulation are interdependent and several maladaptive mechanisms often coexist, for example, vasodilatation, myocardial suppression and relative hypovolaemia may occur simultaneously in sepsis.

Many presentations in this book may be complicated by shock, but, in this chapter, shock is considered the primary presenting problem detected on routine observations or on targeted examination of a severely or non-specifically unwell patient.

Hypovolaemic shock

The physiological process that underlies hypovolaemic shock is decreased intravascular volume which reduces cardiac filling pressures and cardiac output. A compensatory increase in heart rate and systemic vascular resistance occurs. Characteristic clinical findings include tachycardia, ↓pulse volume, ↓JVP, and cool, clammy peripheries. It is important to note that tachycardia may be absent ('masked') in patients on rate-limiting medications, such as beta-blockers or calcium channel antagonists.

Haemorrhage

Blood loss is not always visible; it may be left at the scene of an accident or concealed within surgical drains. The pelvis, retroperitoneum, peritoneum, thorax and thighs can accommodate several litres of extravascular blood. In addition to trauma, important causes of haemorrhagic shock include GI bleeding (see Chapter 8), ruptured abdominal aortic aneurysm (AAA) and ectopic pregnancy. Resuscitation is the top priority. Use Box 8.1 as a framework for evaluating resuscitation needs but tailor your assessment to the individual. Monitoring trends of the patient's vital signs is more important than a single 'snapshot' assessment and is essential for evaluating response to treatment.

Other fluid losses

Hypovolaemia may result from burns, diarrhoea, vomiting, polyuria or prolonged dehydration, particularly in the elderly. Fluid may also be lost into the so-called physiological 'third space' (e.g., in bowel obstruction and acute pancreatitis). Extracellular fluids are normally distributed between the interstitial compartment (75%) and the intravascular compartment (25%). Third spacing refers to the accumulation of fluid in an extracellular and extravascular space.

Cardiogenic shock

Cardiogenic shock occurs when the heart is unable to pump effectively to maintain cardiac output. This occurs most commonly because of damage to the heart muscle (e.g., myocardial infarction [MI]) but can occur because of cardiomyopathy, arrhythmias, valvular problems or inflammatory conditions (e.g., myocarditis). It may also occur due to ineffective pumping because of an external factor, such as overdose.

Clinical signs are similar to those of hypovolaemic shock, but the JVP is usually raised and there may be pulmonary oedema. Features specific to the underlying cause may be present, such as bradycardia in complete heart block. The ECG is often diagnostic.

Myocardial infarction

Shock may result from large infarcts, particularly of the anterior wall; from smaller infarcts in patients with pre-existing ventricular impairment; or from structural complications of MI, such as papillary muscle rupture, ventricular septal defect or tamponade.

Other cardiac and valvular disorders

Tachy- or bradyarrhythmias, severe cardiomyopathy and acute myocarditis may also prevent the heart from pumping effectively. Valvular disorders which may lead to cardiogenic shock include prosthetic valve dysfunction, endocarditis and critical aortic stenosis.

Other causes

Overdose of cardiac medications (e.g., beta blockers, calcium channel blockers) may result in negative inotropy and chronotropy resulting in the physiological features of cardiogenic shock.

Distributive shock

In distributive shock, peripheral vasodilatation causes a drop in systemic vascular resistance, resulting in relative hypovolaemia (↑size of vascular space without a corresponding increase in intravascular volume). The compensatory rise in cardiac output is insufficient to maintain blood pressure and shock occurs. Tachycardia and hypotension are often accompanied by warm peripheries and ↑pulse volume. Sepsis is the most common cause of distributive shock, but it may also be caused by acute pancreatitis, burns or trauma.

Sepsis

Distributive shock may complicate sepsis (Chapter 26), which is a clinical syndrome describing life-threatening organ dysfunction caused by a dysregulated host inflammatory response to infection. Septic shock is a subset of sepsis in which underlying circulatory and cellular-metabolic abnormalities are profound enough to increase mortality. As our understanding of this condition improves, the definitions have been refined, and older terms such as sepsis syndrome or septicaemia are no longer used.[1]

Anaphylaxis

Anaphylaxis is a life-threatening, histamine-mediated, allergic reaction occurring as a result of contact with a precipitant such as foodstuffs, insect stings or drugs (e.g., antibiotics). The reaction produces a very rapid onset of airway obstruction, breathing or circulatory problems either in isolation or in combination. Airway swelling, bronchoconstriction, severe hypotension (because of distributive shock) and rash are possible presenting features. In severe anaphylaxis, severe shock or even cardiac arrest may occur without other preceding symptoms or signs. A related problem is a blood transfusion reaction; ABO incompatibility may present with shock as the only initial sign, particularly in unconscious or sedated patients.

Drug causes

Antihypertensives and anaesthetic agents (particularly epidural and spinal anaesthesia) may cause features of distributive shock through excessive peripheral vasodilatation.

Adrenal crisis

Deficiency of cortisol (e.g., during acute physiological stress in adrenal insufficiency) may lead to inadequate vasoconstriction and distributive shock because of the important role cortisol

1. Singer M, Deutschman CS, Seymour CW, et al. The Third International Consensus Definitions for Sepsis and Septic Shock (Sepsis-3). JAMA. 2016 Feb 23;315(8):801-10.

plays in potentiating the action of angiotensin II and catecholamines in vasoconstriction.

Neurogenic shock

Neurogenic shock is a rare form of distributive shock associated with direct injury to the sympathetic fibres that control vascular tone from a spinal injury.

Obstructive shock

Obstructive shock occurs when there is a physical obstruction in the flow of blood. The physiology is similar to cardiogenic shock with a reduction in cardiac output and subsequent reduction in organ perfusion.

Tension pneumothorax

A tension pneumothorax occurs when air is trapped in the pleural space under positive pressure, displacing mediastinal structures and compromising cardiac function. This is a life-threatening condition necessitating urgent treatment. Typical findings include respiratory distress, ↓ipsilateral breath sounds, tachycardia and hypotension. Tracheal deviation may be absent. Immediate decompression is essential.

Cardiac tamponade

Accumulation of fluid in the pericardial space (pericardial effusion) impedes cardiac filling. As little as 200 mL of fluid may cause tamponade if accumulation is rapid, for example, in trauma, aortic dissection or myocardial rupture. Hypotension, tachycardia, ↑JVP and pulsus paradoxus are usually present. There may also be muffled heart sounds, Kussmaul's sign (a 'paradoxical' rise in JVP on inspiration) and small ECG complexes. Echocardiography will confirm the presence of an effusion, provide evidence of cardiac compromise and guide therapeutic drainage.

Pulmonary embolism

Massive pulmonary embolism (PE) typically presents with sudden-onset chest pain, dyspnoea, syncope and hypoxia with shock. The JVP is usually elevated, and the ECG may show features of right heart strain. In critically unwell patients, bedside echocardiography may assist. CXR is often normal.

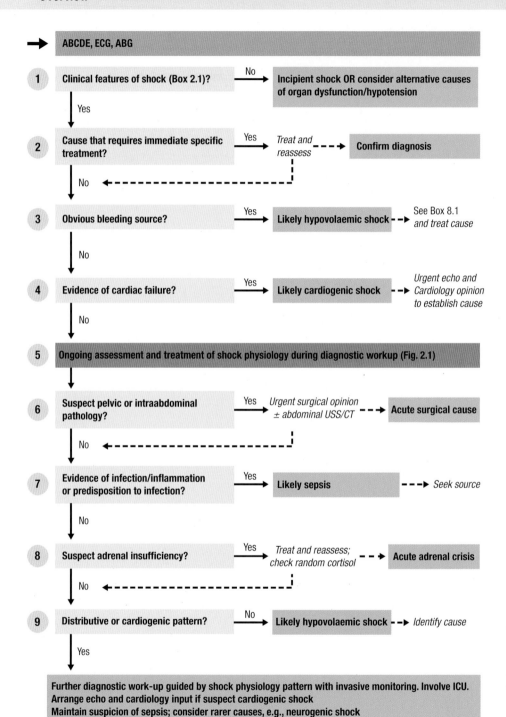

ABCDE, ECG, ABG

1 Clinical features of shock (Box 2.1)? — No → Incipient shock OR consider alternative causes of organ dysfunction/hypotension

Yes

2 Cause that requires immediate specific treatment? — Yes → *Treat and reassess* ----→ Confirm diagnosis

No

3 Obvious bleeding source? — Yes → Likely hypovolaemic shock --→ See Box 8.1 *and treat cause*

No

4 Evidence of cardiac failure? — Yes → Likely cardiogenic shock --→ *Urgent echo and Cardiology opinion to establish cause*

No

5 Ongoing assessment and treatment of shock physiology during diagnostic workup (Fig. 2.1)

6 Suspect pelvic or intraabdominal pathology? — Yes → *Urgent surgical opinion ± abdominal USS/CT* ---→ Acute surgical cause

No

7 Evidence of infection/inflammation or predisposition to infection? — Yes → Likely sepsis ---→ *Seek source*

No

8 Suspect adrenal insufficiency? — Yes → *Treat and reassess; check random cortisol* --→ Acute adrenal crisis

No

9 Distributive or cardiogenic pattern? — No → Likely hypovolaemic shock --→ *Identify cause*

Yes

Further diagnostic work-up guided by shock physiology pattern with invasive monitoring. Involve ICU.
Arrange echo and cardiology input if suspect cardiogenic shock
Maintain suspicion of sepsis; consider rarer causes, e.g., neurogenic shock

2

1   Clinical features of shock (see Box 2.1)?

Use the features in Box 2.1 to identify shock. Tissue hypoperfusion is the diagnostic feature. Absolute values of heart rate and BP are less informative than monitoring trends over time. Some patients may maintain BP within normal limits despite organ dysfunction. If the patient falls short of the criteria in Box 2.1 but you suspect significant circulatory compromise, pursue a working diagnosis of 'incipient shock' and continue to work through the diagnostic pathway.

2   Cause that requires immediate specific treatment?

In some cases, specific interventions to reverse the underlying cause of shock offer the only effective treatment and take precedence over further investigation or supportive measures (Table 2.1). Most will be identified and immediate treatment initiated as part of the initial ABCDE assessment.

3   Obvious bleeding source?

Where shock arises from acute haemorrhage, the initial aims of treatment are to minimize further blood loss and restore adequate circulating volume. Categorize hypovolaemic shock, assess resuscitation requirements and monitor response to treatment as described in Box 8.1. In patients with traumatic haemorrhage, always consider the possibility of multiple causes of shock, such as cardiac tamponade, tension pneumothorax and blood loss.

4   Evidence of cardiac failure?

Pulmonary oedema suggests cardiogenic shock. The most common cause is severe left ventricular dysfunction following an acute MI. Perform an ECG to look for evidence of infarction or ischaemia (see Box 3.2). Serial ECGs are often required to look for dynamic changes. Arrange a bedside echocardiogram to assess left ventricular function and exclude mechanical causes (especially acute mitral regurgitation).

Patients without pulmonary oedema but with ↑JVP ± peripheral oedema may have a cardiogenic component to shock. Those with right ventricular infarction (suspect with inferior or posterior MI in the previous 72 hours), chronic right heart failure or tricuspid regurgitation may be inadequately filled despite ↑JVP and will respond to a fluid challenge. Otherwise, echocardiography is mandatory to look for evidence of right ventricular dysfunction, cardiac tamponade and PE.

Patients with cardiogenic shock require invasive monitoring and specialist interventions; urgent Cardiology and ICU referral is essential.

5   Ongoing assessment and treatment of shock physiology during diagnostic work-up (Fig. 2.1)

In the absence of obvious haemorrhage, major cardiac dysfunction or a rapidly reversible cause of shock (Table 2.1), the next step is to initiate treatment and assess response. As shown in Fig. 2.1, monitoring the effect of fluid challenges on haemodynamic variables and tissue perfusion helps to delineate the mechanism(s) of shock and guide further resuscitation and treatment. Central venous pressure (CVP) monitoring may be required to improve assessment of fluid status. This process should be carried out in parallel with continued evaluation for a specific underlying cause.

It is important to be aware of concealed bleeding because haemorrhagic shock can be missed in the early stages. Haemoglobin

---

Box 2.1 Clinical features of shock

Haemodynamic

- Systolic BP ≤90 mmHg or a drop of ≥40 mmHg from baseline
- Pulse >100/min

Tissue hypoperfusion

- Skin: capillary refill time >2 sec or cold/pale/mottled extremities
- Renal: oliguria (<0.5 mL/kg/hr) or ↑serum creatinine (acute)
- CNS: Confusion, agitation or reduced conscious level in more severe cases
- Global: ↑lactate (>2 mmol/L) in the absence of hypoxaemia

Table 2.1 Rapidly reversible causes of shock

Reversible cause	Suspect if	Test to confirm	Urgent intervention
Tension pneumothorax	Respiratory distress, tracheal deviation towards opposite side, hyperresonance or reduced ↓breath sounds on the same side	Nil – treat immediately	Needle decompression
Tachyarrhythmia	Ventricular tachycardia (VT) or supraventricular tachycardia (SVT) >150 bpm	Nil – treat immediately	DC cardioversion
Bradyarrhythmia	3rd-degree atrioventricular block or HR <40 bpm	Nil – treat immediately	Atropine, adrenaline, external or transvenous pacing
Anaphylaxis	Respiratory distress, stridor, wheeze, angioedema, rash	Nil – treat immediately	Intramuscular adrenaline, IV fluids
ST-elevation myocardial infarction (MI)	Chest pain, nausea, sweating, light-headedness (see Box 3.2)	ECG	Primary angioplasty or thrombolysis
Pulmonary embolism	Dyspnoea, hypoxia (especially with clear lung fields), chest pain, ↑JVP, risk factors, ECG changes (see Fig. 3.11)	CTPA if stable; urgent echocardiogram if unstable; nil if peri-arrest	Thrombolysis
Cardiac tamponade	↑JVP, pulsus paradoxus, small QRS complexes on ECG	Echocardiogram	Pericardiocentesis

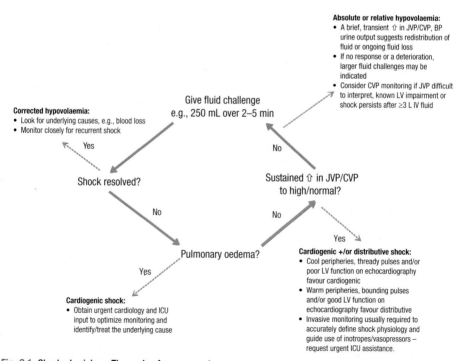

Fig. 2.1 Shock physiology: The cycle of assessment

and/or haematocrit levels may be misleading because they can be normal in acute haemorrhage and fall only following fluid replacement. Lactate clearance (change in blood lactate levels over time) is a proxy for monitoring response to treatment.

6 Suspect pelvic or intra-abdominal pathology?

If an acute abdominal or pelvic pathology is suspected, then an urgent surgical review should be requested together with abdominal imaging with ultrasound and/or CT. A ruptured AAA or ectopic pregnancy require immediate intervention.

Rupture of a AAA should be considered in patients >60 years who present with a pulsatile abdominal mass or sudden-onset, severe abdominal/back pain, particularly if they have a known history of a AAA (Chapter 7). In such patients, urgent imaging should be arranged while contacting a vascular surgeon.

Suspect ruptured ectopic pregnancy in any woman of child-bearing age with recent-onset lower abdominal pain, shoulder-tip pain or PV bleeding (Chapter 7). Confirm pregnancy with an immediate serum or urine pregnancy test and contact the Gynaecology team to arrange urgent review, diagnostic ultrasound, and ongoing management.

Other pointers to an underlying surgical cause include severe abdominal pain ± tenderness/guarding/peritonism, air under the diaphragm on CXR, or ↑amylase. Look for intestinal obstruction on abdominal X-ray in patients with abdominal pain/distension and repeated vomiting. Request an urgent surgical review. See Chapter 7 for further details.

7 Evidence of infection/inflammation or predisposition to infection?

Look for features of sepsis (Chapter 26). If present, perform a full septic screen to identify a likely source, but do not delay administering antibiotics. Assume sepsis in any patient with immunocompromise until proven otherwise.

Investigate and manage as described in Chapter 26.

8 Suspect adrenal insufficiency?

Adrenal insufficiency is often overlooked because many patients have fever and are assumed, at least initially, to have sepsis. Always consider the diagnosis and look for clinical/biochemical features. Useful indicators include prominent GI symptoms (almost always present but non-specific), pigmentation of recent scars, palmar creases and mucosal membranes, vitiligo, and typical metabolic abnormalities including ↓Na$^+$, ↑K$^+$ and hypoglycaemia. Even a blood glucose at the low end of normal (3.5–4.5 mmol/L) suggests an inadequate 'stress response'. If you suspect adrenal insufficiency, treat with IV hydrocortisone immediately and check a random cortisol level. A short ACTH (synacthen) test may be helpful but takes 30 minutes to perform and should not delay empirical treatment in critically unwell patients. Remember that those patients who take systemic steroids for therapeutic purposes are at risk of adrenal insufficiency when acutely unwell. There is no treatment duration or glucocorticoid dose for which adrenal insufficiency can be ruled out, but those receiving higher doses or those who have been on therapy for >1 month are at highest risk and will require an increased dose of steroids while acutely unwell.

9 Distributive or cardiogenic pattern?

Reassess for the presence of relative or absolute hypovolaemia (Fig. 2.1). Look for concealed sources of haemorrhage, dehydration (reduced skin turgor, dry mucous membranes) and causative/contributory factors, such as history of diarrhoea and vomiting, reduced intake, diuretics or antihypertensives. Check for ketonuria and metabolic acidosis to exclude diabetic ketoacidosis. If the patient remains shocked despite adequate IV fluid resuscitation, consider a distributive or cardiogenic element, involve ICU, institute appropriate (invasive) monitoring and consider urgent echocardiography.

Chest pain is one of the most common presentations to acute care settings. The diagnostic approach to acute chest pain is different from that of *intermittent* chest pain and they should be considered as distinct clinical entities.

Acute chest pain

The primary aim is to rapidly identify life-threatening pathologies such as acute coronary syndromes (ACS), aortic dissection and pulmonary embolism (PE). Clinical history and urgent investigations such as ECGs, CXRs and serum biomarkers (e.g., troponin, D-dimer) play a central role in narrowing the differential diagnosis.

Acute coronary syndromes (ACS)

Acute thrombus formation in a ruptured or eroded atheromatous coronary artery plaque causes an ACS. Acute coronary syndromes include ST elevation MI (STEMI), non-ST elevation MI (NSTEMI), and unstable angina. All three conditions typically present with symptoms of acute myocardial ischaemia (Box 3.1), but they can be differentiated from each other using ECG and biochemical parameters.

- STEMI—Sudden total occlusion of a major vessel causes ischaemia of a full-thickness segment of myocardium. STEMI is diagnosed in patients with a presentation consistent with acute myocardial iscaemia with associated diagnostic ECG changes (Box 3.2). Symptoms of chest discomfort are typically abrupt in onset, severe, persistent, unrelieved by glyceryl trinitrate (GTN) spray, and accompanied by autonomic upset (sweating, nausea and vomiting). The mainstay of treatment in these patients is immediate reperfusion by primary angioplasty or fibrinolytic therapy.
- NSTEMI—With incomplete occlusion of a major vessel or a good collateral blood supply there is less extensive ischaemia, but it is still sufficient to cause a degree of cardiomyocyte necrosis. NSTEMI is diagnosed in patients with a presentation consistent with acute myocardial ischaemia with associated biochemical evidence of myocardial necrosis, typically proven by a rise in high-sensitivity cardiac troponin. There may be ECG changes suggesting ischaemia (see Figs 3.7, 3.8 and 3.9), but the changes to do not meet the criteria for a STEMI (Box 3.2).
- Unstable angina—In cases of unstable angina, there are symptoms of acute myocardial ischaemia without biochemical evidence of myocardial necrosis. Unstable angina can be distinguished from stable angina if the pain is new, occurs at rest, or occurs with increasing frequency, duration and intensity in a patient with a previous history of angina. Unstable angina or NSTEMI may also occur in the absence of acute plaque rupture if tissue hypoperfusion occurs, for example, when hypoxaemia, anaemia, tachyarrhythmia or hypotension are superimposed upon stable coronary artery disease (CAD).

Aortic dissection

This is a tear in the inner wall of the aorta, typically causing unrelenting chest pain that radiates through to the back, between the shoulder blades. Indeed, the patient may describe the pain as coming from the back. The character of the pain is often described as 'ripping', 'tearing' or 'sharp' (Box 3.3). Autonomic upset including syncope is common, and neurological deficit may occur due

Box 3.1 Symptoms of acute myocardial ischaemia

Acute myocardial ischaemia tends to be perceived as a diffuse, poorly localized retrosternal discomfort that may radiate to the left (or right) shoulder/arm, throat, jaw or back. Typical descriptions include 'tightness', 'pressure' and 'heaviness', but many others, such as 'burning', are recognized. Patients often illustrate the sensation by placing a hand or fist over their chest. Many patients do not perceive myocardial ischaemia as painful but most feel a sense of 'discomfort'—if you ask about 'pain' only, you may miss the diagnosis. Associated features can include dyspnoea, nausea, light-headedness, diaphoresis, and palpitations. Some patients (e.g., elderly or diabetic) may experience minimal or even no pain, making the diagnosis more challenging. Note that symptoms of myocardial ischaemia are highly variable, and ACS must be considered in patients with suggestive ECG changes even in the absence of typical symptoms.

Box 3.2 ECG abnormalities in acute coronary syndromes

ECG abnormalities in STEMI

1. ≥1 mm ST elevation in at least 2 adjacent limb leads, such as II and III; I and aVL *OR*
2. ≥2 mm ST elevation in at least 2 adjacent precordial (chest) leads, such as V_2 and V_3; V_5 and V_6 *OR*
3. Left bundle branch block of new onset

Major ischaemic ECG changes (strongly suggestive of myocardial ischaemia but not diagnostic of STEMI)

1. ST changes that vary with onset and offset of pain ('dynamic' changes)
2. ≥1 mm horizontal ST depression in ≥2 adjacent leads
3. Deep symmetrical T wave inversion

Minor ischaemic ECG changes (less specific for myocardial ischaemia)

1. <1 mm horizontal ST depression
2. New or evolving T wave inversion or flattening

to occlusion of the carotid, vertebral, spinal, or peripheral arteries, or hypoperfusion due to hypotension. Mortality is high (1% per hour in the initial phase), necessitating rapid diagnosis and management. Aortic dissection must be suspected in any patient presenting with coexisting cardiovascular and neurological symptoms or signs.

Box 3.3 Features suggestive of acute aortic dissection

• Pain reaches maximal intensity within seconds of onset
• Main site of pain is interscapular
• Character of pain described as 'tearing' or 'ripping'
• Syncope or new focal neurological signs
• New early diastolic murmur (aortic regurgitation)
• Asymmetrical pulses (not previously documented)
• Interarm blood pressure differential >20 mmHg
• Marfan's syndrome
• Widened mediastinum on CXR

Pulmonary embolism

Pain due to a pulmonary embolism (PE) depends on the site and size of the embolism. Small emboli causing distal pulmonary infarction may be associated with pleuritic chest pain and few other clinical signs, whereas larger emboli may produce severe, sudden-onset, central chest pain, associated with dyspnoea and potentially haemoptysis, syncope or shock. Most emboli arise from lower limb deep vein thrombosis (DVT), but clinical features of DVT are inconsistent and may be absent.

Acute pericarditis

This typically causes constant retrosternal pain with a sharp, stabbing character that may radiate to the shoulders, arm or trapezius ridge. It is usually more localized than ischaemic pain and may be accompanied by a pericardial rub on auscultation. Pain is often, but not invariably, worsened by inspiration, movement, swallowing, or lying down, and eased by sitting forward.

Gastro-oesophageal disorders

Gastro-oesophageal disorders can commonly present with chest pain and should be considered in the differential diagnosis. Oesophageal spasm can cause severe retrosternal discomfort that mimics cardiac pain. Gastro-oesophageal reflux disease (GORD) usually presents with 'heartburn': a hot or burning retrosternal discomfort that radiates upwards. Oesophageal rupture is often diagnosed late and carries a high mortality rate. It should be suspected in any patient who develops chest pain after vomiting.

Pneumothorax

Pneumothorax causes unilateral, sudden-onset pleuritic chest pain, often associated with breathlessness. In large pneumothoraces there may be unilateral reduced breath sounds and hyperresonance to percussion on examination. Diagnosis is usually confirmed on CXR.

Pneumonia

This may cause pleuritic chest pain, usually accompanied by other clinical features such as fever, cough, purulent sputum and breathlessness.

Musculoskeletal problems

A common cause of chest discomfort that may have a traumatic or atraumatic source. The pain often varies with posture or movement and may be reproduced or exacerbated by local palpation. Rib fracture typically causes severe pain, but most cases are due to minor soft-tissue injuries and may be symptomatic for up to 6 weeks. Malignant chest wall invasion produces constant, unremitting, localized pain that is not related to respiration and may disturb sleep.

Anxiety

Anxiety is a common cause of chest pain but should be a diagnosis of exclusion. Associated features may include breathlessness with 'inability to take enough air' and tingling around the mouth; the onset of symptoms may coincide with stressful situations or emotional distress.

Other causes

- Subdiaphragmatic inflammatory pathology (e.g., intra-abdominal abscess) can mimic pneumonia (pleuritic pain, fever, small pleural effusion).
- Intrathoracic malignancy may involve the pleura and present with pleuritic pain ± pleural effusion.
- Rheumatic diseases (e.g., systemic lupus erythematosus, rheumatoid arthritis) can present with pleuritic chest pain ± pleural effusion due to pleural inflammation.

- Mediastinal masses, for example, thymoma or lymphoma, tend to cause a dull, constant, progressive retrosternal pain that disturbs sleep.
- Herpes zoster may cause severe pain, sometimes preceded by tingling or burning, followed by development of a vesicular rash in a dermatomal distribution. The rash has often not manifested at the time of presentation, making diagnosis difficult.

Intermittent chest pain

Angina pectoris

The term stable angina describes episodes of symptomatic myocardial ischaemia (Box 3.1) that tend to be precipitated by a predictable degree of exertion and rapidly relieved by rest and/or GTN spray, with episodes typically lasting <10 minutes. In patients with angina, myocardial blood flow is adequate under resting conditions but is insufficient to meet metabolic demands during periods of increased cardiac work. It is almost always due to atherosclerotic narrowing in one or more coronary arteries. In considering the likelihood of angina, it is therefore important to consider the underlying risk of coronary artery disease (CAD) (Box 3.4). Less commonly, angina may result from tachyarrhythmias (especially on a background of significant coronary narrowing) or transient coronary artery spasm.

Gastro-oesophageal disorders

As described above, gastro-oesophageal reflux disease can mimic angina as it typically causes a hot, burning retrosternal discomfort which radiates upwards; it is often provoked by bending or lying flat, such as in bed, and there may be a relationship with food. Symptoms are relieved by antacids. Oesophageal spasm can cause severe retrosternal discomfort which may be worsened by exertion and relieved by nitrates.

Musculoskeletal disorders

These are a common cause of chest discomfort with a wide variety of presentations; most are due to minor soft-tissue injuries. The pain typically varies with posture or movement and

Box 3.4 Estimating the likelihood of coronary artery disease (CAD)[1]

High risk

- Previously documented CAD or other vascular disease, for example, stroke or peripheral arterial disease
- Male >60 years *OR* >50 years with ≥2 risk factors *OR* >40 years with ≥3 risk factors
- Female >60 years with ≥3 risk factors

Moderate risk

- All patients not in high-risk or low-risk group

Low risk

- Age <30 years
- Female <40 years with no risk factors

[1]Risk factors: cigarette smoking, diabetes mellitus, hypertension, hypercholesterolaemia (total cholesterol ≥6.5 mmol/L), family history of premature CAD.

may respond to NSAIDs. In costochondritis, there is well-localized tenderness of the costochondral junctions that is exacerbated by local pressure.

Asthma/COPD

Patients with asthma/COPD may describe exertional chest 'tightness' on account of bronchospasm, which may be difficult to distinguish from angina. There is usually an associated history of wheeze, breathlessness and cough, and precipitants other than exertion may be apparent, for example, common allergens or viral upper respiratory tract infection (RTI).

Anxiety

As with acute chest pain, emotional distress can be a common cause of intermittent chest pain but is a diagnosis of exclusion. There may be evidence of hyperventilation with tingling around the mouth and extremities. Episodes tend to arise in the context of stress rather than exertion.

Clinical tool
ECG abnormalities in chest pain

The ECG in STEMI

Acute transmural ischaemia produces ST elevation in leads that 'look at' the affected region of myocardium:
- In anterior MI (Fig. 3.1), V_2–V_5
- In lateral MI, V_5, V_6, I and aVL
- In inferior MI (Fig. 3.2), II, III and aVF.

There may be associated ST depression in the opposing leads ('reciprocal change'). Posterior MI (Fig. 3.3) is recognized by reciprocal anterior ST depression and a dominant R wave (reciprocal Q wave) in V_1.

Further ECG changes occur as the infarct progresses (Fig. 3.4): loss of the R wave, followed by development of Q waves and T wave inversion (TWI). ST segments typically return to baseline. Extensive anteroseptal infarction may cause new left bundle branch block (Fig. 3.5) rather than ST elevation.

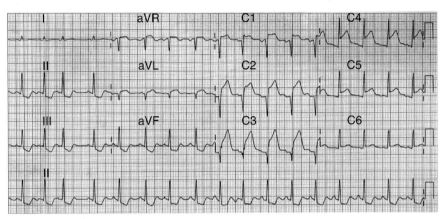

Fig. 3.1 Acute anterior ST elevation MI. (From Douglas G, Nicol F, Robertson C. Macleod's clinical examination, 12th ed. Edinburgh: Churchill Livingstone, 2009.)

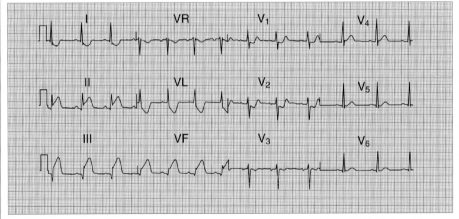

Fig. 3.2 Acute inferior ST elevation MI. (From Hampton JR. The ECG in practice, 5th ed. Edinburgh: Churchill Livingstone, 2008.)

Clinical tool—cont'd
ECG abnormalities in chest pain

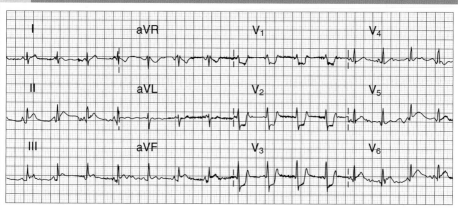

Fig. 3.3 Acute inferoposterior ST elevation MI. (From Grubb NR, Newby DE. Churchill's pocketbook of cardiology, 2nd ed. Edinburgh: Churchill Livingstone, 2006.)

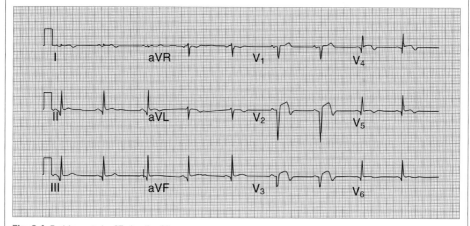

Fig. 3.4 Evolving anterior ST elevation MI.

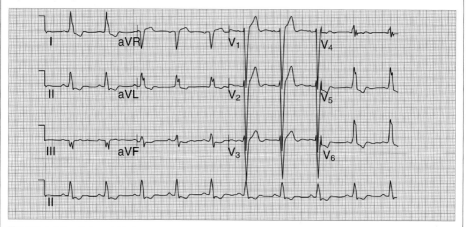

Fig. 3.5 Left bundle branch block.

Continued

Clinical tool—cont'd
ECG abnormalities in chest pain

ST elevation in leads V_2–V_5 can be a normal finding ('high takeoff') and, in the absence of a previous ECG, may cause diagnostic confusion. With high takeoff, the ST elevation is typically concave and frequently associated with notching in the terminal portion of the QRS complex (Fig. 3.6).

The ECG in unstable angina/NSTEMI

New horizontal ST depression suggests active ischaemia (Fig. 3.7); the extent and depth of depression correlate with the severity of ischaemia. 'Dynamic' ST segment changes—those that coincide with pain and normalize with resolution of pain—strongly suggest ischaemia. It is therefore important to repeat the ECG over time and compare these ECGs, as well as any prehospital ECG trace.

TWI may be the only ECG evidence of ischaemia. Biphasic TWI in leads V2–V3 (Fig. 3.8) or deep symmetrical TWI in these leads ± other precordial leads (Fig. 3.9) suggests critical obstruction of the left anterior descending artery. Other patterns of TWI are less specific. Lateral TWI, together with downward-sloping ST depression, is a common feature of left ventricular hypertrophy (Fig. 3.10) or digitalis treatment; comparison with previous ECGs is very helpful. TWI confined to leads V_1–V_3 (Fig. 3.11) suggests right heart strain and favours a diagnosis of PE over ACS. TWI also occurs with cardiomyopathies, pericarditis, myocarditis, cerebrovascular events (especially subarachnoid haemorrhage), electrolyte abnormalities and hyperventilation. However, in the appropriate clinical context, new or evolving TWI supports a diagnosis of ACS.

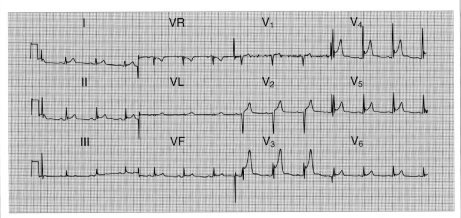

Fig. 3.6 'High takeoff' ST segments. (From Hampton JR. The ECG made easy, 7th ed. Edinburgh: Churchill Livingstone, 2008.)

Clinical tool—cont'd
ECG abnormalities in chest pain

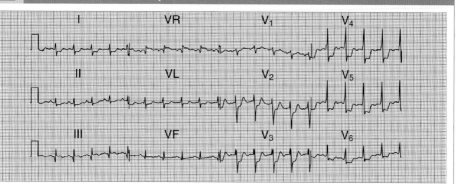

Fig. 3.7 Ischaemic anterolateral ST segment depression. (From Hampton JR. The ECG in practice, 5th ed. Edinburgh: Churchill Livingstone, 2008.)

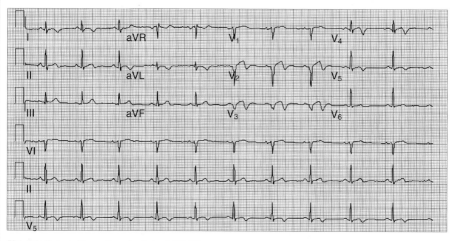

Fig. 3.8 Biphasic T wave inversion in leads V2–V3.

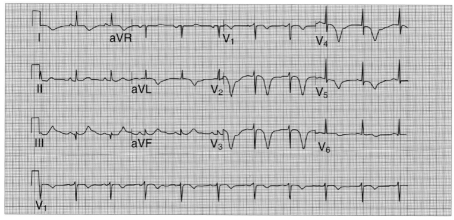

Fig. 3.9 Deep symmetrical T wave inversion.

Continued

Clinical tool—cont'd
ECG abnormalities in chest pain

The ECG in acute pericarditis

Acute pericarditis characteristically produces widespread ST elevation (not corresponding to the territory of a single coronary artery) which is concave (upward-sloping) and associated with ST depression in aVR (Fig. 3.12). Associated PR segment depression (with PR elevation in aVR) is highly suggestive. Unlike STEMI, ST elevation typically persists for many days. T waves are upright during ST changes but subsequently invert.

The ECG in PE

In most cases, the ECG is normal or shows only sinus tachycardia. Specific abnormalities suggestive of PE

include new right axis deviation, a dominant R wave in lead V_1, TWI in leads V_1–V_3 (Fig. 3.11) or right bundle branch block (Fig. 3.13). The 'classic' ECG finding of a deep, slurred S wave in I with a Q wave and TWI in III ('$S_1Q_3T_3$') is rare.

The ECG in aortic dissection

The ECG may be normal or show nonspecific abnormalities. If the dissection flap involves the ostium of a coronary artery, there may be ECG changes of a STEMI (usually inferior). The ECG may change rapidly, for example, changes of STEMI may resolve then recur due to differential changes in blood pressure in the true and false aortic lumens.

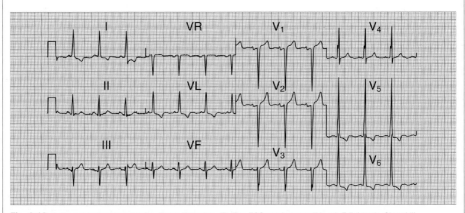
Fig. 3.10 Left ventricular hypertrophy. (From Hampton JR. The ECG made easy, 7th ed. Edinburgh: Churchill Livingstone, 2008.)

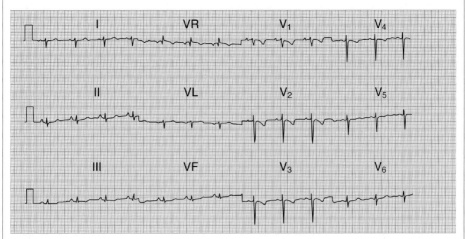
Fig. 3.11 Anterior T wave inversion due to acute right heart strain. (From Hampton JR. The ECG in practice, 5th ed. Edinburgh: Churchill Livingstone, 2008.)

Clinical tool—cont'd
ECG abnormalities in chest pain

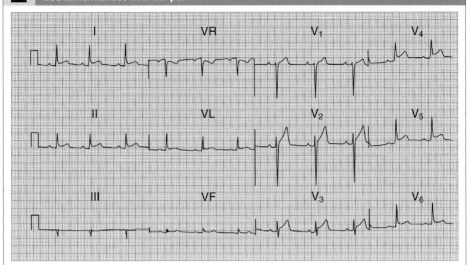

Fig. 3.12 Acute pericarditis. (From Hampton JR. 150 ECG problems, 3rd ed. Edinburgh: Churchill Livingstone, 2008.)

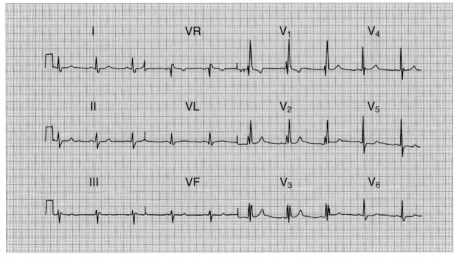

Fig. 3.13 Right bundle branch block. (From Hampton JR. 150 ECG problems, 3rd ed. Edinburgh: Churchill Livingstone, 2008.)

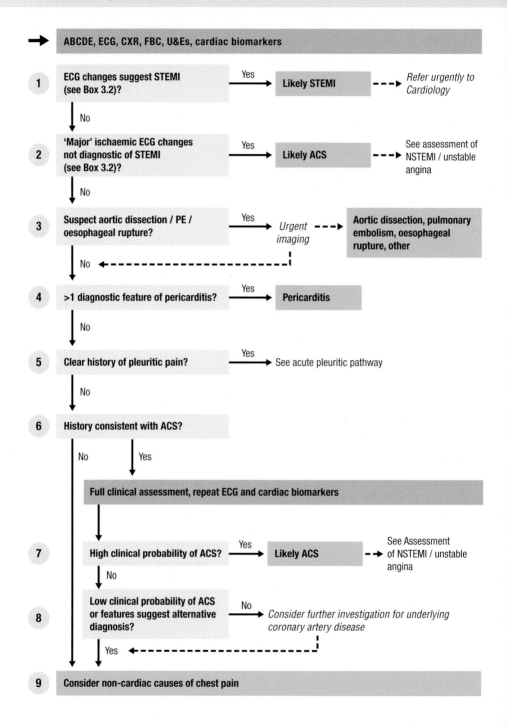

1 ECG changes suggest STEMI (Box 3.2)?

Patients with acute chest pain and ECG changes compatible with STEMI (Box 3.2) require immediate reperfusion therapy, such as primary angioplasty or thrombolysis. Unless ECG changes are old, the history is incompatible with ACS (noting that ischaemia can present atypically or with minimal symptoms) or there is a strong clinical suspicion of aortic dissection (see below), make a diagnosis of STEMI.

- Attach cardiac monitoring and repeat ABCDE regularly.
- Establish the duration of the pain and whether it is ongoing.
- In younger patients with few or no risk factors for CAD (Box 3.4), consider recreational drug misuse (e.g., cocaine, amphetamine).
- Refer urgently to Cardiology for consideration of primary angioplasty
- If angioplasty is not available, confirm eligibility for thrombolysis (Box 14.2).

If ST elevation is present but does not meet the criteria for a STEMI, repeat the ECG at frequent intervals and manage as NSTEMI/unstable angina.

2 'Major' ischaemic ECG changes not diagnostic of STEMI (Box 3.2)?

If the ECG shows 'major' ischaemic changes (Box 3.2), confirm that the history is consistent with ACS. If so, make a provisional diagnosis of NSTEMI/unstable angina, and assess as described below. If the ECG is nondiagnostic (e.g., old left bundle branch block, paced ventricular rhythm), manage as per NSTEMI/unstable angina if clinical features are supportive of ACS. Assessment of NSTEMI/unstable angina Step 1 Identify critically unwell patients

Assessment of NSTEMI/unstable angina

Step 1 Identify critically ill patients

Attach cardiac monitoring to all patients with ongoing chest pain and review regularly with serial ECGs. Admit to a critical care unit/high-dependency unit (CCU/HDU) and arrange urgent Cardiology review if you identify any of the following:

- Shock (Chapter 2)
- ST elevation or refractory pain.
- Pulmonary oedema
- Ventricular arrhythmia or complete heart block

Step 2 Consider all potential factors contributing to myocardial ischaemia

In patients with ongoing pain:

- Give IV morphine (up to 10 mg) and GTN spray.
- Maintain SpO_2 ≥94%.
- Identify and treat tachyarrhythmias.
- If any suspicion of anaemia or acute bleeding (e.g., pallor, haematemesis, melaena) check Hb urgently (prior to giving antiplatelet agents/anticoagulants).
- If tachycardic, assess and treat any ongoing pain, then consider beta blockade (if no contraindications).
- Evaluate the response to GTN spray; if pain improves, consider IV GTN infusion.

Step 3 Identify high-risk patients

Risk-stratify patients using a validated scoring system such as the GRACE (Global Registry of Acute Coronary Events) score. The GRACE score predicts the risk of in-hospital and 6-month mortality in patients with ACS and can be used to aid the selection of patients for clinical and interventional procedures.

Step 4 Use cardiac biomarkers to differentiate unstable angina from NSTEMI

Measure serum troponin. If elevated, a NSTEMI can be diagnosed as there is evidence of myocardial necrosis. If the troponin is not elevated, further action will depend on the time of onset of the chest pain, timing of the initial troponin, the troponin level, and your local protocol. As a general rule, a single troponin test cannot be used to exclude NSTEMI unless the troponin level is very low and the chest pain was not recent in onset (usually ≥3 hours ago). Otherwise, a repeat troponin is required to identify if troponin is rising or has reached the diagnostic threshold for NSTEMI. If serial troponins are negative, NSTEMI can be excluded. In this instance, a diagnosis of unstable angina can be made in patients with symptoms of acute myocardial ischaemia, which is:

- new onset
- duration of <1 hr (a duration longer than this would be expected to result in myocardial necrosis)
- occurring at rest
- associated with ischaemic ECG changes
- increasing in severity, duration, or frequency in a patient with a background of angina

Whether NSTEMI or unstable angina is diagnosed, seek input from Cardiology to plan further assessment and management. If there are no ECG changes, no rises in troponin, and no features consistent with unstable angina, an alternative cause of chest pain must be considered.

3 Suspect aortic dissection, PE or oesophageal rupture?

In the absence of clear ECG evidence of ischaemia/infarction, consider other life-threatening conditions such as aortic dissection, PE and oesophageal rupture. For all of these, a high index of suspicion is vital as a delay in diagnosis may prove fatal and characteristic 'textbook' clinical features are often absent.

It is critical to exclude aortic dissection in any patients with severe acute chest pain and ANY of the features in Box 3.3. In the absence of these features, consider the diagnosis in any patient with a first presentation of severe acute chest pain and no clear alternative diagnosis, especially if:

- There is a background of hypertension, previous aortic surgery, trauma or pregnancy, or
- The pain is described as 'sharp' or radiates to the back.

A normal CXR does not exclude aortic dissection. There are two characteristic age presentation peaks for dissection: patients in their 70s with atherosclerotic disease and patients with connective tissue disorders in their 30s. If aortic dissection is suspected, arrange immediate contrast-enhanced thoracic CT; in unstable patients, consider bedside transthoracic echo, which will identify most type A dissections (but does not exclude the diagnosis).

Consider PE if there is sudden-onset, severe chest pain associated with any of the following features:

- Marked dyspnoea or hypoxaemia in the absence of pulmonary oedema
- High risk of PE, e.g., malignancy, recent surgery, prolonged immobility or clinical evidence of DVT
- Syncope or signs of shock (Box 2.1)— especially with ↑JVP
- Supportive ECG changes (Fig. 3.11).

In patients who are hypotensive or peri-arrest, consider urgent transthoracic echo to look for evidence of acute right heart strain and exclude alternative diagnoses (e.g., cardiac tamponade), and consider thrombolysis (after excluding contraindications; Box 14.2). Otherwise, arrange urgent CT pulmonary angiography.

Suspect oesophageal perforation if acute severe chest pain arises after vomiting/retching or oesophageal instrumentation. Arrange immediate CXR if ≥1 hour after perforation (may show subcutaneous emphysema, pneumomediastinum or pleural effusion). If the patient presents <1 hour after symptom onset or a high index of suspicion remains despite a normal CXR, request water-soluble contrast barium swallow/CT and surgical review.

4 More than one diagnostic feature of pericarditis?

Diagnose pericarditis if more than one of the following features are present:
- Pain radiating to the trapezius ridge (highly specific for pericarditis) or other typical features
- Pericardial friction rub (85% of cases)
- Typical ECG changes (Fig. 3.12; present in 80% of cases).

Request an echocardiogram to detect any associated effusion (urgently if any features of tamponade) and assess left ventricular (LV) function (may be impaired if associated myocarditis).

5 Clear history of pleuritic pain?

If the patient reports pain that clearly and consistently varies with respiratory movements, especially if described as 'sharp', 'knifelike', 'stabbing' or 'catching', and particularly if associated with dyspnoea, then proceed to the acute pleuritic pain pathway later in this chapter. If there is any doubt, continue the diagnostic pathway for nonpleuritic pain initially and reconsider if no clear diagnosis emerges or the patient's description becomes more suggestive of pleuritic pain.

6 History consistent with ACS?

Further assessment for ACS is generally not required in patients with:
- A single, short-lived episode of pain, for example, <10 minutes
- A typical episode of stable exertional angina
- A clear alternative cause for pain, such as herpes zoster; recent chest wall injury with tenderness on palpation; GORD
- An atypical history with very low risk of for CAD, for example, <30 years with no risk factors.

Otherwise, continue to investigate for an ACS.

7 High clinical probability of ACS?

If the clinical features are highly suggestive of ACS in a patient with risk factors for CAD, work through the assessment of NSTEMI/unstable angina described above even in the absence of diagnostic ECG findings. Note that ECGs should be repeated regularly in patients with suspected ACS, especially during further episodes of pain. Discuss any patients where there is significant concern about ACS, but without any classic diagnostic criteria, with Cardiology, who can advise about necessary further investigation and management.

8 Low clinical probability of ACS or features suggest alternative diagnosis?

Symptoms are less likely to represent ACS if the patient has a low likelihood of CAD (Box 3.4), there are no ECG changes, and the pain is atypical. However, atypical presentations are common, and if the cause of chest pain is unclear, send serial troponins to exclude NSTEMI. If troponins are raised but the clinical probability of ACS is felt to be low, then consider alternative causes of raised troponin (Box 3.5). In the absence of an alternative cause, continue to treat as ACS.

> **Box 3.5 Conditions associated with elevation of serum troponin other than acute coronary syndrome**
>
> - Prolonged severe hypotension/cardiac arrest
> - Acute decompensated heart failure
> - Tachy- or bradyarrhythmias
> - Myocarditis/myopericarditis
> - Aortic dissection
> - Pulmonary embolism
> - Severe sepsis or burns
> - Cardiac trauma/surgery/ablation
> - Acute neurological disease, such as stroke, subarachnoid haemorrhage
> - Congestive cardiac failure
> - Infiltrative cardiac diseases, such as sarcoidosis, amyloidosis
> - End-stage renal failure
>
> If serial troponins are normal and the symptoms are not felt to represent acute myocardial ischaemia, then ACS is unlikely. Nonetheless, if there is any doubt as to whether the symptoms represent acute myocardial ischaemia, and they meet the criteria for unstable angina, then seek Cardiology input for consideration of further investigation (Box 3.6)

Box 3.6 Investigations in suspected angina

- Investigations are used to seek evidence of myocardial ischaemia during cardiac stress or to confirm and/or refute underlying CAD.
- Exercise ECG and other 'stress tests' seek to establish whether increases in cardiac work induce myocardial ischaemia. During exercise, the development of typical symptoms with ST segment shift >1 mm suggests angina. Absence of symptoms and ECG changes at high workload argues against angina.
- Exercise ECG is often inconclusive and has a high 'false-positive' rate in low-risk patients. Other forms of stress testing, for example, myocardial perfusion scan or dobutamine stress echocardiogram, offer higher sensitivity/specificity and are particularly useful when the resting ECG is abnormal, for example, in left bundle branch block, or if the patient is unable to perform treadmill exercise.
- Stress tests are contraindicated in unstable angina, decompensated heart failure or severe hypertension.
- Coronary angiography is the definitive test for defining the presence, extent and severity of CAD. Severe stenosis in one or more vessels strongly suggests ischaemia as the cause of pain whilst the absence of significant coronary stenosis effectively excludes angina.
- In patients with a relatively low risk of CAD, CT coronary angiography is a useful, noninvasive method to rule out stable angina by excluding the presence of significant CAD.

9 Consider noncardiac causes of chest pain

- Evaluate and investigate for GORD if dyspeptic features dominate.
- Consider musculoskeletal pain or herpes zoster if there are typical features.
- Consider paroxysmal tachyarrhythmia if the pain was accompanied by rapid palpitation, particularly if an ECG was not obtained during symptoms to exclude this possibility.
- Reevaluate for aortic dissection or PE and consider echocardiogram/thoracic CT if ongoing pain, haemodynamic compromise or other clinical concern.
- Consider thoracic or respiratory review if there is an unexplained CXR abnormality, such as mediastinal/hilar mass.
- Reassess for pericarditis and arrange an echocardiogram to look for pericardial effusion if there are any suggestive features (step 4, above) or cardiomegaly on CXR.

Consider hyperventilation or anxiety if there are suggestive clinical features and PE has been excluded. If an ABG test has been performed, $PaCO_2$ will be reduced, but PaO_2 will be normal in the presence of hyperventilation.

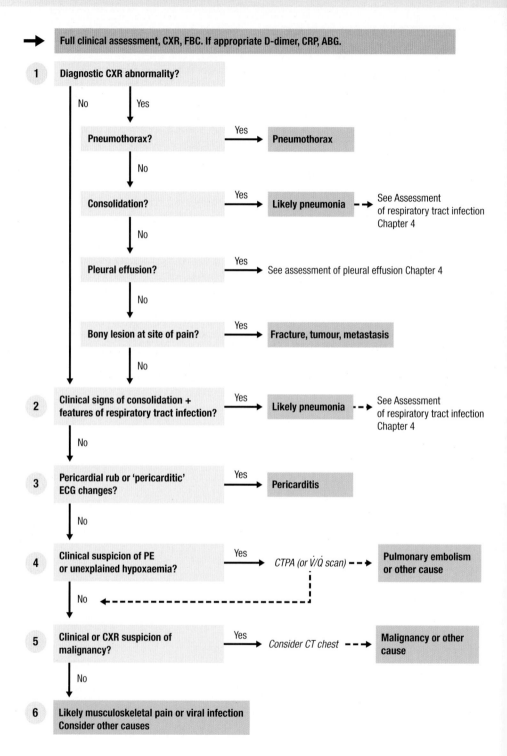

Full clinical assessment, CXR, FBC. If appropriate D-dimer, CRP, ABG.

1 Diagnostic CXR abnormality?

No / Yes

Pneumothorax? — Yes → **Pneumothorax**

No

Consolidation? — Yes → **Likely pneumonia** - - ► See Assessment of respiratory tract infection Chapter 4

No

Pleural effusion? — Yes → See assessment of pleural effusion Chapter 4

No

Bony lesion at site of pain? — Yes → **Fracture, tumour, metastasis**

No

2 Clinical signs of consolidation + features of respiratory tract infection? — Yes → **Likely pneumonia** - - ► See Assessment of respiratory tract infection Chapter 4

No

3 Pericardial rub or 'pericarditic' ECG changes? — Yes → **Pericarditis**

No

4 Clinical suspicion of PE or unexplained hypoxaemia? — Yes → *CTPA (or V̇/Q̇ scan)* - - ► **Pulmonary embolism or other cause**

No

5 Clinical or CXR suspicion of malignancy? — Yes → *Consider CT chest* - - ► **Malignancy or other cause**

No

6 Likely musculoskeletal pain or viral infection
Consider other causes

1 Diagnostic CXR abnormality?

Look carefully for:
- Pneumothorax (Fig. 4.5)—small pneumothoraces are easily missed.
- Consolidation (Figs 4.3 and 4.4)—if present, go to further assessment of respiratory tract infection (RTI—see Chapter 4), especially if accompanied by cough, purulent sputum, dyspnoea or fever.
- Pleural effusion (Fig. 4.2)—if present, assess as per Chapter 4.
- Rib fractures or metastatic deposits—if the latter are present, investigate for a primary lung cancer, metastatic disease or multiple myeloma.

2 Clinical signs of consolidation and features of respiratory tract infection?

Even in the absence of definitive CXR changes, pneumonia is the likely diagnosis if pleuritic pain is accompanied by:
- Focal chest signs, such as crackles, bronchial breathing, and
- Symptoms of RTI: productive cough, acute dyspnoea or fever.
  If present, assess as Chapter 4.

3 Pericardial rub or 'pericarditic' ECG changes?

Diagnose pericarditis if pleuritic pain is accompanied by typical ECG features of pericarditis (Fig. 3.12) or a pericardial rub. Request an echocardiogram to detect any associated effusion (urgently if any features of tamponade—and assess LV function (may be impaired if associated myocarditis).

4 Clinical suspicion of PE or unexplained hypoxaemia?

Consider a PE in any patient presenting with pleuritic chest pain. Clinical suspicion should be high, and PE must be excluded, in patients with:
- Relevant risk factors, such as active malignancy, history of PE/DVT, recent surgery or prolonged immobility

- Haemoptysis or dyspnoea, in the absence of an alternative explanation (e.g., RTI)
- Evidence of DVT
- Unexplained hypoxaemia
- ECG features of PE Fig. 3.11
- No clear alternative diagnosis

Use the history and examination findings, Wells score and a D-dimer test to guide investigation for PE. Note that D-dimer is less useful for investigating PE in hospitalized patients. In this situation, perform a CT pulmonary angiogram (CTPA) if there is clinical suspicion and the Wells score is ≥2. As well as being a sensitive investigation for PE, CTPA may demonstrate an alternative cause of pleuritic chest pain.

5 Clinical or CXR suspicion of malignancy?

Consider further investigation with CT chest ± a respiratory opinion in patients >40 years or with a history of smoking/asbestos exposure if pain is accompanied by:
- A history of weight loss
- Recurrent or unexplained haemoptysis
- Recent change in voice
- Persistent cervical lymphadenopathy
- Finger clubbing
- Night sweats
- Suspicious CXR changes (Box 6.1).

6 Likely musculoskeletal pain or viral infection. Consider other causes

Seek a respiratory opinion and consider further imaging in patients with dyspnoea or a new CXR abnormality other than those described above. Rarer causes of pleuritic chest pain include drug-induced pleuritis (e.g., amiodarone, methotrexate) or pleurisy secondary to a rheumatic disease (e.g., systemic lupus erythematosus, rheumatoid arthritis).

Otherwise, the most likely diagnoses are viral pleurisy or musculoskeletal pain. Suspect the former if there is fever, coryzal or 'flu-like' symptoms or a pleural rub; suspect the latter if there is any recent injury, prolonged severe coughing, unusually strenuous upper body activity, marked exacerbation of pain on movement or obvious tenderness on palpation.

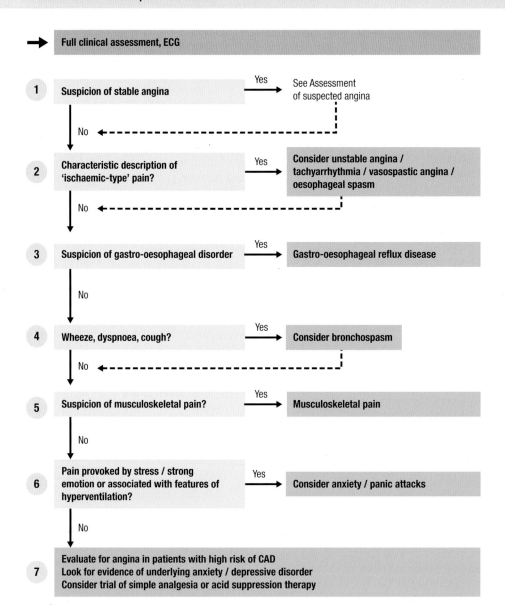

Full clinical assessment, ECG

1 Suspicion of stable angina — Yes → See Assessment of suspected angina

No

2 Characteristic description of 'ischaemic-type' pain? — Yes → Consider unstable angina / tachyarrhythmia / vasospastic angina / oesophageal spasm

No

3 Suspicion of gastro-oesophageal disorder — Yes → Gastro-oesophageal reflux disease

No

4 Wheeze, dyspnoea, cough? — Yes → Consider bronchospasm

No

5 Suspicion of musculoskeletal pain? — Yes → Musculoskeletal pain

No

6 Pain provoked by stress / strong emotion or associated with features of hyperventilation? — Yes → Consider anxiety / panic attacks

No

7 Evaluate for angina in patients with high risk of CAD
Look for evidence of underlying anxiety / depressive disorder
Consider trial of simple analgesia or acid suppression therapy

1   Suspicion of stable angina?

The hallmark of stable angina is a correlation between symptoms and alterations in cardiac work. Retrosternal discomfort that consistently arises during exertion and is rapidly relieved (<5 minutes) by rest strongly suggests angina. The quality of the discomfort may vary widely and is frequently vague or nonspecific. The likelihood of angina also depends on the risk of underlying CAD. With rare exceptions, coronary atherosclerosis is central to the pathogenesis of angina, so patients with a low risk of CAD have a correspondingly low risk of angina.

Assessment of suspected angina

Step 1 Consider unstable angina and structural heart disease
An abrupt onset, sudden worsening, or increase in duration and frequency of exertional chest pain indicates unstable angina.

If the patient has an ejection systolic murmur, exertional syncope or ECG features of left ventricular hypertrophy (Fig. 3.10), arrange echocardiography to exclude aortic stenosis and hypertrophic cardiomyopathy.

Step 2 Confirm or refute the diagnosis
In patients >40 years with a typical history and moderate/high likelihood of CAD (Box 3.4), make a clinical diagnosis of stable angina and proceed to step 3.

If the risk of CAD is low, consider CT coronary angiography, if available, as a first-line investigation. If negative, return to the algorithm for intermittent chest pain (reenter at step 3). If positive, proceed to a stress test or invasive angiography.

Otherwise, consider a stress test (Box 3.6). If positive, diagnose stable angina and proceed to step 3. If negative (i.e. no evidence of inducible ischaemia at high stress), return to the algorithm for intermittent chest pain (reenter at step 3). Seek input from Cardiology if you have a high clinical suspicion and are unable to identify a clear alternative cause.

If results are equivocal (e.g., suboptimal test, minor abnormality, or typical symptoms without ECG changes), consider an alternative stress test or coronary angiography to clarify the diagnosis.

Step 3 Assess symptom severity and risk
The severity of angina is based not on the intensity of pain but the frequency of symptoms, impairment of exercise capacity, and consequent functional limitation. This information is used to guide treatment and monitor response, quantify symptoms accurately and determine their impact on work, hobbies, and daily activities. The persistence of limiting symptoms despite antianginal therapy is an indication for angiography with a view to revascularization. Exercise ECG may be used to identify high-risk patients whose prognosis could be improved by angiography and revascularization.

2   Characteristic description of 'ischaemic-type' pain (Box 3.1)?

Intermittent episodes of myocardial ischaemia unrelated to exertion may occur with critical coronary obstruction due to plaque rupture and thrombus formation (unstable angina), coronary artery spasm (vasospastic angina) or paroxysmal tachyarrhythmia (especially in the presence of an underlying coronary stenosis). Oesophageal spasm may closely mimic ischaemic-type discomfort and lacks a consistent relationship to exertion. Consider these diagnoses in patients with intermittent characteristic ischaemic-type discomfort that lacks a predictable relationship to exertion or (with the exception of unstable angina) in whom stress testing fails to demonstrate inducible myocardial ischaemia.

Suspect paroxysmal arrhythmia if any of the following:
- Palpitation preceding or during symptoms
- Previously documented tachyarrhythmia
- Infrequent episodes of variable duration.

If suspected, attempt to document the rhythm during a typical episode of symptoms.

Suspect vasospastic angina if any of the following:
- No apparent triggers
- Sudden onset of intense symptoms ± autonomic features
- Short duration of episodes (2–5 minutes)
- Episodes occurring in clusters.

If suspected, consider a trial of Holter ECG monitoring to look for evidence of ST elevation during symptomatic episodes.

Suspect oesophageal spasm if any of the following:

- Intermittent dysphagia
- History or typical symptoms of GORD (below)
- Discomfort occurring predominantly at night or after eating.

If the history suggests GORD, consider reassessment after a trial of a proton pump inhibitor; otherwise, refer to the GI team for consideration of upper GI endoscopy/oesophageal manometry.

3 Suspicion of gastro-oesophageal disorder?

If the pain is unlikely to be cardiac, seek typical features of other disorders. GORD is typically associated with a hot burning retrosternal discomfort which radiates upwards and is often provoked by bending or lying flat or aggravated by food. Symptoms are often relieved by acid suppression therapy (e.g., proton pump inhibitor) and this can be useful to confirm the diagnosis. Upper GI endoscopy may be indicated if symptoms are refractory or there is concern of an underlying malignancy (evaluate as described in Chapter 10).

4 Wheeze, dyspnoea, cough?

Chest pain associated with asthma and COPD may be difficult to distinguish from angina on clinical grounds if symptoms are provoked by exertion and produce a sensation of chest 'tightness'. Helpful diagnostic features may include a history of cough or wheeze (especially nocturnal), diurnal variation in symptoms, the presence of wheeze on auscultation, a history of atopy and absence of risk factors for CAD. If asthma or COPD is suspected, evaluate as described in Chapter 4.

5 Suspicion of musculoskeletal pain?

Musculoskeletal pain may present in a multitude of ways but is usually localized, induced by specific movements and reproduced by palpation. A history of recent injury, strain or vigorous activity would also support the diagnosis. Further investigation is rarely necessary; a symptomatic response to simple analgesia helps to confirm the diagnosis.

6 Pain provoked by stress/strong emotion or associated with features of hyperventilation?

Attributing episodes of chest pain to anxiety can be challenging and should be a diagnosis of exclusion. Emotional distress increases cardiac work and may provoke angina, but symptoms that occur exclusively in this context are more likely to have a psychological origin. Associated features of panic or hyperventilation during episodes (e.g., breathlessness with 'inability to take in enough air', choking sensation, tingling in the extremities, light-headedness) support the diagnosis. Seek specialist input before attributing a new presentation of chest pain to anxiety in patients with a high risk of CAD.

7 Evaluate for angina in patients at high risk of CAD. Consider other causes

In many patients, it is not possible to reach a definite diagnosis. Reassess those with inconclusive investigations for angina or with a high likelihood of CAD (Box 3.4) if symptoms persist. Where a cardiac cause has been ruled out and no other cause is apparent, patients often respond to simple reassurance. However, a minority experience severe, refractory symptoms and may merit specialist assessment for underlying psychological factors and/or management of chronic pain.

Dyspnoea is the subjective sensation of breathing discomfort. It is an important predictor of quality of life, exercise tolerance and mortality in many conditions, such as COPD and heart failure. It occurs when ventilatory signals from the brainstem are misaligned to sensory feedback from the thorax. It is important to remember that severity of dyspnoea is highly subjective, and some individuals may not experience breathlessness despite severe impairment of gas exchange.

Acute dyspnoea

Acute dyspnoea is defined here as new or abruptly worsening breathlessness within the preceding 2 weeks. Concomitant objective signs of severe hypoxaemia, hypercapnia, exhaustion or ↓GCS may herald life-threatening pathology. The diagnosis can be made by combining clinical evaluation with key investigations including CXR, ECG, pulse oximetry and arterial blood gas (ABG) analysis. In the initial phase of assessment, diagnosis and treatment should be conducted in parallel, and the cycle of intervention and reassessment should continue until the patient is stable. Important causes of acute dyspnoea are listed below.

Upper airway obstruction

- Inhaled foreign body
- Anaphylaxis
- Epiglottitis
- Extrinsic compression, e.g., rapidly expanding haematoma

Lower airway disease

- Acute bronchitis
- Asthma
- Acute exacerbation of chronic obstructive pulmonary disease (COPD)
- Acute exacerbation of bronchiectasis
- Anaphylaxis

Parenchymal lung disease

- Pneumonia
- Lobar collapse
- Acute respiratory distress syndrome (ARDS)

Other respiratory causes

- Pneumothorax
- Pleural effusion
- Pulmonary embolism (PE)
- Acute chest wall injury

Box 4.1 MRC dyspnoea scale

Grade 1 Not troubled by breathlessness except on strenuous exercise

Grade 2 Short of breath when hurrying or walking up a slight hill

Grade 3 Walks slower than contemporaries on level ground because of breathlessness, or has to stop for breath when walking at own pace

Grade 4 Stops for breath after walking about 100 m or after a few minutes on level ground

Grade 5 Too breathless to leave the house, or breathless when dressing or undressing

Adapted from Fletcher CM, Elmes PC, Fairbairn MB et al. 1959. The significance of respiratory symptoms and the diagnosis of chronic bronchitis in a working population. Br Med J. 2:257–266.

Cardiovascular causes

- Acute cardiogenic pulmonary oedema
- Acute coronary syndrome
- Cardiac tamponade
- Arrhythmia
- Acute valvular heart disease

Other causes

- Metabolic acidosis
- Psychogenic breathlessness (acute hyperventilation)

Chronic dyspnoea

Chronic dyspnoea is defined here as breathlessness of >2 weeks' duration. Use the Medical Research Council (MRC) dyspnoea scale (Box 4.1) to assess the severity of breathlessness.

Important causes of chronic dyspnoea are listed below.

Respiratory causes

- Asthma
- COPD
- Pleural effusion
- Lung cancer: bronchial carcinoma, mesothelioma, lymphangitis carcinomatosis
- Interstitial lung disease (ILD): classified according to whether the cause is unknown

(e.g., idiopathic pulmonary fibrosis) or known (e.g., sarcoidosis, hypersensitivity pneumonitis).

- Chronic pulmonary thromboembolism
- Bronchiectasis
- Cystic fibrosis
- Pulmonary hypertension (primary or secondary)
- Pulmonary vasculitis
- Tuberculosis (TB)
- Laryngeal/tracheal stenosis, e.g., extrinsic compression, malignancy

Cardiovascular causes

- Chronic heart failure
- Coronary artery disease ('angina equivalent')
- Valvular heart disease

- Paroxysmal arrhythmia
- Constrictive pericarditis
- Pericardial effusion
- Cyanotic congenital heart disease

Other causes

- Anaemia
- Obesity hypoventilation syndrome (OHS)
- Chest wall disease, e.g., kyphoscoliosis
- Physical deconditioning
- Diaphragmatic paralysis
- Psychogenic hyperventilation
- Neuromuscular disorder, for example, myasthenia gravis, muscular dystrophies
- Cirrhosis (hepatopulmonary syndrome)
- Tense ascites

4

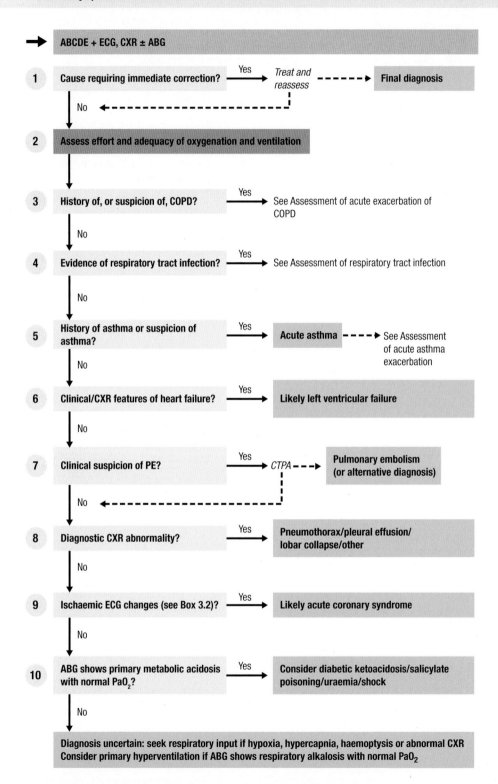

ABCDE + ECG, CXR ± ABG

1   Cause requiring immediate correction?   **Yes** → *Treat and reassess* - - - - → **Final diagnosis**

    No

2   **Assess effort and adequacy of oxygenation and ventilation**

3   History of, or suspicion of, COPD?   **Yes** → See Assessment of acute exacerbation of COPD

    No

4   Evidence of respiratory tract infection?   **Yes** → See Assessment of respiratory tract infection

    No

5   History of asthma or suspicion of asthma?   **Yes** → **Acute asthma** - - - → See Assessment of acute asthma exacerbation

    No

6   Clinical/CXR features of heart failure?   **Yes** → **Likely left ventricular failure**

    No

7   Clinical suspicion of PE?   **Yes** → *CTPA* - - → **Pulmonary embolism (or alternative diagnosis)**

    No

8   Diagnostic CXR abnormality?   **Yes** → **Pneumothorax/pleural effusion/ lobar collapse/other**

    No

9   Ischaemic ECG changes (see Box 3.2)?   **Yes** → **Likely acute coronary syndrome**

    No

10   ABG shows primary metabolic acidosis with normal PaO_2?   **Yes** → **Consider diabetic ketoacidosis/salicylate poisoning/uraemia/shock**

    No

Diagnosis uncertain: seek respiratory input if hypoxia, hypercapnia, haemoptysis or abnormal CXR
Consider primary hyperventilation if ABG shows respiratory alkalosis with normal PaO_2

1 Cause requiring immediate correction?

Identify and provide immediate corrective treatment for:

- Airway obstruction
- Tension pneumothorax
- Anaphylaxis
- Arrhythmia with cardiac compromise

Seek specialist input if necessary and repeat the assessment following intervention.

2 Assess effort and adequacy of oxygenation and ventilation

This is fundamental to the assessment of acute respiratory compromise and should be reassessed frequently to monitor progress and evaluate the effect of interventions.

Assess the effort of breathing by repeated clinical observation of rate, depth and pattern of respiration; look for use of accessory muscles, ability to complete full sentences, and features of exhaustion. Monitor the SpO_2 by pulse oximetry in all patients and perform ABG analysis if any of the following features are present:

- A need for airway or ventilatory support
- SpO_2 <92% (or unreliable), central cyanosis or high O_2 requirements (>4 L/min)
- Features of hypercapnia: drowsiness, confusion, asterixis
- Severe, prolonged or worsening respiratory distress
- Background of COPD and/or chronic type 2 respiratory failure

Correct hypoxia by administration of supplemental O_2. Titrate the inspired O_2 concentration (FiO_2) to the minimum required to achieve a target SpO_2:

- 94–98% for previously well patients.
- 88–92% for patients with chronic type 2 respiratory failure. Use a controlled O_2 delivery device, that is, a venturi mask. Target saturations may be lower in patients with lower baseline SpO_2. Monitor FiO_2 requirements carefully to maintain the target SpO_2.

Use the $PaCO_2$ to assess adequacy of ventilation (see Clinical tool Interpretation of arterial blood gases). In patients with a high or rising $PaCO_2$, look for reversible factors contributing to ventilatory impairment, for example, bronchospasm, sedation or respiratory depressants. Be vigilant for loss of hypoxic drive-in patients with chronic type 2 respiratory failure receiving supplemental O_2, particularly if the patient is becoming drowsy. Suspect an alternative cause, e.g., exhaustion, airways obstruction, if no reversible factors are identified or if there is no improvement despite treatment.

It is imperative to seek early input from the critical care team and consider the need for respiratory support (e.g., noninvasive ventilation or tracheal intubation and mechanical ventilation) when any of the following features are present:

- Impending exhaustion
- Acute/acute-on-chronic ventilatory failure not resolving with correction of reversible factors
- Progressively rising $PaCO_2$
- SpO_2 <90% or PaO_2 <8 kPa despite maximal respiratory assistance
- Progressively rising FiO_2 requirements to maintain target SpO_2

3 History of, or suspicion of, COPD?

In the absence of a preexisting diagnosis, suspect COPD in any patient with a history of smoking and:

- Clinical (Fig. 4.1) or CXR features of hyperinflation
- Persistent respiratory symptoms including exertional dyspnoea, cough with or without productive sputum, and wheeze

Assessment of acute exacerbation of COPD

Step 1 Clarify cause for acute deterioration

- Ensure that there are no new CXR abnormalities: look carefully for evidence of collapse, consolidation, pneumothorax or pleural effusion. If there are features of consolidation, treat as pneumonia rather than 'infective exacerbation of COPD'.
- Ask about cough and sputum: treat as an infective exacerbation of COPD when there is an increase in sputum volume or purulence but no evidence of consolidation.
- If wheeze is predominant and there are no features of infection, the likely diagnosis is noninfective exacerbation of COPD. Look

Clinical tool
Interpretation of arterial blood gases

An ABG measurement is obtained for two primary reasons: assessment of oxygenation and ventilation, and assessment of acid-base status. PaO_2 reflects oxygenation, and a reduction in PaO_2 (type 1 respiratory failure) indicates impairment of oxygenation. By contrast, $PaCO_2$ is determined by alveolar ventilation (i.e., the volume of air transported between the alveoli and the outside world in any given time) and increased $PaCO_2$ (hypercapnia) implies ventilatory failure (type 2 respiratory failure).

An acidosis is any process that acts to lower blood pH ($\uparrow H^+$); an alkalosis is one that acts to raise blood pH ($\downarrow H^+$). A respiratory or metabolic acid-base disturbance usually triggers an adjustment by the other system to limit the change in blood pH (compensation). Respiratory compensation happens over minutes; metabolic compensation, which is regulated by the kidneys, takes days to weeks.

Increasingly, venous blood gas (VBG) samples are being used instead of ABG measurements as they are far less painful to obtain. While VBG samples provide sufficient assessment of acid-base status, ABG measurements are required for accurate determination of oxygenation and ventilation.

Assessment of oxygenation

To assess if oxygenation is impaired, it is necessary to assess whether the PaO_2 is appropriate for the FiO_2. The administration of supplemental O_2 makes ABG analysis more complex. A useful rule of thumb is that the difference between FiO_2 (%) and PaO_2 (in kPa) should be ≤10. A patient breathing room air (FiO_2 of 21%) should have a PaO_2 of at least 11 kPa, while a patient receiving supplementary oxygen with a FiO_2 of 40% should have a PaO_2 of at least 30 kPa.

Assessment of ventilation

A rise in $PaCO_2$ indicates ventilatory failure of the alveoli and type 2 respiratory failure. When this process occurs over a long period (e.g., a patient with a long history of COPD), it is usually accompanied by an increase in HCO_3^- that serves to maintain acid-base balance within normal range. This is chronic (compensated) type 2 respiratory failure. However, in the presence of an acute rise in $PaCO_2$ (e.g., acute exacerbation of COPD), a rise in H^+ and acidosis will occur as metabolic compensation cannot occur quickly enough to maintain normal acid-base balance. This is acute or acute-on-chronic (decompensated) type 2 respiratory failure (Table 4.1). In type 2 respiratory failure, the rate of rise in $PaCO_2$ and the associated increase in H^+ provide a better guide to severity than the absolute value of $PaCO_2$.

A $\downarrow PaCO_2$ implies hyperventilation. If PaO_2 is also lowered (or just within normal limits), the hyperventilation is probably an appropriate response to hypoxia. Alternatively, if HCO_3^- is decreased, it may reflect respiratory compensation for a primary metabolic acidosis, for example, diabetic ketoacidosis. A $\downarrow PaCO_2$ with normal PaO_2 and HCO_3^- (on room air) suggests primary (psychogenic) hyperventilation, but this is a diagnosis of exclusion (see below).

Assessment of acid-base status

If the presence of an acidosis or alkalosis has been established, the next step is to establish whether the process is predominantly respiratory or metabolic. A rise in $PaCO_2$ indicates a respiratory acidosis, while a reduction in $PaCO_2$ indicates a respiratory alkalosis. By contrast, a reduction in HCO_3^- indicates a metabolic acidosis, while a rise in HCO_3^- indicates a metabolic alkalosis.

Primary respiratory acidosis (ventilatory failure) and alkalosis (hyperventilation) are dealt with above.

Causes of metabolic acidosis and alkalosis are shown in Box 4.2. If there is a primary metabolic acidosis, calculate the anion gap (anion gap = $[Na^+ + K^+] - [Cl^- + HCO_3^-]$; normal, 12–16 mmol/L). The anion gap measures the difference between the positively and negatively charged electrolytes in the blood. It is useful to narrow the differential diagnosis of the cause of the metabolic acidosis.

Table 4.1 Arterial blood gases in different patterns of respiratory failure

Type	Failure	PaO_2	$PaCO_2$	HCO_3^-	pH
Type 1 Respiratory Failure	—	$\downarrow$	$\rightarrow / \downarrow$	$\rightarrow$	$\rightarrow / \uparrow$
Type 2 Respiratory Failure	Acute	$\downarrow$	$\uparrow$	$\rightarrow$	$\downarrow$
	Chronic	$\downarrow$	$\uparrow$	$\uparrow$	$\rightarrow$
	Acute-on-chronic	$\downarrow$	$\uparrow$	$\uparrow$	$\downarrow$

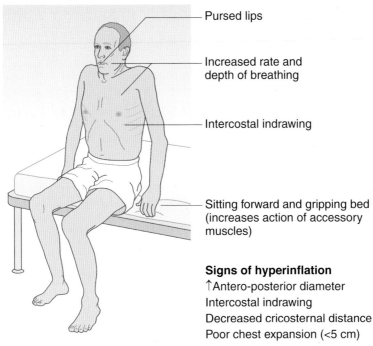

Pursed lips

Increased rate and depth of breathing

Intercostal indrawing

Sitting forward and gripping bed (increases action of accessory muscles)

Signs of hyperinflation
↑Antero-posterior diameter
Intercostal indrawing
Decreased cricosternal distance
Poor chest expansion (<5 cm)

Fig. 4.1 Clinical features of COPD.

Box 4.2 Causes of metabolic acidosis and alkalosis

Metabolic acidosis (low HCO$_3^-$)

With raised anion gap (mnemonic: MUDPILES)
- Methanol
- Uraemia
- Diabetic/alcoholic/starvation ketoacidosis
- Paracetamol/propylene glycol/paraldehyde
- Iron/isoniazid
- Lactic acidosis
- Ethylene glycol
- Salicylates

With normal anion gap
- Renal tubular acidosis
- Diarrhoea
- Ammonium chloride ingestion
- Adrenal insufficiency

Metabolic alkalosis (high HCO$_3^-$)
- Vomiting
- Potassium depletion, for example, diuretics
- Cushing syndrome
- Conn's syndrome (primary hyperaldosteronism)

---

for precipitants e.g., an environmental trigger, noncompliance with inhalers or recently commenced beta-blocker therapy. Often a precipitant cannot be identified.
- Evaluate for PE (see Fig. 4.6) when there is a sudden increase in breathlessness or hypoxia without wheeze, change in sputum or new CXR abnormality.

Step 2 Establish preexacerbation status and details of previous exacerbations
This provides a comprehensive picture of underlying e.g., disease severity, helping to guide the goals and limits of therapy.
- Baseline performance: quantify normal exercise tolerance, ask about activities that provoke dyspnoea and ascertain ability to perform/limitations to activities of daily living (ADLs).
- Baseline lung function: refer to previous ABG/SpO$_2$ measurements and PFTs to provide an objective estimate of disease

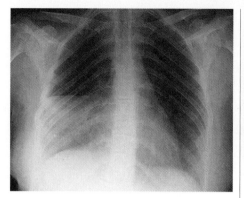

Fig. 4.2 Pneumonia of the right middle lobe.

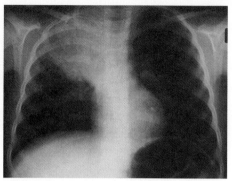

Fig. 4.3 Right upper lobe pneumonia containing air bronchograms.

severity and look for evidence of chronic hypercapnia (see above).

- Trajectory of disease: consider changes in the above severity measures over time, the frequency of admissions and previous requirement for respiratory support, for example, noninvasive and invasive ventilation.
- Previous sputum cultures: antibiotic prescribing should be guided by local protocols, but knowledge of previous pathogens may permit more effective tailored therapy; discuss with the Microbiology team if unusual or resistant organisms have been grown on previous cultures.

Step 3 Compare current status to baseline and monitor response to treatment

- Oxygenation and ventilation: compare current ABG values and SpO$_2$ to previous records. Give supplemental O$_2$ to return SpO$_2$/PaO$_2$ to baseline. If the patient has chronic type 2 respiratory failure, monitor for loss of ventilatory drive and repeat an ABG analysis after any increase in FiO$_2$.
- Functional reserve: assess overall work of breathing (rate, depth, use of accessory muscles). Very high respiratory work cannot be maintained for long; refer to critical care if there is impending exhaustion and escalation of care is appropriate.
- Airways obstruction: assess PEFR and the presence/extent of wheeze; monitor changes to gauge response to bronchodilator therapy.

- Following recovery, record predischarge PEFR, SpO$_2$ and ABG on air.

4 Evidence of respiratory tract infection (RTI)?

Consider respiratory tract infection if any of the following features are present:
- New cough with purulent sputum or significant increase in purulent sputum
- Temperature ≥38°C or <35°C
- Acute illness with sweating, rigors and myalgia
- Clinical/CXR signs of consolidation (Figs 4.2 and 4.3) with ↑WBC/CRP

Assessment of respiratory tract infections

Step 1 Classify the type of RTI

In patients with features of RTI, distinguish pneumonia from nonpneumonic infection by the presence of focal chest signs, e.g., crepitations, bronchial breathing and/or new CXR opacification (see Figs 4.2 and 4.3). Classify as community-acquired pneumonia (CAP) if infection has been acquired out of hospital, and hospital-acquired pneumonia (HAP) if the onset of illness occurred ≥48 hours after hospital admission, or within 90 days of discharge from hospital following an admission of 2 or more days. In previously well patients without focal chest signs or CXR abnormalities, the likely diagnosis is nonpneumonic RTI, e.g., acute bronchitis. In patients with known bronchiectasis, consider an infective exacerbation if the sputum becomes more purulent or offensive; assessment of patients with underlying COPD is described above.

Step 2 Assess severity

The CURB-65 score (Table 4.2) can help risk-stratify patients with CAP based on predicted mortality. This can be used as a guideline to inform whether a patient requires inpatient or outpatient treatment. Patients with CURB-65 scores ≥2 will require admission to hospital for IV antibiotics and monitoring. There may be situations where a low mortality score may not reflect true mortality risk and clinical judgment is required. For example, patients with a low CURB-65 score may still require admission to hospital if they require supplementary oxygen or are deemed to be at high risk of deterioration due to comorbidity.

Step 3 Look for predisposing factors

Assess for factors associated with immuno-compromise, e.g., chronic disease (diabetes, cirrhosis, malnutrition, AIDS), acute disease (any critical illness), drugs (steroids, immunotherapy, chemotherapy) or previous splenectomy. Suspect aspiration in patients with a history of swallowing difficulty, reduced consciousness level, stroke, or alcohol/drug misuse. Preceding viral infection, especially influenza, may predispose to severe secondary bacterial infection. Consider endocarditis in patients with multiple discrete or flitting shadows on CXR, especially if they are high risk. Consider testing for blood-borne viruses in all patients who present with pneumonia, and be aware that ≥2 presentations with pneumonia in 12 months is considered an AIDS-defining condition. Pneumonia may occur distal to a bronchial carcinoma. Repeat the CXR 4 to 6 weeks after treatment to ensure resolution of changes in patients with risk factors, and consider further investigation (e.g., bronchoscopy if there are persistent symptoms/CXR features or recurrent pneumonia at the same site).

Step 4 Gather information to inform antimicrobial choice

In any patient requiring hospitalization for RTI, culture blood and sputum, perform serological assessment for atypical pathogens

Table 4.2 CURB-65 score

Feature	Score
Confusion	Abbreviated Mental Test <8/10 or new disorientation in time, place or person
Urea	>7 mmol/L
RR	≥30/min
BP	Systolic <90 or diastolic <60 mmHg
Age	≥65 years
Total score	**30-day mortality risk**
0 or 1	Low risk; <3% mortality risk
2	Intermediate risk; 3–15% mortality risk
3–5	High risk; >15% mortality risk

Adapted from Lim W, et al. 2003. Defining community acquired pneumonia severity on presentation to hospital: an international derivation and validation study. Thorax. 58(5):377–382.

and take a viral throat swab. In patients with severe pneumonia (CURB-65 >2), send pneumococcal and Legionella urine antigen tests. Legionella urine antigen testing allows for rapid results early in the illness. Pneumococcal urine antigen testing shows greater sensitivity than blood or sputum samples. Discuss with the Respiratory physicians regarding the requirement for an aspiration of pleural fluid for microscopy and culture if there is an associated parapneumonic effusion. If there is a suspicion of TB, send multiple sputum samples (induced with nebulized hypertonic saline if possible) for Ziehl–Neelsen staining and TB culture. Factors which raise the suspicion of TB may include:

- Significant immunocompromise or debility
- Previous residence in an endemic TB area
- Recent close contact with a smear-positive TB patient
- CXR evidence of previous TB
- A background of persistent productive cough with weight loss, night sweats or other constitutional symptoms

5 History of asthma or suspicion of asthma?

Acute dyspnoea with worsening wheeze in a patient with a preexisting diagnosis of asthma suggests an acute exacerbation. In the absence of a preexisting diagnosis, suspect asthma in any patient with widespread generalized wheeze and reduced PEFR with no evidence of COPD, anaphylaxis or pulmonary oedema. Consider other causes of acute dyspnoea, for example, pneumothorax or PE, if neither of these features are present.

Assessment of acute asthma exacerbation

Step 1 Assess severity and need for hospital admission

Assess severity in any patient with suspected acute asthma according to Table 4.3; perform an ABG analysis when there are life-threatening features or SpO_2 <92%. Admit patients to hospital if they have:

- Life-threatening features
- Features of a severe attack persisting after initial treatment
- PEFR <75% or significant ongoing symptoms after 1 hour of treatment
- Other features causing concern, for example, previous near-fatal asthma or poor compliance with treatment

If there are ongoing features of a severe attack, monitor in a critical care environment with repeated assessment of SpO_2, PEFR, RR, HR, work of breathing and ABG. Refer urgently to the intensive care unit if $PaCO_2$ is >6 kPa or rising, or if there is worsening hypoxia, exhaustion or ↓GCS.

Step 2 Look for treatable precipitants

Seek evidence of infection (e.g., pyrexia, purulent sputum, ↑WBC, physical/CXR signs of consolidation (see Figs 4.2 and 4.3)) and flitting upper lobe infiltrates, suggesting allergic bronchopulmonary aspergillosis. Culture sputum if this is purulent and obtain blood cultures if temperature is ≥38°C. Carefully review the CXR to exclude pneumothorax (Fig. 4.4).

Step 3 Assess baseline control

Establish:

- Frequency and severity of exacerbations
- Baseline symptoms between exacerbations
- Best PEFR
- Current inhaler regimen, technique and compliance

Table 4.3 Clinical features of severe asthma		
Severity	**PEFR**	*or* **Other features**
Moderate	50–75% best or predicted	Increased symptoms No features of acute severe asthma
Severe	33–50% best or predicted	Any of: RR >25 breaths per minute HR >110 bpm Inability to complete sentences in one breath
Life-threatening	<33% best or predicted	Any of: PaO_2 <8 kPa 'Normal' $PaCO_2$ (4.6–6.0 kPa) SpO_2 <92% Silent chest Cyanosis Exhaustion/altered conscious level Poor respiratory effort Arrhythmia Hypotension
Near-fatal	—	$PaCO_2$ >6 kPa and/or requiring mechanical ventilation with raised inflation pressures

Modified from British Thoracic Society, Scottish Intercollegiate Guidelines Network 158 2019. British guideline on the management of asthma.

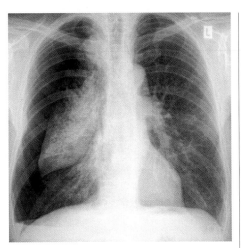

Fig. 4.4 Right pneumothorax.

- Frequency of PRN inhaler use
- Frequency of oral steroids (consider bone protection if prolonged or frequent use of steroids)
- Current smoking status

Look for avoidable precipitants e.g., pollen, pets, cold air, exercise, smoking, occupational triggers, beta blockers, NSAIDs.

Step 4 Recovery

Assess with pulmonary function tests (PFTs) ± PEFR diary following resolution of the acute episode.

6   Clinical/CXR features of heart failure?

Acute decompensated heart failure is the likely cause of breathlessness if any of the following are present:

- CXR evidence of pulmonary oedema or congestion (Fig. 4.5)
- A recent history of orthopnoea or nocturnal dyspnoea with progressively worsening exertional dyspnoea
- Signs of fluid overload, such as peripheral oedema or a raised JVP

Always suspect the diagnosis in patients with a background of chronic heart failure or other predisposing cardiac condition (e.g.,

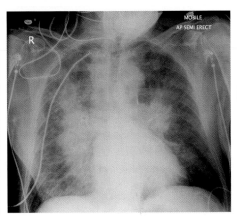

Fig. 4.5 Left ventricular failure. Note the hazy perihilar shadowing ('bat's wings'), the prominent, dilated upper lobe veins and the basal Kerley B lines, all characteristic of pulmonary oedema. There is also cardiomegaly.

previous MI or valvular disease), but assess carefully for alternative causes of acute decompensation (especially if the above features are absent), and remember that acute heart failure can also present de novo.

Difficulty may arise when the CXR is not diagnostic (e.g., in early or mild cases) and when auscultatory findings resemble those heard in other disorders (e.g., pulmonary fibrosis, bilateral pneumonia). A therapeutic trial may assist diagnosis: rapid improvement of symptoms with vasodilators/diuretics is strongly suggestive of heart failure as the aetiology of dyspnoea. Consider noncardiogenic pulmonary oedema in acutely dyspnoeic patients with bilateral pulmonary infiltrates but no other evidence of heart failure. ARDS is a well-recognized form of noncardiogenic pulmonary oedema associated with lung inflammation that occurs in the setting of severe acute pathology such as trauma, burns, pancreatitis or sepsis.

Echocardiography to assess ventricular and valvular function is a key diagnostic test and is particularly useful in patients without a preexisting diagnosis of heart failure or in those with possible noncardiogenic pulmonary oedema.

If available, brain-type natriuretic peptide (BNP) testing can help to rule out acute heart failure. Low plasma BNP makes the diagnosis unlikely; however, BNP is also raised in a wide variety of other cardiac and noncardiac conditions, so elevated levels do not automatically confirm a diagnosis of acute heart failure.

7 Clinical suspicion of PE?

PE is often underdiagnosed. Clinical and CXR findings, in isolation, lack diagnostic sensitivity and specificity. Use a clinical decision tool such as that shown in Fig. 4.6 and Table 4.4 to evaluate for PE in patients with acute dyspnoea and any of the following:
- Relevant risk factors, such as active malignancy, history of PE/DVT, recent surgery or prolonged immobility
- Haemoptysis, pleuritic chest pain or evidence of deep vein thrombosis (DVT)
- Unexplained hypoxaemia
- ECG features of right heart strain (Fig. 3.11)
- No clear alternative diagnosis

D-Dimer is less useful in hospitalized patients, so in this setting consider further investigation when the Wells score is ≥2 or when clinical suspicion is high. Have a low threshold for performing ABG analysis as subtle oxygenation

Table 4.4 Wells score (pulmonary embolism)

Clinical variable	Points
Clinical signs and symptoms of DVT[a]	3
No alternative diagnosis is more likely than PE	3
Heart rate >100 bpm	1.5
Immobilization for more than 3 days or surgery in the previous 4 weeks	1.5
Previous DVT/PE	1.5
Haemoptysis	1
Active malignancy (treatment within last 6 months or palliative)	1
Score >4: PE likely; ≤4: PE unlikely	

[a]Minimum of leg swelling and pain elicited upon palpation of the deep veins.

abnormalities may not be detected by SpO_2. Where imaging is performed to exclude PE, CTPA is considered first line as it offers greater sensitivity than a ventilation/perfusion (V/Q) scan and additionally may demonstrate an alternative diagnosis in the absence of a PE.

8 Diagnostic CXR abnormality?

CXR may be more sensitive than clinical examination for detecting some lung abnormalities, for example, pneumothorax (Fig. 4.4), pleural effusion (Fig. 4.7) or lobar collapse (Figs 6.3 and 6.4).

While a patient may present with acute dyspnoea secondary to a pleural effusion, it is more commonly associated with chronic dyspnoea. If the patient has lobar collapse, consider further investigation (e.g., CT thorax, bronchoscopy) to exclude a proximal obstructing lesion.

If CXR appearances are nonspecific or uncertain, continue through the diagnostic process and attempt to correlate with clinical findings. Consider further imaging, such as CT thorax, or specialist Respiratory input if no firm diagnosis emerges.

9 Ischaemic ECG changes (Box 3.2)?

Dyspnoea may be the predominant manifestation of myocardial ischaemia/infarction.

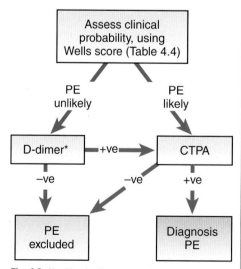

Fig. 4.6 Algorithm for the assessment of suspected pulmonary embolism using the Wells score.*Highly sensitive assay.

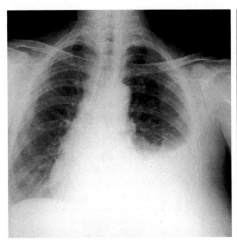

Fig. 4.7 Left pleural effusion.

If there is ECG evidence of ischaemia (Box 3.2) and no obvious alternative cause for breathlessness, assess as described in Chapter 3.

10 **ABG analysis shows primary metabolic acidosis with normal PaO_2?**

In the presence of a metabolic acidosis, patients can have an increased respiratory rate (and therefore appear dyspnoeic) as they 'blow off' CO_2 in an attempt to normalize the pH and compensate for the metabolic acidosis. Identify the presence of metabolic acidosis by ABG/VBG analysis (see Clinical tool Interpretation of arterial blood gases). If present, look for an underlying cause (Box 4.2). Do not attribute dyspnoea solely to metabolic acidosis when there is evidence of hypoxaemia.

4

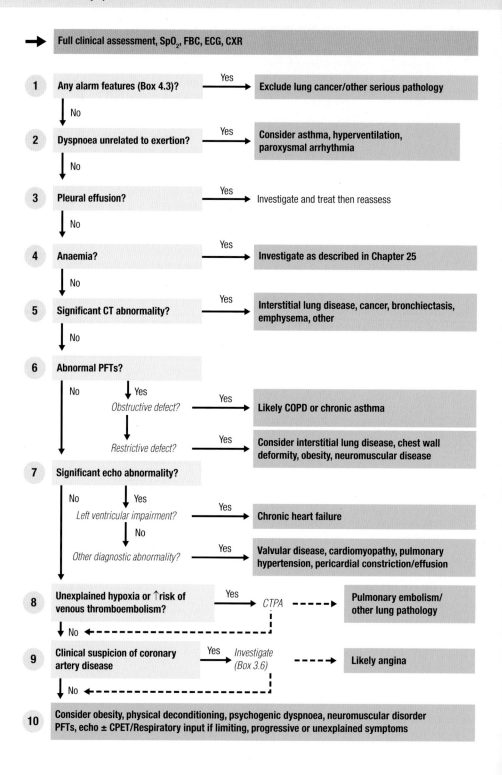

1 Any alarm features (Box 4.3)?

Change in voice or stridor may indicate laryngeal/tracheal obstruction secondary to intrinsic cancer or extrinsic compression (e.g., lymphoma, thyroid tumour or retrosternal goitre); if present, refer the patient urgently for endoscopic evaluation, for example, fibre optic bronchoscopy/nasoendoscopy.

Refer for urgent specialist evaluation with CT ± bronchoscopy to exclude lung cancer if the patient has risk factors (>40 years old or smoking history) accompanied by any suspicious clinical or CXR features (Box 4.3); these include lobar collapse, which may indicate a proximal obstructing tumour.

In younger non-smokers consider initial further evaluation with CT thorax; refer for specialist assessment if CT suggests malignant disease, fails to reveal a clear alternative cause or is not readily available. Evaluate patients with haemoptysis, as described in Chapter 6.

2 Dyspnoea unrelated to exertion?

Chronic dyspnoea arising from organic disease is almost always provoked or exacerbated by exertion. In patients who report episodic dyspnoea unrelated to exertion, the range of diagnoses is more limited.

Asthma is associated with episodic periods of symptoms with no (or minimal) symptoms between episodes. The diagnosis of asthma requires a history of clinical features and objective evidence of variable airflow obstruction. Suspect asthma if there is:

- More than one of wheeze, dyspnoea, chest tightness or cough with or without sputum
- A reproducible precipitant for episodes, such as cold air, pollen, house dust or pets
- Diurnal variation in symptoms with prominent nocturnal or early morning symptoms
- A history of atopy

Seek objective evidence of airflow reversibility or variability to confirm the diagnosis: the former by spirometry (≥15% improvement in FEV_1 following inhaled bronchodilators), the latter by asking the patient to keep a diary of peak-flow recordings (look for >20% diurnal variation on ≥3 days/week for 2 weeks). Consider specialist assessment if the diagnosis is uncertain, especially if occupational asthma is suspected.

Paroxysmal tachyarrhythmia may present with discrete episodes of breathlessness without any clear precipitant (although dyspnoea, when present, is usually aggravated by exertion). Consider this if:

- Dyspnoea is accompanied by palpitations
- Episodes arise 'out of the blue' with an abrupt onset, or
- The ECG shows evidence of preexcitation (Fig. 5.3).

If paroxysmal tachyarrhythmia is suspected, attempt to document the rhythm during symptoms if necessary, using an ambulatory recorder or smart phone ECG monitor.

Dyspnoea that occurs predominantly at rest with no consistent relationship to exertion may be functional. Suspect this if the patient exhibits typical features (Box 4.4) in the absence of objective evidence of cardiorespiratory disease.

Box 4.3 Alarm features in chronic dyspnoea

Clinical features

- Stridor
- Haemoptysis
- Weight loss
- Change in voice
- Persistent or nontender cervical lymphadenopathy
- Finger clubbing

CXR features (see also Box 6.1)

- Lung mass
- Cavitation
- Hilar enlargement
- Lobar collapse (persistent)

N.B. These features are especially worrying if the patient is a smoker, is >40 years or has had asbestos exposure.

Box 4.4 Features suggestive of psychogenic dyspnoea

- Provoked by stressful situations
- Inability to take a deep breath or 'get enough air'
- Frequent deep sighs
- Digital/perioral tingling
- ↓$PaCO_2$ with normal PaO_2 on ABG analysis
- Short breath-holding time

3   Pleural effusion?

A pleural effusion (Fig. 4.7) is a common cause of chronic dyspnoea and will be detected on clinical examination and/or the CXR. Box 4.5 lists the causes of abnormal collections of fluid in the pleura. Further action will depend on the likely aetiology of the effusion. Most cases of bilateral pleural effusion will be transudative effusions caused by fluid overload or hypoalbuminaemia. In this case, next steps involve identifying and managing the underlying cause. In cases of unilateral effusion where the cause is unclear, consultation with the Respiratory physicians and consideration of pleural fluid aspiration is required. Laboratory analysis of the fluid will suggest the underlying diagnosis.
- Use Light criteria to distinguish exudative from transudative effusions (Box 4.6).

Box 4.5 Causes of abnormal pleural fluid collections

Serous effusions

Transudate
- Cardiac failure
- Hepatic failure
- Renal failure
- Nephrotic syndrome
- Hypoalbuminaemia
- Peritoneal dialysis
- Hypothyroidism
- Meigs' syndrome (pleural effusion, benign ovarian fibroma and ascites)

Exudate
- Parapneumonic (usually bacterial)
- Bronchial carcinoma
- TB
- Connective tissue disease
- Pancreatitis
- Mesothelioma
- Post-MI syndrome
- Sarcoidosis

Other fluids

Pus
- Empyema; most commonly caused by acute bacterial infection of the pleura

Chyle
- Chylothorax; caused by lymphatic obstruction, most commonly by metastatic cancer

Blood
- Haemothorax; causes acute dyspnoea, usually following trauma

---

Box 4.6 Light's criteria for differentiation of pleural exudate and transudate

The pleural fluid is likely to be an exudate if ≥1 of the following criteria is present:
- Pleural fluid protein:serum protein ratio >0.5
- Pleural fluid LDH:serum LDH ratio >0.6
- Pleural fluid LDH >two-thirds of the upper limit of normal serum LDH

- Review pleural fluid biochemistry. The presence of amylase indicates pancreatitis; pH <7.3 suggests bacterial infection or cancer; rheumatoid factor suggests connective tissue disease.
- Identify evidence of infection. Send all samples for microscopy and culture, including samples for microscopy with Ziehl–Neelsen staining to identify acid-fast bacilli. If suspicious of TB, send a sample for culture but note that cultures may take several months.
- Send a sample of pleural fluid to cytology to investigate for malignancy.

4   Anaemic?

Always check Hb in patients with exertional dyspnoea. If Hb is decreased, evaluate as described in Chapter 25 but consider other causes—especially if Hb is only slightly decreased or symptoms persist despite correction.

5   Significant CT abnormality?

Arrange high-resolution CT to look for evidence of ILD if the patient has any of the relevant features listed in Box 4.7.

Refer for specialist evaluation if CT shows evidence of ILD or other serious pathology, e.g., cancer, bronchiectasis. Arrange further investigation with PFTs, if these have not been performed already, if the CT shows features of emphysema.

6   Abnormal PFTs?

In any patient with chronic dyspnoea without an obvious diagnosis from the initial assessment, arrange PFTs to investigate lung function (see Box 4.7 and Tables 4.5 and 4.6).

Diagnose COPD if FEV_1/FVC is <70% (indicating airway obstruction) with a post-bronchodilator FEV_1 <80% predicted (indicating incomplete

PFTs if there is:

- Wheeze
- Prominent nocturnal or early morning symptoms
- Symptoms precipitated by cold weather or common allergens
- History of atopy
- Clinical or CXR features of hyperinflation
- Smoker aged >40 years
- Chronic productive cough (≥3 consecutive months for ≥2 successive years)
- Occupational dust exposure, treatment with methotrexate/amiodarone or previous radiotherapy
- ↓SpO2 (at rest or on exertion) with no apparent alternative cause
- Major or progressive decrease in effort tolerance without other obvious cause.

Echocardiogram if there is:

- Significant ECG abnormality, e.g., left bundle branch block, evidence of left ventricular hypertrophy (LVH), pathological Q waves, frequent ventricular ectopics, atrial fibrillation
- Previous MI or chronic hypertension (especially if target organ damage)
- ↑JVP or peripheral oedema
- Murmur (not previously investigated)
- Clinical/CXR evidence of pulmonary congestion, cardiomegaly or pulmonary hypertension
- Elevated BNP

High-resolution CT thorax if there is:

- Interstitial shadowing on CXR (Fig. 4.8)
- Unexplained restrictive lung defect or ↓gas transfer
- Strong clinical suspicion of interstitial lung disease, such as hypoxia or end-inspiratory crackles in a patient with previous exposure to birds, dust or hay

reversibility). Look for other characteristic abnormalities, including ↑total lung capacity (TLC) and residual volume (RV) (which helps to differentiate from ILD in borderline cases) and ↓diffusion capacity (indicative of significant emphysema). Exclude alpha$_1$-antitrypsin deficiency in younger patients. If SpO$_2$ is ≤92%, perform an ABG analysis to identify patients with type 2 respiratory failure or those who might qualify for home oxygen therapy.

Diagnose asthma if there is an obstructive ventilatory defect with ≥15% improvement in FEV$_1$ following inhaled bronchodilators. If not, consider further assessment with repeat spirometry, PEFR diary or specialist evaluation if there is high clinical suspicion or borderline spirometry results.

In patients with a restrictive lung defect (Table 4.5), evaluate for an underlying cause:

- Arrange echocardiography and reassess following treatment if there is evidence of heart failure
- Look for major chest wall deformity, for example, severe kyphoscoliosis. Identify history and/or examination findings consistent with neuromuscular disease. Investigate ILD with high-resolution CT if there are suggestive clinical/CXR features (Fig. 4.8) or there is no clear alternative cause.
- Consider obesity—measure and document BMI.

Suspect extrapulmonary compression (e.g., neuromuscular disorder, chest wall deformity) if there is a decrease in TLC with normal

Table 4.5 Pulmonary function tests			
Test	**Description**	**Measures**	**Examples of relevant diagnoses**
Spirometry	Airflow at the mouth is measured during a forced exhalation	FEV$_1$, FVC	Obstructive lung disease: disproportionate reduction in FEV$_1$ (FEV$_1$:FVC ratio <0.8)
			Restrictive lung disease: proportionate reduction in FEV$_1$ and FVC
Reversibility	Spirometry is repeated after giving bronchodilators	FEV$_1$, FVC	Complete reversibility of obstruction is common in asthma, incomplete reversibility common in COPD
Lung volumes	Gas dilution or whole-body plethysmography	TLC, RV	COPD (normal or increased TLC), restrictive lung disease (reduced TLC and RV)
Diffusion capacity	Carbon monoxide uptake from alveoli is measured	DLCO, Dm	Interstitial pneumonitis, emphysema (low DLCO), pulmonary haemorrhage (high DLCO)

DLCO—lung diffusion of carbon monoxide; Dm—mean lung density; FEV$_1$—forced expired volume in 1 second; FVC—forced vital capacity; RV—residual volume; TLC—total lung capacity.

Table 4.6 Severity of airflow obstruction

Severity	FEV$_1$
Mild	50–80% predicted
Moderate	30–49% predicted
Severe	<30% predicted

Source: Modified from Boon NA, Colledge NR, Walker BR, Hunter JAA. Davidson's principles and practice of medicine, 20th ed. Box 19.30. Edinburgh: Churchill Livingstone, 2006; 680.

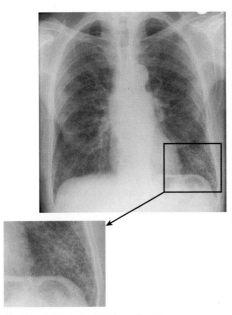

Fig. 4.8 CXR in interstitial lung disease.

RV, and an intrapulmonary cause, e.g., ILD, if there is a proportionate decrease in TLC and RV.

7 Significant echocardiographic abnormality?

Refer for Cardiology evaluation if the echo shows major valvular abnormality (e.g., severe mitral regurgitation or aortic stenosis) or pericardial effusion.

In chronic heart failure, exertional dyspnoea may be the sole presenting feature, but significant cardiac dysfunction is unlikely in the absence of the indications for echocardiogram listed in Box 4.7. The presence and severity of left ventricular systolic dysfunction can be determined by echocardiography. Consider Cardiology referral if left ventricular systolic function is normal but the patient has clinical features suggestive of heart failure, for example, elevated JVP, oedema or CXR evidence of pulmonary congestion—especially if there is left ventricular hypertrophy/left atrial dilatation (heart failure with preserved ejection fraction) or a history of previous cardiac surgery/radiotherapy (constrictive pericarditis).

If the echo suggests pulmonary hypertension without significant LV impairment or valvular disease, evaluate fully for underlying chronic lung disease (e.g., PFTs, high-resolution CT chest, sleep studies, CTPA) and refer for specialist assessment.

8 Unexplained hypoxia or ↑risk of venous thromboembolism?

Exclude chronic thromboembolic disease in any patient with unexplained hypoxia or risk factors for thromboembolic disease. CT pulmonary angiography is the first line investigation and in the absence of thromboembolic disease, should also help to identify alternative lung pathology, e.g., ILD, emphysema.

9 Clinical suspicion of coronary artery disease?

Angina occasionally manifests as a sensation of breathlessness without chest discomfort. Evaluate for angina with an exercise ECG or other stress test (Box 3.6) if the patient has risk factors for coronary artery disease (Box 3.4) and symptoms are consistently provoked by exertion and relieved within 5 minutes by rest. Relief of symptoms with anti-anginal therapy or coronary revascularisation confirms the diagnosis.

10 **Consider other causes. Further investigation if limiting, progressive or unexplained symptoms**

At this stage, review any abnormalities detected and determine whether they are sufficient to account for the presentation. In patients with multiple possible causes for dyspnoea (e.g., obesity, left ventricular impairment and airways disease), cardiopulmonary exercise testing (in which ECG, respiratory gas exchange and minute ventilation are recorded during exercise) may help to establish the predominant mechanism. Patients with a major change or progressive decline in exercise capacity without adequate explanation require further evaluation; arrange an echocardiogram and PFTs if

these have not yet been performed, and consider referral for specialist evaluation, for example, cardiac catheterisation or cardiopulmonary exercise testing.

Obesity and/or physical deconditioning may be responsible for exertional breathlessness and reduced exercise capacity; suspect this in patients with ↑BMI (especially >30), recent weight gain or a sedentary lifestyle. OHS is defined as the presence of hypercapnia in an obese individual in the absence of concomitant pulmonary or neuromuscular disease that could otherwise explain the hypercapnia. PFTs are often normal but can confirm a mild–moderate restrictive defect. Nearly 90% of patients diagnosed OHS also have obstructive sleep apnoea.

4

5 Palpitation

Palpitation is an unpleasant awareness of the heartbeat. Patients may describe the sensation as skipping, fluttering, racing, pounding, thudding or jumping. Most causes of palpation are benign and often not due to a heart rhythm abnormality, but episodes can be frightening to an individual. In most cases, the key to diagnosis lies in documenting the cardiac rhythm during symptoms. It is important to establish the frequency, intensity and impact of symptoms as this is essential to guide treatment.

Heightened awareness of normal heartbeat

Awareness of the normal heartbeat is common but may be a source of anxiety in patients, particularly those with health concerns. It is most commonly noted when lying awake in bed or sitting at rest.

Sinus tachycardia/↑stroke volume

Sinus tachycardia is defined as a heart rate above 100 bpm. Causes of sinus tachycardia are shown in Box 5.1; anxiety is the most frequent cause. Patients typically report episodes of a fast, regular, pounding heartbeat that builds up and resolves over minutes. Increased stroke volume due to aortic regurgitation or vasodilator drugs may produce a forceful heartbeat without tachycardia.

Extrasystoles

Atrial or ventricular extrasystoles (ectopics or premature beats) do not usually cause symptoms but, in some patients, produce a sensation of dropped beats (due to ↓ stroke volume of the ectopic beat) or 'thumps' (due to ↑ stroke volume of the postectopic sinus beat), or, if frequent, an irregular heartbeat. Extrasystoles are common in healthy individuals and usually benign, but frequent ventricular extrasystoles, particularly in older patients, may indicate underlying structural or coronary heart disease.

Paroxysmal supraventricular tachycardia

Supraventricular tachycardia (SVT) refers to atrioventricular nodal reentry tachycardia (AVNRT) and AV reentry tachycardia (AVRT).

- AVNRT is due to right atrial and AV node reentry, usually in structurally normal hearts.
- AVRT (known as *Wolff–Parkinson–White syndrome*) is caused by a reentry circuit formed from the AV node and an 'accessory pathway'—an abnormal band of conducting tissue connecting atria and ventricles (Fig. 5.1).

Both AVNRT and AVRT produce episodes of regular tachycardia (± light-headedness and breathlessness) with an abrupt onset and offset. The ECG shows a regular narrow-complex tachycardia at 140–220 bpm (Fig. 5.2).

In patients with an accessory pathway, the ECG in sinus rhythm can either be normal or show a short PR interval and slurring of the QRS upstroke ('delta wave') due to premature activation of ventricular tissue by the accessory pathway—'preexcitation' (Fig. 5.3).

Atrial arrhythmias (atrial tachycardia, flutter and fibrillation)

Atrial tachycardia produces symptoms similar to SVT; the ECG shows a narrow-complex tachycardia with abnormal P waves. Diagnoses include atrial fibrillation and atrial flutter.

- *Atrial fibrillation* (AF) is common and becomes increasingly common with older age. Underlying causes are shown in Box 5.2. In AF, atrial activity is chaotic and the ventricles are activated rapidly and

Box 5.1 Causes of sinus tachycardia

- Anxiety or panic disorder
- Stress or strong emotion
- Drugs: beta2-agonists, anticholinergics, cocaine, amphetamines
- Anaemia
- Thyrotoxicosis
- Fever
- Pregnancy
- Phaeochromocytoma

irregularly. Patients with AF experience an erratic or irregular heartbeat that is usually fast. AF may be asymptomatic or associated with breathlessness, light-headedness or ↓ exercise tolerance. The ECG shows an irregular narrow-complex tachycardia with no P waves (Fig. 5.4). AF may manifest as paroxysmal or persistent depending upon permeance and response to treatment.

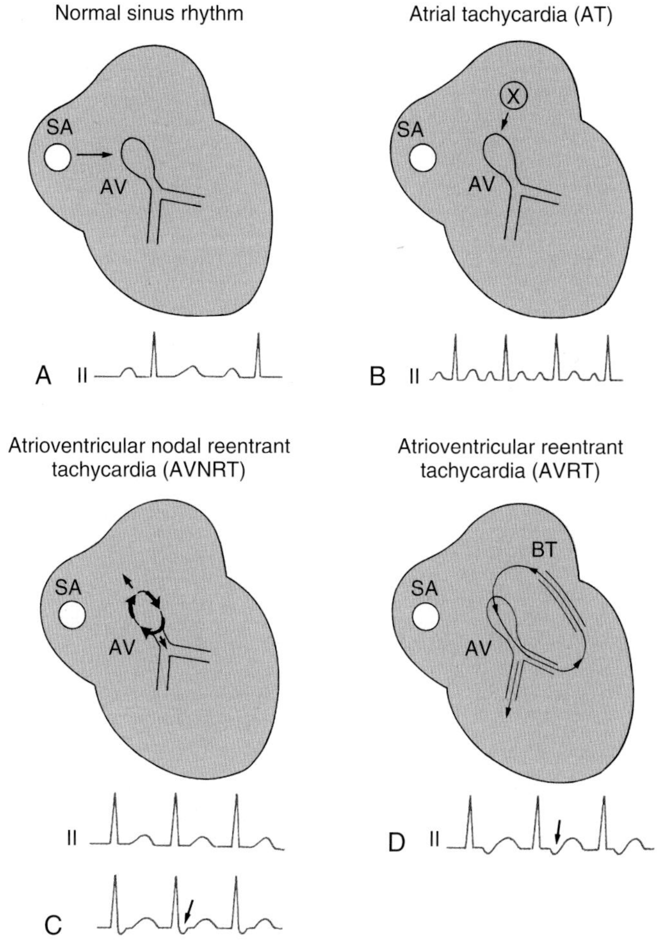

Fig. 5.1 Types of paroxysmal supraventricular tachycardias (PSVTs). (A) The reference is normal sinus rhythm. (B) With (unifocal) atrial tachycardia (AT), a focus (X) outside the sinoatrial (SA) node fires off automatically at a rapid rate. (C) With atrioventricular (AV) nodal reentrant tachycardia (AVNRT), the cardiac stimulus originates as a wave of excitation that spins around the AV nodal (junctional) area. As a result, retrograde P waves may be buried in the QRS or appear just after the QRS complex (arrow) because of nearly simultaneous activation of the atria and ventricles. Rarely, they appear just before the QRS. (D) A similar type of reentrant (circus-movement) mechanism may occur with a manifest or concealed bypass tract (BT) of the type found in Wolff–Parkinson–White syndrome. This mechanism is referred to as atrioventricular reentrant tachycardia (AVRT). Note the negative P wave (arrow) in lead II, somewhat after the QRS complex. (From Goldberger's clinical electrocardiography: a simplified approach, 10th ed. Fig. 14.7. Elsevier, 2024.)

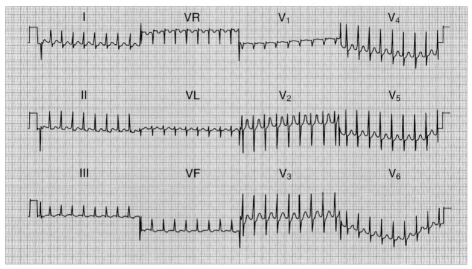

Fig. 5.2 **Supraventricular tachycardia.** (From Hampton JR. 150 ECG problems, 3rd ed. Edinburgh: Churchill Livingstone, 2008.)

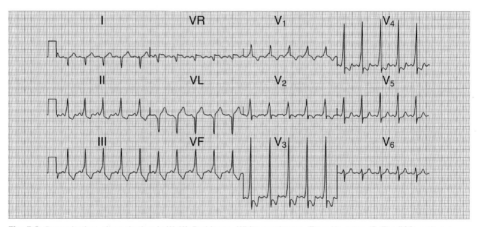

Fig. 5.3 **Preexcitation: sinus rhythm in Wolff–Parkinson–White syndrome.** (From Hampton JR. The ECG made easy, 7th ed. Edinburgh: Churchill Livingstone, 2008.)

<table>
</table>

Box 5.2 Common causes of atrial fibrillation
• Hypertension
• Ischaemic heart disease
• Valvular heart disease (especially mitral stenosis)
• Alcohol (acute or chronic)
• Sepsis
• Electrolyte abnormality
• Cardiomyopathy
• Sick sinus syndrome
• Congenital heart disease
• Constrictive pericarditis
• Hyperthyroidism
• Idiopathic ('lone' AF)

• *Atrial flutter* is caused by a large reentry circuit within the right atrium that generates an atrial rate of 300bpm. This is usually associated with AV block, resulting in a ventricular rate of 150 bpm (2:1 block) or 100 bpm (3:1 block). Symptoms are similar to those of SVT, and the ECG shows a regular narrow-complex tachycardia with 'saw-toothed' flutter waves (Fig. 5.5). With 2:1 block these may be obscured, so suspect atrial flutter in any patient with a regular narrow-complex tachycardia of 150bpm.

5

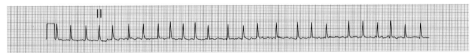

Fig. 5.4 AF with a rapid ventricular response. (From Hampton JR. The ECG in practice, 5th ed. Edinburgh: Churchill Livingstone, 2008.)

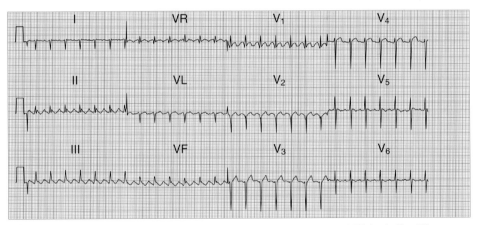

Fig. 5.5 Atrial flutter with 2:1 AV block. (From Hampton JR. The ECG in practice, 5th ed. Edinburgh: Churchill Livingstone, 2008.)

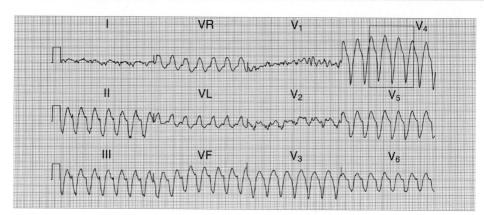

Fig. 5.6 Ventricular tachycardia. (From Hampton JR. The ECG in practice, 5th ed. Edinburgh: Churchill Livingstone, 2008.)

Patients with AF or flutter are at greater risk of thromboembolic complications, including stroke.

Ventricular tachycardia

Ventricular tachycardia (VT) is a potentially life-threatening arrhythmia that most frequently occurs in patients with previous MI or cardiomyopathy. It can also arise spontaneously in structurally normal hearts or be provoked (e.g., poisoning). Rapid palpitation is often accompanied by presyncope (a feeling of faintness and near-collapse), syncope, dyspnoea or chest pain. In patients with significant underlying left ventricular impairment, palpitation is frequently absent. The ECG shows a regular broad-complex tachycardia (Fig. 5.6). A variant, torsades de pointes (polymorphic VT), with a characteristic ECG appearance (Fig. 5.7), may occur in patients with a prolonged QT interval.

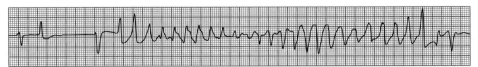

Fig. 5.7 **Torsades de pointes.** (From Boon NA, Colledge NR, Walker BR. Davidson's principles and practice of medicine, 20th ed. Edinburgh: Churchill Livingstone, 2006.)

5

Bradyarrhythmia, such as sick sinus syndrome, intermittent AV block

Bradyarrhythmias more commonly present with light-headedness or syncope, but the patient may report intermittent episodes of a slow but forceful heartbeat. Associated ECG findings include sinus pauses, junctional bradycardia and intermittent second- or third-degree AV block (Figs 24.1 and 24.2).

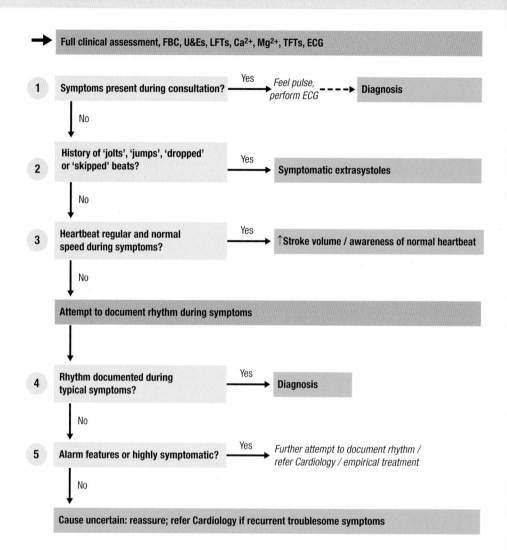

1 Symptoms present during consultation?

If the patient has symptoms during the consultation, feel the pulse immediately and perform an ECG. This may sound overly simple, but much of the difficulty in diagnosing palpitation lies in trying to document the rhythm during a typical episode of symptoms.

2 History of 'jolts', 'jumps', 'dropped' or 'skipped' beats?

It is not always possible to distinguish frequent extrasystoles from sustained arrhythmias such as AF on the history alone. However, a clear history of an occasional 'jump' in the chest or isolated 'dropped' or 'skipped' beats is highly suggestive.

3 Heartbeat regular and normal speed during symptoms?

Many patients with palpitation describe the heartbeat as 'forceful' or 'strong' rather than fast, slow or irregular. This argues against an arrhythmic cause; it may reflect ↑ stroke volume, e.g., aortic regurgitation, anaemia, vasodilators, or simply awareness of the normal heartbeat. Look for underlying physical and psychosocial factors, but further investigation is usually unnecessary unless there is a specific additional concern.

Attempt to document rhythm during symptoms

This is a key diagnostic step. The chosen method will be dictated predominantly by the frequency of symptoms.
- Consider inpatient telemetry if the patient has experienced a recent episode, such as in the last 72 hours, particularly if the patient has had associated syncope or presyncope or has other high-risk features (Box 24.3).
- Use Holter monitoring if symptoms are occurring frequently but intermittently. Monitoring duration should be informed by symptom frequency (up to 1 week). If symptoms are occurring less than weekly, consider more prolonged ambulatory monitoring through a wireless ECG patch recorder or an external patient-activated recorder. Ambulatory smart phone monitors

are now available that are patient activated and allow an ECG to be recorded and sent to the clinician.
- If symptoms are very infrequent, ask the patient to phone for an ambulance, report to their family doctor or to an emergency department during an episode (advise not to drive). Depending on symptom severity, consider referral for insertion of an implantable loop recorder.
- If symptoms are induced by physical exertion refer for a supervised exercise ECG.

4 Rhythm documented during typical symptoms?

Diagnose arrhythmia as the cause of palpitation if symptoms correlate to ECG recording findings.

Assess the frequency and intensity of symptoms and the impact on occupation and lifestyle. Establish the efficacy and side effects of previous treatments.

Sinus tachycardia

- Review all prescribed medications and ask about any recreational drugs, screen for anaemia and hyperthyroidism and, where appropriate, perform a pregnancy test.
- If ↑BP or if episodes are associated with headache, flushing or GI upset, measure 24-hour urinary metanephrines to exclude phaeochromocytoma.
- Request an echocardiogram if there are any features to suggest structural heart disease, such as unexplained murmur or signs of heart failure.
- Look for evidence of an anxiety or panic disorder.

Extrasystoles

- Seek potential exacerbating factors including metabolic disturbance (e.g., $\downarrow K^+$, $\downarrow Mg^{2+}$), drugs (e.g., tricyclic antidepressants, digoxin, alcohol) or caffeine consumption.
- Consider further investigation (e.g., echocardiography, exercise ECG) if frequent or associated with other signs/symptoms of cardiovascular disease.

5

Table 5.1 CHA$_2$DS$_2$-VASc thromboembolic risk score

Thromboembolic risk factor	Points
Congestive heart failure: clinical evidence of heart failure or reduced LV ejection fraction	1
Hypertension	1
Age: ≥75 years	2
Diabetes mellitus	1
Stroke: previous stroke, TIA or systemic embolism	2
Vascular disease: history of MI, peripheral arterial disease or aortic atheroma	1
Age: 64–75 years	1
Sex: female sex	1
Risk of thromboembolic events (event rate/100 person years) according to score Score 0 = low risk (0.78) Score 1 = intermediate risk (2.01) Score ≥2 = high risk (8.82)	

Modified from Kirchhof P et al. 2016 ESC Guidelines for the management of atrial fibrillation developed in collaboration with EACTS. Eur Heart J. 2016;37(38):2893–2962 and Olesen JB et al. Validation of risk stratification schemes for predicting stroke and thromboembolism in patients with atrial fibrillation: nationwide cohort study. Br Med J 2011;342:d124.

Table 5.2 ORBIT bleeding risk score[a]

Criteria	N/Y	Points
Haemoglobin <13g/dL for males and <12g/dL for females, or haematocrit <40% for males and <36% for females	No	0
	Yes	2
Age > 74 years	No	0
	Yes	1
Bleeding history (GI bleeding, intracranial bleeding, haemorrhagic stroke)	No	0
	Yes	2
GFR < 60 mL/min/1.73m^2	No	0
	Yes	1
Treatment with antiplatelet agents	No	0
	Yes	1

[a]Risk of bleed (event per 100 patient-years):
Score 0–2: low risk, 2.4 bleeds per 100 patient-years
Score 3: medium risk, 4.7 bleeds per 100 patient-years
Score 4–7: high risk, 8.1 bleeds per 100 patient-years

From NICE guidelines: atrial fibrillation: diagnosis and management (NG196). Published 27 April 2021. Primary reference: O'Brien E et al. The ORBIT bleeding score: a simple bedside score to assess bleeding risk in atrial fibrillation. Eur Heart J 2015;36(46):3258–3264.

Supraventricular tachycardia

- Look for preexcitation on a resting ECG (Fig. 5.3) to suggest an accessory pathway-mediated tachycardia.
- Refer to cardiology for electrophysiology study ± radiofrequency ablation if symptoms are frequent, disabling or unpleasant or if there are side effects on medical therapy.

Atrial flutter/fibrillation

- Perform echocardiography to exclude structural heart disease, e.g., cardiomyopathy, left ventricular hypertrophy, valvular disease.
- Seek causative or exacerbating factors: measure BP, electrolytes and thyroid function; enquire about alcohol intake and symptoms of angina. In acute presentations, screen for infection.
- Use the CHA$_2$DS$_2$-VASc score (Table 5.1) to assess thromboembolic risk in patients with nonvalvular AF (all patients with mitral stenosis are at high risk). Offer anticoagulation with a direct-acting oral anticoagulant to people with AF and a CHA$_2$DS$_2$-VASc score of ≥2 (men) or ≥3 (women). Aspirin monotherapy is not supported by current evidence. It is important when initiating anticoagulation to consider the risk of bleeding. This supports shared decision making between clinician and patient and improves confidence and compliance. A number of clinical tools to assess bleeding risk have been developed, with HAS-BLED being the most well-known. The most recent guidelines published by NICE support the use of the ORBIT bleeding risk score (Table 5.2) due to its higher accuracy in predicting absolute bleeding risk.
- Refer to Cardiology if symptoms are frequent, distressing or disabling despite first-line medical therapy, such as beta blockers.

Ventricular tachycardia

- Perform an ECG to look for evidence of underlying structural heart disease, e.g., cardiomyopathy.
- Enquire about previous MI and symptoms of/risk factors for ischaemic heart disease.
- Measure the QT interval on the ECG in sinus rhythm.
- Measure electrolytes—especially K^+, Mg^{2+} and Ca^{2+}.
- Urgently refer all patients to Cardiology for further investigation and treatment.

Bradyarrhythmia

- Seek an underlying cause: check thyroid function and review drugs for rate-limiting agents, e.g., digoxin, beta blockers, calcium channel blockers.

Refer symptomatic bradyarrhythmia or asymptomatic second-degree AV block (Mobitz type II), complete heart block or sinus pauses >3 seconds to Cardiology. Clear documentation of sinus rhythm during a typical attack excludes an arrhythmic cause for symptoms.

Continue to step 5 if the patient did not experience a typical episode of palpitation during the period of rhythm monitoring.

5 Alarm features or highly symptomatic?

The lengths to which you should go to document the ECG during symptoms depends on both the severity of symptoms and the estimated risk of a life-threatening arrhythmia, for example, VT or complete heart block.

Consider reassurance without further investigation for patients with mild, infrequent symptoms and no high-risk features (Box 24.3). Reasses if symptoms subsequently become more frequent or intrusive. Persist with attempts to document the rhythm in patients with symptoms that are frequent, unpleasant or which interfere with occupation or lifestyle.

Irrespective of symptom frequency and intensity, refer patients with any of the following features to Cardiology for further investigation:

- Palpitation associated with syncope or presyncope.
- Family history of sudden cardiac death or inheritable cardiac conditions.
- Significant abnormality on resting ECG.
- Risk factors for VT, such as previous MI, ventricular surgery or cardiomyopathy.
- Where the underlying diagnosis has significant implications for occupation (e.g., professional driver).

5

6 Haemoptysis

The term haemoptysis describes the coughing up of blood. Haemoptysis requires evaluation to exclude serious pathology such as lung cancer, TB and PE; many patients will require detailed imaging and specialist assessment. Massive haemoptysis (>500 mL/24 hours) may be life-threatening.

Respiratory tract infections

Respiratory tract infections (RTIs) are the most common cause of haemoptysis. They typically cause blood-stained purulent sputum rather than frank blood and have associated features such as cough, fever and dyspnoea. In acute bronchitis, mucosal inflammation can rupture superficial blood vessels; patients with chronic obstructive pulmonary disease may have haemoptysis during an infective exacerbation. Pneumonia may cause frank haemoptysis, especially with invasive bacteria, such as *Staphylococcus aureus*, *Klebsiella* spp. or fungi; patients are usually profoundly unwell. TB produces chronic cough with small volumes of haemoptysis, fever, night sweats, weight loss and characteristic CXR changes.

Lung cancer

Haemoptysis is common in primary bronchial malignancy but rare in lung metastases. Risk factors are smoking (especially ≥40 pack-years) and age >40 years; repeated small haemoptyses or blood-streaked sputum for ≥2 weeks in this group strongly suggests malignancy. Massive haemoptysis may occur if the tumour erodes into a large vessel. Weight loss, cough, lymphadenopathy and finger clubbing are well-recognized features. CXR may show a variety of abnormalities (Box 6.1) but may be normal.

Pulmonary embolism

Frank haemoptysis may be caused by pulmonary infarction secondary to pulmonary embolus. Associated clinical features include sudden-onset dyspnoea and pleuritic chest pain. A pleural rub or signs of DVT may be present in a minority of cases. The CXR is often normal but may show a wedge-shaped peripheral opacity or pleural effusion.

Bronchiectasis

Haemoptysis may occur in bronchiectasis where there is typically a background of chronic cough with copious foul-smelling purulent sputum. Finger clubbing and coarse inspiratory crackles may be evident on examination.

Other causes

Pulmonary oedema may cause pink, frothy sputum which can appear like blood, but dyspnoea is almost always the dominant complaint. Other causes include pulmonary hypertension (especially associated with mitral stenosis), coagulopathies, foreign-body inhalation, chest trauma or granulomatosis.

Box 6.1 The CXR in lung cancer

Common abnormalities on CXR in patients with lung cancer include:
- A discrete mass (Fig. 6.1) or cavitating lesion (Fig. 6.2).
- Collapse of a lobe secondary to tumour obstruction (Figs. 6.3 and 6.4).

- Unilateral hilar enlargement or pleural effusion (Fig. 4.2).
- Consolidation (Figs. 4.3 and 4.4) that fails to resolve or recurs in the same lobe.

In a substantial proportion of cases, the CXR is normal.

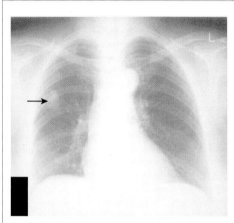

Fig. 6.1 A solitary lung mass *(arrow).* (From Douglas G, Nicol F, Robertson C. Macleod's clinical examination, 12th ed. Edinburgh: Churchill Livingstone, 2009.)

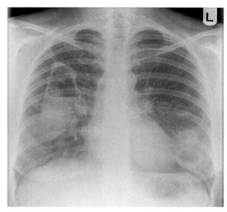

Fig. 6.2 A cavitating lung lesion. (From Corne J, Pointon K. Chest x-ray made easy, 3rd ed. Edinburgh: Churchill Livingstone, 2010.)

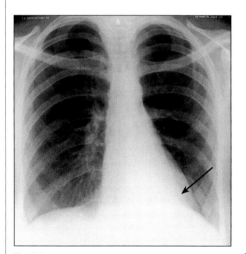

Fig. 6.3 Left lower lobe collapse. The changes in left lower lobe collapse may be subtle and easily overlooked; note the triangular opacification behind the heart, giving the appearance of an unusually straight left heart border *(arrow).* (From Boon NA, Colledge NR, Walker BR. Davidson's principles and practice of medicine, 20th ed. Edinburgh: Churchill Livingstone, 2006.)

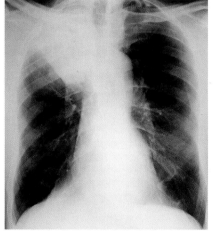

Fig. 6.4 Right upper lobe collapse. Note the right upper zone opacification, loss of volume in the right lung field and tracheal deviation. (From Corne J, Pointon K. Chest x-ray made easy, 3rd ed. Edinburgh: Churchill Livingstone, 2010.)

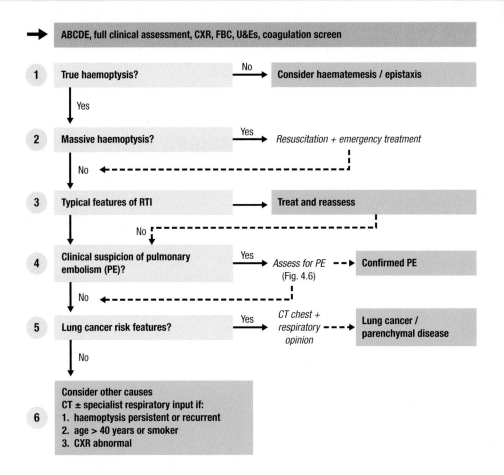

ABCDE, full clinical assessment, CXR, FBC, U&Es, coagulation screen

1 True haemoptysis? — No → Consider haematemesis / epistaxis

Yes

2 Massive haemoptysis? — Yes → *Resuscitation + emergency treatment*

No

3 Typical features of RTI — → Treat and reassess

No

4 Clinical suspicion of pulmonary embolism (PE)? — Yes → *Assess for PE (Fig. 4.6)* --→ Confirmed PE

No

5 Lung cancer risk features? — Yes → *CT chest + respiratory opinion* ---→ Lung cancer / parenchymal disease

No

6 Consider other causes
CT ± specialist respiratory input if:
1. haemoptysis persistent or recurrent
2. age > 40 years or smoker
3. CXR abnormal

1 True haemoptysis?

Depending on the patient history provided, it can sometimes be difficult to distinguish between blood originating from the respiratory, GI or ENT systems. A clear history of blood being coughed up or mixed with sputum reliably indicates haemoptysis. Blood that suddenly appears in the mouth without coughing suggests a nasopharyngeal origin; ask about nosebleeds and look for epistaxis or a bleeding source within the mouth.

Blood originating from the GI tract is typically dark, acidic (test pH) and may contain food particles (Chapter 8); blood that is frothy, alkaline and bright red or pink suggests a respiratory source.

2 Massive haemoptysis?

Bleeding is difficult to quantify clinically but estimate the volume and rate of blood loss, for example, by direct observation with a graduated container. The major risk in patients with massive haemoptysis is asphyxiation through flooding of alveoli or airway obstruction. Seek immediate anaesthetic help if there is any sign of airway compromise.

3   Typical features of RTI?

Small amounts of haemoptysis which has appeared acutely (<1 week) with purulent sputum and/or fever suggests acute RTI; assess as described in Chapter 4 and arrange follow-up with a repeat CXR after 6 weeks to ensure that both the symptoms (including haemoptysis) and the radiographic consolidation have resolved.

4   Clinical suspicion of PE?

PE can be underdiagnosed as physical and CXR findings may be unreliable. A high index of suspicion is required. Consider PE and assess as shown in Fig. 4.7 and Table 4.4 if haemoptysis is acute and accompanied by any of the following:

- Rapid-onset pleuritic pain or dyspnoea.
- Symptoms or signs of DVT.
- Specific risk factors, such as active malignancy or recent surgery.
- New-onset frank haemoptysis with no other obvious cause (e.g., no typical features of RTI).

5   Lung cancer risk features?

Even if another diagnosis appears likely, it is imperative to exclude lung cancer in any patient with persistent haemoptysis (>2 weeks) as a cancer may coexist. Particular risk factors to consider include:

- History of cigarette smoking.
- Weight loss, finger clubbing, Horner's syndrome or cervical lymphadenopathy.
- Mass, cavitating lesion, persistent consolidation/collapse or unilateral hilar adenopathy/pleural effusion on CXR (Box 6.1).

Thoracic CT is a useful first-line investigation and may reveal a tumour or other cause for haemoptysis, such as bronchiectasis. Urgently refer the patient to a Respiratory specialist for further assessment ± bronchoscopy even if CT is normal.

6   Consider other causes/further investigation

A coagulation screen should be performed on all patients with haemoptysis, but particularly those on anticoagulant therapy, with a history of bleeding disorder or with evidence of bleeding elsewhere.

Chronic cough with daily mucopurulent sputum production or persistent coarse inspiratory crackles suggests bronchiectasis— confirm the diagnosis with high-resolution thoracic CT.

Consider TB if any of the following features are present:

- Prior residence in an endemic area.
- Immunosuppression (HIV, malnutrition, general debility).
- Suggestive clinical features, e.g., night sweats, fever, weight loss.
- Suggestive CXR findings, e.g., a cavitating lesion (Fig. 6.2), persistent consolidation, miliary TB.

If suspected, obtain ≥3 sputum samples for acid-fast bacilli and mycobacterial culture, and seek expert Respiratory input.

If there is evidence of renal involvement (e.g., haematuria, proteinuria, ↓ glomerular filtration rate) consider anti-glomerular basement membrane disease and granulomatosis with polyangiitis; seek urgent renal input and check anti-GBM and ANCA antibodies.

If the cause is still unclear, consider CT and specialist Respiratory input—especially if >40 years, smoking history, ongoing symptoms or any CXR abnormality.

Gastrointestinal System

Acute abdominal pain

The spectrum of diagnoses manifesting as acute abdominal pain is extensive, ranging from the life-threatening to the innocuous. Effective initial assessment and triage requires the rapid recognition of critically unwell patients requiring urgent intervention by utilizing history, examination and, where appropriate, targeted investigations. Proceed with caution on making diagnoses based purely on history and examination as the specificity in diagnosis based on these alone is often poor. In tandem with targeted investigations, however, the diagnostic yield is far higher, especially for the more serious pathologies.

Chronic/episodic abdominal pain

Chronic abdominal pain is common and challenging to assess. Careful evaluation with targeted investigation is required to exclude organic pathology. Most younger patients will have a functional disorder, such as irritable bowel syndrome (IBS), but this should only be a diagnosis of exclusion. Chronic pelvic pain in women should be carefully investigated for a gynaecological cause before a functional diagnosis is made. In older patients with new, persistent abdominal pain, the priority is to exclude underlying pathology, with a focus on malignancy.

It is standard practice to break down the differential diagnoses of abdominal pain by the nine abdominal regions (Fig. 7.1).

Generalized or umbilical abdominal pain

- Perforation
- Intestinal obstruction
- Mesenteric ischaemia
- Ectopic pregnancy
- Testicular torsion
- Pancreatitis
- Ruptured abdominal aortic aneurysm (AAA)
- Aortic dissection
- Gastroenteritis
- Diabetic ketoacidosis/hypercalcaemia/adrenal crisis (diffuse)
- Constipation
- Nonorganic bowel disease (may affect any region)

Epigastric pain

Abdominal
- Peptic ulcer disease/gastritis/gastroesophageal reflux disease (GORD)
- Gastric or pancreatic cancer
- Pancreatitis
- Aortic aneurysm

Referred pain
- Acute coronary syndrome
- Pneumonia

Right hypochondrium

- Gall bladder disease, e.g., biliary colic, cholecystitis, cholangitis
- Liver disorders, e.g., hepatitis, hepatomegaly, trauma, abscess
- Appendicitis with high appendix
- Subphrenic abscess
- Right lower lobe disease, e.g., pneumonia

Left hypochondrium

- Pancreatitis
- Splenic disease, e.g., rupture, aneurysm
- Subphrenic abscess
- Left lower lobe disease, e.g., pneumonia

Right and left lumbar region including loin pain

- Pyelonephritis/perinephric abscess
- Renal colic, e.g., calculus
- Polycystic kidney disease
- Renal tumour
- Adrenal haemorrhage

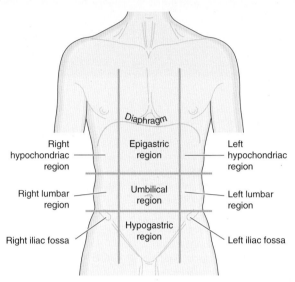

Fig. 7.1 **Regions of the abdomen.** See text for typical sites of pain. (From Gray J, Smith R, Homer C. Illustrated dictionary of midwifery, 3rd ed. New York: Elsevier; 2022.)

Iliac fossa pain

Right iliac fossa pain
- Appendicitis
- Terminal ileitis, e.g., Crohn's disease, *Yersinia*
- Mesenteric adenitis

Iliac fossa pain on either side
- Diverticulitis
- Colitis
- Colon cancer
- Renal colic
- Ectopic pregnancy or acute ovarian pathology
- Pelvic inflammatory disease/endometriosis
- Ovarian torsion/cyst rupture
- Testicular torsion/trauma/orchiditis
- Hip pathology
- Inguinal hernia
- Psoas abscess

Hypogastric and suprapubic region

- Lower urinary tract infection (UTI)/cystitis
- Urinary retention
- Uterine pathology, e.g., pelvic inflammatory disease, fibroid

Key questions

What are the characteristics of the pain?

Careful consideration of a patient's abdominal pain symptoms will yield immeasurable information to aid targeting investigations. The mnemonic 'SOCRATES' is often helpful: consider the Site, Onset, Character, Radiation, Associated features, Timing, Exacerbating and relieving factors and Severity of the pain.

Visceral pain is conducted by autonomic nerve fibres, so its location corresponds to the embryological origin of the affected structure (Fig. 7.2). The pain may arise from distension or excessive contraction (spasm) of hollow organs. It also arises from tissue damage (inflammation), ischaemia or direct chemical stimulation of pain receptors in organs. It is typically described as dull, is poorly localized and is not associated with abdominal guarding or rigidity. Visceral pain may be constant, e.g., in bowel ischaemia, or 'colicky'. Colicky pain reflects intermittent episodes of intense smooth muscle contraction that produce spasms of discomfort, lasting seconds to minutes before subsiding. Some disorders are described as 'colic' but are actually pseudocolic (e.g., renal or biliary colic). In these cases, the pain builds

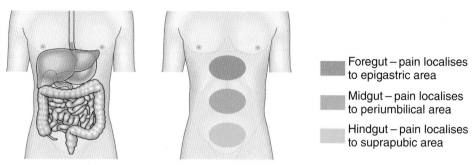

Foregut – pain localises to epigastric area

Midgut – pain localises to periumbilical area

Hindgut – pain localises to suprapubic area

Fig. 7.2 Abdominal pain. Perception of visceral pain is localized to the epigastric, umbilical or suprapubic region, according to the embryological origin of the affected organ. (From Douglas G, Nicol F, Robertson C. Macleod's clinical examination, 12th ed. Edinburgh: Churchill Livingstone, 2009.)

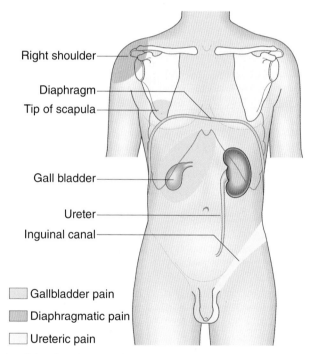

Right shoulder

Diaphragm

Tip of scapula

Gall bladder

Ureter

Inguinal canal

Gallbladder pain

Diaphragmatic pain

Ureteric pain

Fig. 7.3 Characteristic radiation of pain from the gallbladder, diaphragm and ureter. (From Douglas G, Nicol F, Robertson C. Macleod's clinical examination, 12th ed. Edinburgh: Churchill Livingstone, 2009.)

to a crescendo over several minutes before reaching a steady peak that may last for several hours before easing.

Somatic pain arises from irritation and inflammation of the parietal peritoneum and is conducted by somatic nerves. It is described as sharp, well localized, constant and often associated with local tenderness and guarding. Widespread inflammation of the parietal peritoneum produces generalized peritonitis.

Referred pain is perceived at a site remote from its source and arises due to convergence of nerve fibres at the same spinal cord level (Fig. 7.3).

Is there a systemic inflammatory response?

Many, but not all, serious causes of acute abdominal pain either stem from or provoke an inflammatory process within the abdominal cavity. The presence of fever, ↑CRP or

- Fever (>38°C)
- ↑CRP (>10 mg/L)[a]
- WBC >11 × 10⁹/L or <4 × 10⁹/L

[a]The significance of the result depends on the clinical context—see text.

↑WBC with neutrophilia suggests that the patient is mounting an acute systemic inflammatory response (Box 7.1) and may inform the differential diagnosis. In some patients, the presence of inflammatory features may assist the interpretation of uncertain physical signs (e.g., mild localized abdominal tenderness), reinforcing suspicion of local peritonitis. In patients without a clear cause for pain, these features may suggest the need for admission and further investigation. By the same token, the absence of these features can, when used correctly, help to exclude important inflammatory pathology. Finally, recognizing and grading the presence of a systemic inflammatory response are central to the assessment of illness severity.

Note that the significance of an individual result depends on the clinical context, particularly with respect to CRP. In general, the higher the result, the greater the extent of systemic inflammation. A marginal rise in CRP (e.g., <30 mg/L) does not provide compelling evidence of a major inflammatory process. However, if the test is being used to help 'rule out' a condition, then it is safer to regard any limit above the upper range of normal as elevated. Caution should be exercised with frail or immunocompromised populations as classic signs of systemic or peritoneal inflammation may be attenuated, resulting in misdiagnosis.

Gastroduodenal disorders

Peptic ulcer disease is a common cause of chronic upper abdominal pain. Almost all duodenal ulcers and 70% of gastric ulcers are attributable to *Heliobacter pylori* infection. The majority of peptic ulcers are asymptomatic. Typical features when they do occur include recurrent episodes of burning or gnawing epigastric discomfort (radiation to the back may occur); relationship to food (variable); associated dyspeptic symptoms, such as nausea and belching; and relief with antacids or proton pump inhibitors.

Gastritis without frank ulceration may produce similar symptoms.

Gastric cancer occurs more frequently in patients >55 years. In addition to pain, associated symptoms include early satiety, unintentional weight loss and vomiting. All of the above disorders are best diagnosed by upper gastrointestinal endoscopy (UGIE).

Gallstone disease

Gallstones are common in the Western population, and most are asymptomatic.

Biliary colic occurs when the gallbladder contracts, forcing a gallstone to the cystic duct opening, leading to gallbladder distension and spasm. It tends to be postprandial and may be exacerbated by fatty foods, manifesting as intense, dull, RUQ or epigastric pain± radiation to the back or scapula (Fig. 7.3). As the biliary tree is not permanently obstructed, it does not cause jaundice, deranged LFTs or abdominal signs. USS should confirm the presence of gallstones or, rarely, demonstrate pathological gallbladder changes. In *cholecystitis*, infection of the gallbladder due to gallstones obstructing the cystic duct occurs. Pain may be accompanied by fever, LFT derangement and RUQ tenderness.

Choledocholithiasis (stone in the common bile duct, (CBD)) causes cholestatic jaundice (Chapter 12) with less severe upper abdominal pain, or indeed no pain. In ascending cholangitis, infection of the biliary tree occurs upstream from a blockage in the CBD (gallstone, tumour, liver fluke). Patients present with significant sepsis, jaundice and abdominal discomfort (Charcot triad).

Pancreatic pain

Acute and chronic pancreatitis are often considered as two parts of a disease spectrum of pancreatic disorder. Acute pancreatitis causes severe upper abdominal pain that radiates to the back, often with repeated vomiting. It is associated with a systemic inflammatory response and may progress to multiorgan failure. Diagnosis is made on the basis of history, examination findings, and blood tests, in particular a raised serum amylase. The majority of cases are caused by gallstones passing down the common bile duct and irritating the pancreas or by alcohol directly injuring the pancreas. Chronic pancreatitis develops in a subset of patients with recurrent episodes of acute pancreatitis. In some patients, the pain is constant and unremitting, while in others, episodes are provoked by drinking alcohol or eating. Associated features relate to the disordered structure and function of the pancreas and include weight loss, anorexia and, in advanced disease, diabetes mellitus (endocrine deficiency) and steatorrhoea (exocrine insufficiency). The majority of cases are due to chronic alcohol excess. Diagnosis is usually made by CT, but endoscopic ultrasound with biopsy may be required to rule out malignancy. Unlike acute pancreatitis, serum amylase is usually unhelpful; ↓faecal elastase indicates pancreatic exocrine insufficiency.

Pancreatic cancer is often painless but may cause unrelenting pain in the upper abdomen that radiates to the back, which is usually associated with cachexia ± cholestatic jaundice.

Bowel ischaemia

Ischaemia of the bowel can be classified into ischaemia of the small bowel (known as mesenteric ischaemia) and ischaemia of the large bowel (known as ischaemic colitis). This can be caused by occlusive (arterial embolism or thrombosis) or nonocclusive (hypoperfusion in septic shock) aetiologies, and both conditions can be acute or chronic.

Mesenteric ischaemia

Acute mesenteric ischaemia presents with acute, severe, constant, diffuse abdominal pain with minimal examination findings (poor localization, no peritonism), systemic upset and, usually, lactic acidosis. Diagnosis can be difficult due to the nonspecific nature of the symptoms. Nevertheless, it is a surgical emergency with a high mortality. 50% of cases are caused by mesenteric embolism (patients may have atrial fibrillation), 25% by thrombosis in situ (atherosclerotic disease), 5% by congestive venous infarction due to

mesenteric vein thrombosis, and 20% by nonocclusive causes such as cardiac failure or septic shock. Diagnosis relies on a high index of suspicion. CT mesenteric angiography is the investigation of choice as plain abdominal CT carries a low sensitivity and specificity.

Chronic mesenteric ischaemia, also called mesenteric angina, is a rare cause of chronic abdominal pain occurring in patients with widespread atherosclerotic disease. Dull periumbilical or lower abdominal pain develops approximately 30 minutes after eating and may be associated with bloody diarrhoea. Weight loss is common as a consequence of food avoidance due to pain or poor absorption. An abdominal bruit may be heard on examination and the diagnosis is made by CT mesenteric angiography.

Ischaemic colitis

Ischaemic colitis is the most common form of bowel ischaemia. The splenic flexure and sigmoid colon are watershed areas between the arterial supply from the superior and inferior mesenteric arteries and therefore susceptible to becoming ischaemic in the presence of hypoperfusion. Ischaemic colitis typically occurs in older patients who present with left-sided abdominal pain and bloody diarrhoea. Diagnosis is confirmed by direct visualization at colonoscopy, but CT is often used as the initial diagnostic test.

Inflammatory bowel disease

Colitis due to either Crohn's disease or ulcerative colitis may cause cramping lower abdominal pain, usually in association with bloody diarrhoea. Small bowel inflammation in Crohn's disease is often manifest by persistent cramping periumbilical or RLQ pain ± diarrhoea (nonbloody) and constitutional upset. Toxic dilatation may occur in both conditions, though is more common with ulcerative colitis and is a surgical emergency. Subacute small bowel obstruction due to oedema or fibrosis causing strictures may lead to colicky postprandial abdominal discomfort. Both disorders are also associated with a range of extraintestinal features (Box 9.3).

Colon cancer

Patients with colon cancer may present with colicky lower abdominal pain from partial or complete bowel obstruction. Other important features include a history of weight loss, change in bowel habit (alternating between constipation and diarrhoea), rectal bleeding and iron deficiency anaemia. Tenesmus is a feature of low rectal tumours. Right-sided cancers present insidiously with vague pain and iron deficiency anaemia. This is because the proximal colon is more distensible and contains liquid faeces, so obstructive features are not seen and blood loss is occult. Screening programmes are in place in many countries due to the outcomes associated with late diagnosis of this common tumour. Tissue diagnosis is usually made by colonoscopy, but CT colonography may be used for frail patients who are unfit for colonoscopy.

Nonorganic bowel diseases

These are extremely common, particularly in younger adults. Diagnosis is based on typical clinical features in the absence of apparent organic disease.

Nonulcer dyspepsia causes symptoms that may be indistinguishable from peptic ulcer disease. UGIE and mucosal biopsies are normal.

Irritable bowel syndrome (IBS) is a collective term for a group of abdominal symptoms for which no organic cause has been found, including disorders affecting motility and enhancing visceral perception. Diagnostic criteria are shown in Box 9.1. Symptoms tend to follow a relapsing and remitting course, and are often exacerbated by psychosocial stress, menstruation and gastroenteritis. It is essential to make a positive diagnosis after ruling out other organic causes of these symptoms, including inflammatory bowel disease, malignancy, coeliac disease and infection.

Renal tract disorders

Infrequent, discrete attacks of pain ± haematuria suggest colic caused by renal calculi or clot. Renal colic is severe and may radiate anteriorly and/or to the groin. Classically renal colic causes patients to writhe in pain and they are unable to find a comfortable position. This is in contrast to patients with peritonitis, who lie very still. Chronic dull, aching or 'dragging' discomfort may be due to cancer, adult polycystic kidney disease (APKD), loin pain–haematuria syndrome or chronic obstruction/pyelonephritis. Frank haematuria requires urological investigation, primarily to rule out malignancy.

Gynaecological conditions

Abdominal pain in women requires additional consideration, with careful correlation to gynecological history. Sudden-onset lower abdominal pain in women of reproductive age may represent surgical emergencies, such as ovarian torsion or ruptured ectopic pregnancy. Endometriosis (endometrial tissue outside the uterus) and pelvic inflammatory disease (PID) are common causes of chronic lower abdominal pain in women of reproductive age. Uterine fibroids, ovarian cancer or cysts may present with nonspecific persistent lower abdominal discomfort ± evidence of a pelvic mass on abdominal/PV examination.

Other diagnostic possibilities

- Constipation
- Small bowel ulcers/tumours
- Atypical infection: giardiasis, abdominal tuberculosis, parasites
- Coeliac disease
- Medical causes of abdominal pain: hypercalcaemia, acute intermittent porphyria, diabetic ketoacidosis (DKA)

7

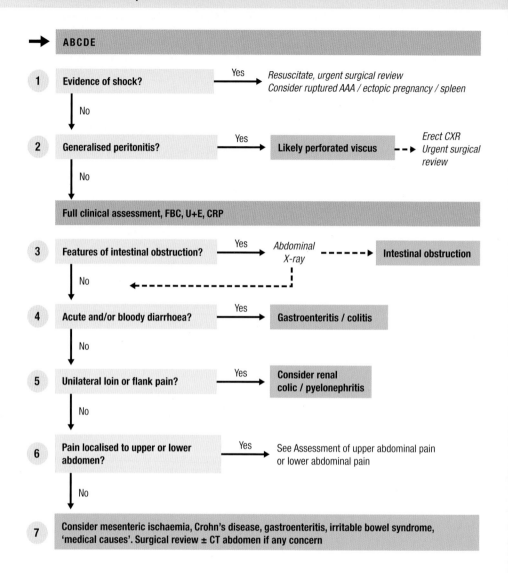

1 Evidence of shock?

Rapidly identify patients who are shocked with evidence of hypovolaemia (↑heart rate,↑ respiration rate, ↓BP) and tissue hypoperfusion (Box 2.1).

If the patient has clinical features of shock, secure two large-bore IV lines; send blood for cross-match, FBC, U+Es, LFTs, coagulation, amylase and arterial/venous blood gas; and begin resuscitation.

The potentially life-threatening diagnoses to consider first include ruptured organs (e.g., AAA, ectopic pregnancy or ruptured spleen) as these require immediate surgical intervention. Peritonism may not be present with these conditions.

- Suspect ruptured AAA in any patient with known AAA, a pulsatile abdominal mass or risk factors (e.g., male >60 years old, positive family history, cigarette smoker) who experiences sudden-onset, severe abdominal/back or loin pain followed rapidly by haemodynamic compromise.
- Suspect ruptured ectopic pregnancy in any pregnant woman or woman of child-bearing age with recent-onset lower abdominal pain or PV bleeding; perform an immediate urine and/or serum hCG test.
- Consider splenic rupture in any shocked patient with abdominal pain who has a history of recent trauma, e.g., road traffic accident.

If any of these diagnoses is suspected, arrange urgent surgical/gynaecological review and appropriate imaging.

In the absence of these conditions, continue to assess for an underlying cause while arranging an ECG, CXR, urinalysis and ABG and refer for surgical review. Other important diagnoses to consider include:

- Perforated viscus.
- Acute mesenteric ischaemia.
- Acute inflammatory conditions, such as pancreatitis, colitis, cholangitis.
- Any condition associated with repeated vomiting, such as intestinal obstruction, gastroenteritis.
- Medical conditions that may 'mimic' a surgical presentation, such as DKA, MI, adrenal crisis, pneumonia.

2 Generalized peritonitis?

Generalized peritonitis is usually caused by leaking enteric fluid from a perforated abdominal viscus, e.g., stomach, duodenum, gallbladder or colon. Pancreatitis may also present in a similar manner. Suspect peritonitis when there is severe, persistent abdominal pain that is worse on movement, coughing or deep inspiration, and generalized abdominal rigidity. The patient will likely be lying still, taking shallow breaths, and will be in obvious distress or discomfort. Inflammatory features are often present but these may be masked/blunted in elderly or immunocompromised patients.

Patients require urgent resuscitation, broad-spectrum antibiotics and immediate surgical referral. Free air under the diaphragm on an erect CXR may been seen (present in 50–75% of cases, Fig. 7.4) though many centres with ready access now consider CT the gold standard due to diagnostic accuracy. Again, maintain a high index of suspicion in the elderly or immunocompromised patient as signs are often subtle, so reassess frequently.

Localized peritonitis occurs where the parietal peritoneum is irritated, for example by an inflamed appendix or diverticular abscess. This results in focal abdominal rigidity over the area affected and may precede progression to generalized peritonitis.

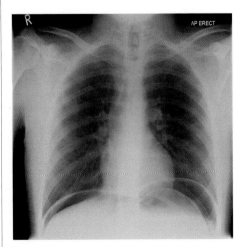

Fig. 7.4 Free air under the diaphragm.

3 Features of intestinal obstruction?

Suspect intestinal obstruction if abdominal pain is colicky and accompanied by vomiting, absolute constipation (no flatus), (no flatus) with or without abdominal distension. The predominant symptoms will vary, depending on the site of obstruction; in high small-bowel obstruction, vomiting and pain are preeminent, whereas in low colonic lesions, constipation and distension are more pronounced. If any of these features are present, perform an abdominal X-ray (AXR, Fig. 7.5) to confirm the diagnosis and estimate the level of the obstruction.

Examine for an incarcerated hernia in any patient with suspected bowel obstruction. Consider further imaging and rectal examination to confirm an obstructing lesion and differentiate it from pseudo-obstruction in patients with large bowel obstruction.

'Drip and suck' is the traditional immediate management: large-bore nasogastric (NG) tube placement to decompress the bowel, and IV fluid and electrolyte replacement. Commence careful monitoring for hypovolaemia and refer to Surgery for further assessment and management.

4 Acute and/or bloody diarrhoea?

Suspect colitis (infective, inflammatory or ischaemic) if the patient has bloody diarrhoea with cramping lower abdominal pain ± tenesmus and features of systemic inflammation (Box 7.1). If clinically unwell, further imaging in the acute setting may be indicated, particularly if toxic colon is suspected, e.g., inflammatory bowel disease (IBD) or pseudomembranous colitis secondary to *Clostridium difficile*. Otherwise, send stool for culture, ensure appropriate hydration and assess as described in Chapter 9. Always consider the possibility of ischaemic colitis if the patient is elderly or has known vascular disease/atrial fibrillation.

5 Unilateral loin or flank pain?

Consider renal tract obstruction (e.g., stones) in severe, colicky loin pain that radiates to the groin. Patients will typically writhe in pain and be unable to find a comfortable position (in contrast to patients with peritonitis, who lie very still). Visible (macroscopic) or dipstick (microscopic) haematuria is present in 90% of cases and nausea/vomiting is common. AAA can mimic this presentation and should

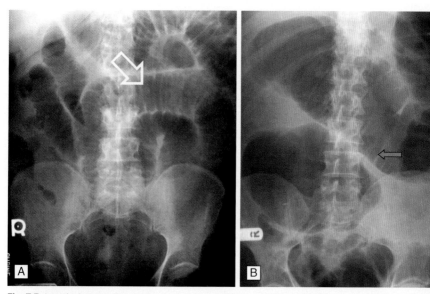

Fig. 7.5 Intestinal obstruction. (A) Small bowel (arrow). (B) Large bowel (arrow). (From Garden OJ, Parks RW, Wigmore SJ. Principles and practice of surgery, 8th ed. New York, Elsevier; 2022.)

be ruled out if a patient is high risk (e.g., male >60 years, positive family history, cigarette smoker) or if the presentation is atypical (e.g., absence of haematuria/restlessness/radiation to groin): arrange an urgent USS and, if this confirms the presence of an AAA, arrange immediate surgical review. Otherwise, organize noncontrast abdominal CT to confirm the presence of a stone (visible in 99% of cases).

In patients with a confirmed stone, check renal function and electrolytes, including acid-base balance, and look for features of infection proximal to the obstruction including ↑temperature/WBC/CRP or leukocytes/nitrites on urinalysis. If you suspect proximal infection, take urine and blood cultures, give IV antibiotics and refer urgently to Urology.

Suspect pyelonephritis if flank pain is non-colicky and associated with inflammatory features (Box 7.1), leukocytes and nitrites (produced by bacteria) on urine dipstick, or loin/renal angle tenderness ± lower urinary tract symptoms. Consider renal USS to exclude a perinephric collection or renal obstruction.

Consider alternative diagnoses (e.g., acute cholecystitis, appendicitis) if there are prominent clinical abdominal signs or if urinalysis is negative for both leukocytes and nitrites. Take blood and urine cultures, start IV antibiotics, arrange US imaging and consult colleagues.

6 Pain localized to upper or lower abdomen?

The localization of pain within the abdomen can be very helpful in narrowing the differential diagnosis (Figs. 7.1 and 7.2).

- If the patient has predominantly RUQ, LUQ, epigastric or generalized upper abdominal pain, proceed to *Acute upper abdominal pain*.
- If the patient has RIF, LIF, suprapubic or bilateral lower abdominal pain, proceed to *Acute lower abdominal pain*.

7 Consider other causes ± surgical review or further imaging if any concern

Organize CT angiography to look for features of mesenteric ischaemia in any patient with severe, diffuse pain, shock or unexplained lactic acidosis—especially when patients are elderly or have vascular disease/atrial fibrillation. The abdominal examination may be unremarkable until advanced stages.

Consider atypical presentations of common disorders such as acute appendicitis or inflammatory bowel disease. For example, a retrocaecal appendix may present with flank pain, while any area of the gut may develop a Crohn's inflammatory mass.

Several medical conditions may present with abdominal discomfort, usually associated with conspicuous vomiting and minimal abdominal signs, e.g., DKA, Addison's disease, hypercalcaemia, migraines and MI. It is important to maintain an open mind to these potential causes and undertake appropriate investigations if a surgical cause is not forthcoming.

Nonorganic bowel disease (e.g., IBS or cyclical vomiting) is a frequent cause of acute abdominal pain. The diagnosis of IBS is discussed in Chapter 9, but enquire about a background of longstanding intermittent abdominal pain with altered bowel habit, and review the notes for previous similar admissions.

A period of observation with repeated clinical evaluation is very often the key to successful diagnosis. For example, abdominal pain that was originally central and non-specific may, on repeat examination, have migrated to the RIF, suggesting a diagnosis of acute appendicitis. Patients who remain systemically well and whose pain appears to be settling can usually be discharged safely, with outpatient review. Those with marked systemic upset or other features causing concern but no clear underlying cause require further investigation ± surgical review.

7

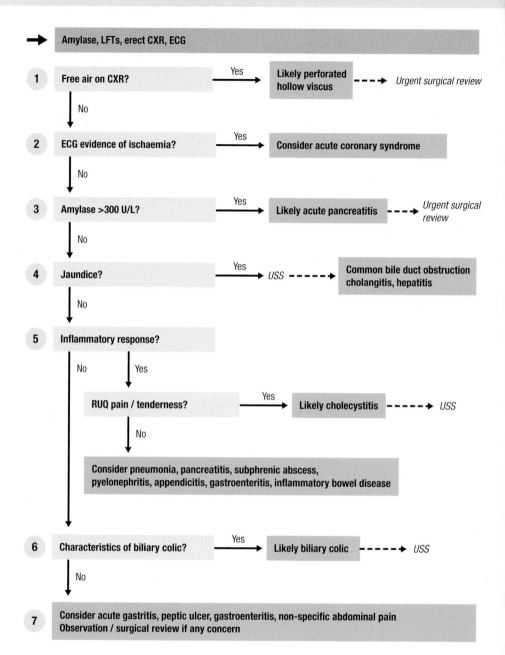

1 Free air on CXR?

Perform an erect CXR in all unwell patients with acute upper abdominal pain; the presence of free air under the diaphragm (Fig. 7.4) indicates perforation of a hollow viscus (present in 50–75% of perforations). Abdominal CT may be the preferred initial diagnostic modality in unwell patients, as long as speed of access doesn't cause delay. Secure wide-bore IV access, cross-match for blood, resuscitate with IV fluids and refer immediately to Surgery.

If a CXR fails to demonstrate free air or is equivocal but clinical suspicion is high (e.g., sudden-onset severe pain with epigastric tenderness and guarding), consider an abdominal CT, but first check amylase and ECG, as described in steps 2 and 3.

2 ECG evidence of ischaemia?

Acute coronary syndromes, particularly inferior myocardial infarction (MI), may present atypically with epigastric pain. Careful clinical consideration is required with this atypical presentation; myocardial ischaemia in patients with stable coronary artery disease may be provoked by severe bleeding, and administration of powerful antithrombotic agents may have catastrophic consequences.

- Perform an ECG in all patients.
- Refer immediately to cardiology if there are features of an ST-elevation MI (Box 3.2).
- In patients with ST depression or other dynamic changes, evaluate carefully for hypotension, sepsis, hypoxia and bleeding before attributing changes to an acute coronary event.
- In patients with nonspecific T-wave changes (Box 3.2), measure cardiac biomarkers to assist diagnosis and continue to search for alternative causes.
- Seek Cardiology input if there is any diagnostic doubt.

3 Amylase >300 U/L?

Measure serum amylase in any patient with acute severe epigastric pain. Patients with an amylase >3× the reference range have a 95% likelihood of having pancreatitis; levels >1,000 U/L are considered diagnostic. Amylase levels are not considered to correlate to disease severity.

If amylase levels are normal or equivocal, continue to suspect the diagnosis if the history is characteristic and:

- There has been a delay in presentation OR
- Pancreatic insufficiency is suspected, that is, there is a history of alcoholism, previous episodes of pancreatitis or known chronic pancreatitis.

In these patients, consider CT with IV contrast (provided renal function is satisfactory) to look for evidence of pancreatic inflammation.

This unpredictable disease is associated with a high rate of mortality (12%) and complications. Once the diagnosis has been made, evaluate repeatedly for evidence of complications such as shock, sepsis, hypoxia (ARDS), and disseminated intravascular coagulation (DIC). Calculate the Glasgow prognostic criteria score (Box 7.2) or another validated

---

Box 7.2 Modified Glasgow criteria[a] for predicting severity of acute pancreatitis

- **P**aO$_2$ <8 kPa (60 mmHg)
- **A**ge >55 years
- **N**eutrophilia WBC >15 × 10^9/L
- **C**alcium (corrected, serum) <2.00 mmol/L (8 mg/dL)
- **R**enal function Urea >16 mmol/L (45 mg/dL) (after rehydration)
- **E**nzymes ALT >200 U/L or LDH > 600 U/L
- **A**lbumin <32 g/L
- **S**ugar Glucose >10 mmol/L (180 mg/dL)

[a]Severity and prognosis worsen as the number of these factors increases. More than three implies severe disease.

prognostic score. Refer patients with severe or high-risk acute pancreatitis (shock, organ failure, Glasgow score ≥3) to a critical care unit. Refer all patients with pancreatitis to Surgery so that further investigation and management can be determined.

4 Jaundice?

Organize an urgent abdominal USS for all patients with acute upper abdominal pain and jaundice to look for evidence of biliary obstruction or hepatitis.

Assume biliary sepsis, at least initially, if the jaundiced patient is unwell with evidence of an inflammatory response (Box 7.1), sepsis or cholestatic jaundice (Chapter 12); give IV antibiotics and, if the USS confirms a dilated CBD, refer immediately to Surgery for further investigation (MRCP) and biliary decompression (ERCP).

Assess as described in Chapter 12 if there are clinical or USS features of acute hepatitis.

5 Inflammatory response?

At this stage, use the presence or absence of a systemic inflammatory response (Box 7.1) to narrow the differential diagnosis.

Arrange prompt abdominal USS to confirm or exclude acute cholecystitis in any patient with inflammatory features accompanied by any of the following:
- Localized RUQ pain.
- Direct tenderness to palpation in the RUQ.
- Positive Murphy sign (sudden arrest of inspiration while taking a deep breath during palpation of the gallbladder).

In the absence of acute cholecystitis, the USS may reveal an alternative cause for the presentation, such as pyelonephritis, hepatitis or a subphrenic collection.

If none of these features are present, consider alternative disorders:
- Basal pneumonia if there is clinical or CXR evidence of basal consolidation especially if accompanied by productive cough or dyspnoea.
- Gastroenteritis in patients with an acute vomiting illness and no abdominal guarding or rigidity (reassess regularly).
- Acute pyelonephritis if urinalysis is positive for leucocytes/nitrites.

Otherwise, consider USS/CT to exclude atypical presentations of acute appendicitis/pancreatitis/cholecystitis, Crohn's disease or other acute inflammatory pathology.

6 Characteristics of biliary colic?

Biliary colic is a common cause of acute upper abdominal pain in patients who are otherwise well and do not exhibit evidence of a systemic inflammatory response. Abdominal USS can assist the diagnosis by demonstrating the presence of gallstones. However, asymptomatic gallstones are very common, and so the history is critical to making an accurate diagnosis.

Look for the following suggestive features:
- Nocturnal or postprandial pain.
- Duration ≤6 hours followed by complete resolution of symptoms.
- The main site is the epigastrium or RUQ ± radiation to the back.
- Constant, vague, aching or cramping discomfort.
- History of previous similar episodes.

Arrange abdominal USS only in patients with a suggestive history.

7 Consider other causes ± observation/ surgical review if any concern

Systemically well patients with an acute vomiting illness and recent infectious contact or ingestion of suspicious foodstuffs are likely to have gastroenteritis.

Suspect acute gastritis if the patient reports new-onset gnawing, burning or vague epigastric discomfort ± mild tenderness, especially if this is associated with dyspeptic symptoms, for example, nausea, belching, heartburn or a history of recent alcohol excess/NSAID use. Consider peptic ulcer disease if there is a background history of similar symptoms.

In many cases, no definite diagnosis is reached. Admit for observation ± surgical review if symptoms are not improving or there are worrying features on examination. Otherwise, patients can usually be discharged, with further outpatient assessment if symptoms recur or persist.

7

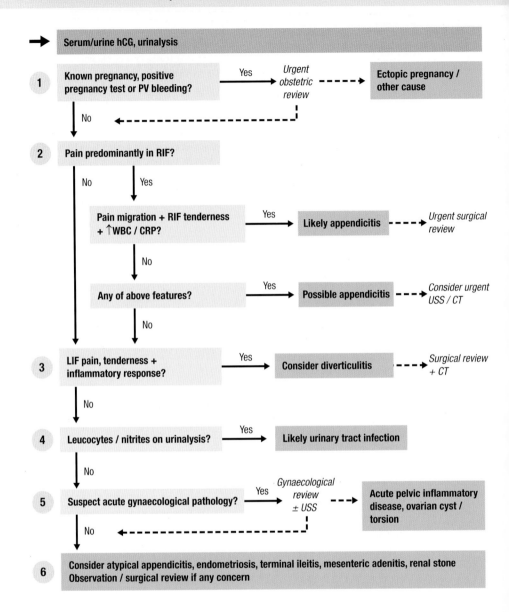

1 Known pregnancy, positive pregnancy test or PV bleeding?

Perform a bedside urine pregnancy test in any pre- or perimenopausal woman with acute lower abdominal pain. If the urine pregnancy test is negative but there is ongoing suspicion of pregnancy (e.g., missed period, vaginal bleeding) send blood for formal laboratory measurement of hCG. If urine or serum hCG are positive, request an urgent gynaecological review with transabdominal ± transvaginal USS to exclude ectopic pregnancy.

Request an obstetric review for assessment of pregnancy-related complications in any woman with known intrauterine pregnancy who develops acute lower abdominal pain, but consider alternative diagnoses, including UTI and acute appendicitis.

2 Pain predominantly in RIF?

Stereotypical clinical characteristics of pain secondary to acute appendicitis are:
- Migration of pain from the periumbilical region to the RIF.
- RIF tenderness or signs of local peritonism.

Several clinical signs may be sought, including Rovsing sign (pain felt in right lower abdomen on palpation of left side) or the psoas sign (pain elicited by lifting the right leg against resistance when in the supine position), but diagnostic accuracy is significantly influenced by a clinician's experience. Systemic upset may also be present (nausea, vomiting, anorexia) alongside evidence of systemic inflammation (Box 7.1). High degree of suspicion should be maintained as clinical signs may be subtle early in the disease course or in frail patients. An ↑WBC and ↑CRP are not specific for appendicitis, but the diagnosis is unlikely if both are within normal limits. Nevertheless, a surgical review is mandatory if the presentation is otherwise typical—especially if <12 hours from onset of symptoms.

Request prompt surgical review if high index of suspicion and consider urgent imaging to assist diagnosis. Abdominal USS may help to confirm the diagnosis rapidly or, in females, identify pelvic pathology, such as ovarian cyst/torsion. CT offers greater diagnostic accuracy and may be considered in males or if diagnostic uncertainty persists after USS.

3 LIF pain, tenderness + inflammatory response?

Exclude sigmoid diverticulitis in any patient with acute LIF pain and tenderness (± guarding) with evidence of systemic inflammation (Box 7.1)—especially if >40 years. Even in the absence of overt tenderness or inflammatory features, maintain a high degree of suspicion if the patient is elderly or has known diverticular disease. Arrange urgent CT to confirm the diagnosis and identify complications (e.g., abscess) or to seek an alternative cause for the presentation.

4 Leukocytes/nitrites on urinalysis?

Suprapubic pain/tenderness is common in UTI, but the absence of nitrites and leukocytes on urinalysis makes the diagnosis unlikely.

Acute appendicitis may cause dysuria, frequency and urgency with positive urinalysis (e.g., haematuria, leukocytes) if the inflamed appendix lies adjacent to the bladder or ureter; always consider this possibility, particularly in males (in whom cystitis is rare). However, in the absence of other worrying features, a positive urinalysis for both leukocytes and nitrites, especially in women, suggests UTI; send an MSU and start empirical treatment.

5   Suspect acute gynaecological pathology?

Have a high index of suspicion for acute gynaecological pathology in any woman of child-bearing age with acute pelvic or lower abdominal pain. There are no definitive signs for clinical diagnosis. Organize an urgent transabdominal/transvaginal USS in patients <35 years who present with abrupt-onset, severe, unilateral pelvic or lower abdominal pain with associated nausea, adnexal tenderness or a palpable adnexal mass. The principal aim of USS is to look for evidence of ovarian torsion, but it may reveal an alternative diagnosis, such as ovarian cyst. Request a Gynaecology review if you have a strong clinical suspicion of torsion or the USS result is positive/equivocal.

In the absence of features suggesting ovarian torsion, consider acute PID. Suspect the diagnosis if there is bilateral lower abdominal pain and tenderness ± fever associated with either of the following features:

- Abnormal vaginal or cervical discharge.
- Acute cervical motion, uterine or adnexal tenderness during bimanual vaginal examination.

The diagnosis is often one of exclusion and, in the emergency setting, it is prudent to seek formal gynaecological input; in difficult cases, diagnostic laparoscopy may be required as imaging studies have low sensitivity. Most laboratory findings are inconclusive in patients with acute pelvic inflammatory disease as many have no systemic inflammatory response, that is, WCC and CRP are within the normal range. A presumptive diagnosis can be made in sexually active females presenting with lower abdominal pain and cervical motion/uterine/adnexal tenderness on examination. Take endocervical swabs for chlamydia and gonorrhoea, and treat in all cases if positive. HIV and syphilis testing should be discussed.

6   Consider other causes ± observation/ surgical review if any concern

Consider atypical presentations of appendicitis resulting from variations in the position of the appendix; e.g., an inflamed appendix that lies within the pelvis may only be tender on rectal examination. Alternative diagnoses in patients with inflammatory features include terminal ileitis and mesenteric adenitis. Seek a formal surgical opinion if the diagnosis is uncertain.

Consider mesenteric ischaemia in any patient who appears unwell or has an unexplained lactic acidosis—especially if they have known vascular disease or atrial fibrillation.

An obstructed renal stone most commonly presents with loin pain but, once descended to the ureter, may cause more localized tenderness in the RIF or LIF; suspect this if the pain radiates to the testes/labia or is associated with visible/dipstick haematuria.

The diagnosis of acute urinary retention is usually obvious but should be excluded in confused patients with lower abdominal tenderness and distress. Clinical examination should be diagnostic but a bladder scan may be helpful.

In female patients, consider the possibility of alternative pelvic pathology, such as endometriosis, especially if there is a relationship to the menstrual cycle.

7

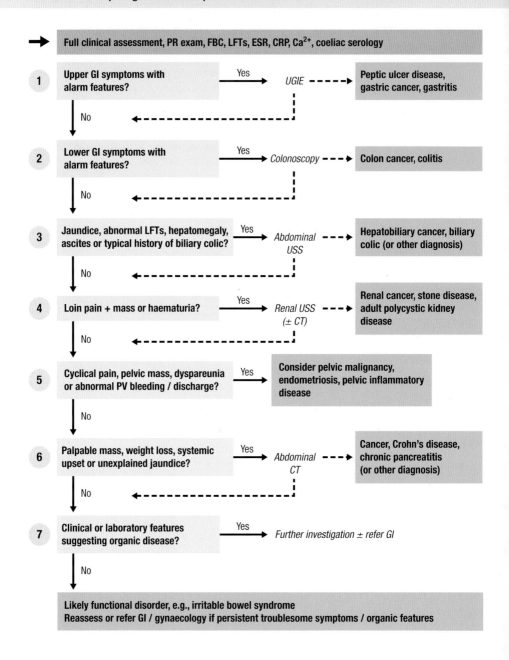

1 Upper GI symptoms with alarm features?

Arrange a prompt UGIE to rule out oesophageal or gastric tumour if there is upper abdominal discomfort with any of the following:

- Weight loss
- Dysphagia
- Persistent vomiting
- Early satiety
- Anorexia
- Haematemesis or malaena
- Iron-deficiency anaemia
- ≥55 years with new-onset persistent symptoms

If a gastric or duodenal ulcer is identified, ensure that a biopsy is negative for malignancy. Prescribe *H pylori* eradication therapy if the CLO test is positive. Assess for risk factors for peptic ulcer disease: recheck the patient's smoking history (smoking is associated with acquisition and increased persistence of *H pylori* infection), alcohol use and medication use (e.g., NSAIDs, bisphosphonates). Confirm successful eradication of *H pylori* with a urea breath test if patient remains symptomatic after 4 weeks.

In patients with macroscopic appearances of an upper GI tumour, obtain the formal biopsy result and discuss urgently with Oncology.

2 Lower GI symptoms with alarming features?

Arrange urgent investigation in any patient with chronic abdominal pain and:

- Rectal bleeding
- Positive faecal occult blood test
- A palpable rectal mass
- Iron-deficiency anaemia
- Change in bowel habit
- Age >45 years
- Recent weight loss

Organize a flexible sigmoidoscopy as the first-line investigation in patients <45 years and a colonoscopy if >45 years. CT colonoscopy may be considered in frail patients or when colonoscopy is unlikely to be well tolerated.

3 Jaundice, abnormal LFTs, hepatomegaly, ascites or typical history of biliary colic?

The combination of new-onset jaundice and persistent/recurrent abdominal discomfort suggests hepatitis, choledocholithiasis or malignancy, e.g., biliary, ampullary, pancreatic or hepatocellular cancer or biliary metastases. Conduct blood testing for liver disorders (Box 7.3) and a transabdominal USS. If the above is inconclusive, further investigation (e.g., CT or MRCP) is mandatory. Discuss with a GI specialist.

Arrange USS and perform a diagnostic ascitic tap in any patient with ascites (send for biochemistry, microbiology and cytology). If the ascites is exudative (serum-ascites albumin gradient (SAAG) <1.1 g/dL) and USS fails to reveal an underlying cause, arrange an abdominal CT scan.

The features of biliary colic are described above. If present, arrange abdominal USS to look for gallstones. Note that gallstones are a very frequent finding in asymptomatic patients so, unless the history is typical or there is evidence of a complication (e.g., dilated CBD, chronic cholecystitis), they are unlikely to explain the presentation.

Refer to a GI specialist if there is a convincing history of biliary pain in the absence of gallstones, especially if associated with abnormal LFTs or a dilated CBD.

4 Loin pain + mass or haematuria?

You must exclude upper renal tract cancer in any patient presenting with persistent loin

---

Box 7.3 Blood tests to assess liver disorders

- ALT, AST, ALP, GGT
- Albumin
- Viral serology for hepatitis A, B, C
- Ferritin
- Immunoglobulins
- Autoantibodies (ANA/AMA/SMA)
- Alpha fetoprotein
- Caeruloplasmin
- Alpha-1 antitrypsin

7

pain associated with a mass or haematuria (visible or dipstick). Renal USS is a first-line investigation and may reveal alternative causes, such as APKD or chronic hydronephrosis. Consider CT ± Urology referral if the cause remains unclear.

5 Cyclical pain, pelvic mass, dyspareunia or abnormal PV bleeding/discharge?

Arrange a pelvic USS in any patient with a pelvic mass or any postmenopausal patient with PV bleeding or recent onset, persistent lower abdominal pain. The features of PID are described above.

Consider endometriosis in any woman of reproductive age with chronic lower abdominal pain and any of the following features:
- Variation with menstrual cycle
- Deep dyspareunia
- Other prominent cyclical or perimenstrual symptoms

Establishing a definitive diagnosis of endometriosis may be challenging—refer to Gynaecology for further assessment.

6 Palpable mass, weight loss, systemic upset?

At this stage, organize an abdominal CT if the patient has weight loss, systemic upset or any palpable masses. Patients with a palpable mass may have been investigated with other modalities in steps 1–5 above, but CT is more likely to identify certain masses (e.g., pancreas, small bowel, renal tract and omental) and should be performed if the cause remains uncertain. In patients with abdominal pain and significant weight loss or other major constitutional upset (e.g., fevers, night sweats, ↑ESR), CT may reveal evidence of lymphoma, solid-organ malignancy or inflammatory disease, for example, chronic pancreatitis, abscess, Crohn's disease.

7 Clinical or laboratory features suggest organic disease?

Further investigation is usually required if the patient is >45 years with recent-onset symptoms, weight loss, constitutional upset or abnormal screening investigations. Important organic causes of pain that may easily be missed include chronic pancreatitis, chronic mesenteric ischaemia and Crohn's disease.

Consider chronic pancreatitis in any patient with a background of chronic alcohol excess or steatorrhoea. Check faecal elastase, perform an abdominal CT and consider specialist referral for further assessment.

Exclude mesenteric ischaemia (CT mesenteric angiography) if there is a close relationship between eating and the onset of pain, especially if there is evidence of vascular disease elsewhere, such as angina or intermittent claudication.

Assess for IBD in any patient with chronic abdominal pain and associated diarrhoea. Check faecal calprotectin to assess for luminal inflammation and, if positive, discuss with Gastroenterology about further investigation

If none of the above is present, a functional cause (e.g., IBS) is likely—particularly when typical symptoms are present (Box 9.1). It is important to make a positive diagnosis and provide initial management. Patients with persistent, troublesome symptoms may require specialist assessment and investigation to exclude organic disease.

Haematemesis describes vomiting blood and indicates bleeding from the upper GI tract. The appearance of blood in the vomit can vary; fresh, red blood is consistent with a brisk, active bleed; altered blood with a dark, granular appearance ('coffee-grounds') suggests the blood has been partially digested and is consistent with a slower or intermittent bleed. Melaena is the passage of black, tarry stools with a characteristic smell; it is usually due to upper GI bleeding but occasionally due to bleeding within the small bowel or right side of the colon.

Haematochezia is the passage of fresh red or maroon blood per rectum; it is usually due to colonic bleeding, but 15% of cases result from profuse upper GI bleeding.

Haematemesis, melaena or haematochezia in the presence of shock imply active bleeding and are medical emergencies.

Haematemesis

With major upper GI haemorrhage, resuscitation to compensate for ongoing blood loss determines survival and must take place alongside assessment. All hospitals have a major haemorrhage protocol with which you should be familiar. Ensure adequate resuscitation while arranging urgent upper GI endoscopy (UGIE) so that the source of bleeding can be identified and the bleeding stopped.

Peptic ulcer disease

Peptic ulcer disease is the most common cause of upper GI bleeding (estimated 50%) and an important cause of massive haemorrhage. It is often accompanied by dyspepsia and/or epigastric pain. Important aetiological factors include *Helicobacter pylori* infection, medications (e.g., NSAIDs/aspirin), gastro-oesophageal reflux disease (GORD) and excess alcohol consumption.

Oesophagitis

An increasing proportion of upper GI bleeding is due to oesophagitis. This is usually due to GORD, but other risk factors include medications (e.g., NSAIDs, bisphosphonates, tetracyclines) or infections (e.g., *Candida*, Herpes simplex). There may be a history of heartburn, indigestion or painful swallowing. Upper GI bleeding secondary to oesophagitis is associated with fewer complications and less mortality than bleeding secondary to peptic ulcer disease.

Mallory–Weiss tear

This is a longitudinal mucosal tear of the distal oesophagus and/or proximal stomach following increased gastric pressure. 90% of these bleeds stop spontaneously. The history is characteristic: forceful retching with initially non-bloody vomit, followed by haematemesis.

Portal hypertension with varices

Portal hypertension describes increased pressure within the portal venous system. In Western countries, the most common cause is cirrhosis, most frequently associated with excessive alcohol consumption. However, some non-cirrhotic conditions are associated with portal hypertension, such as schistosomiasis, portal vein thrombosis or idiopathic portal hypertension. Collateral veins form in response to portal hypertension, allowing portal blood to bypass the liver and enter the systemic circulation directly, for example, at the gastro-oesophageal junction. These oesophageal/gastric varices are superficial and liable to rupture, causing massive GI haemorrhage. Bleeding can be catastrophic, particularly if coagulopathy and thrombocytopenia are present. It is difficult clinically to distinguish variceal bleeding from other causes of massive upper GI bleeding (e.g., peptic ulcer disease), even if the patient has known cirrhosis.

Upper GI malignancy

In patients with upper GI malignancy, there is often a background of weight loss, anorexia, early satiety and/or dysphagia. Rarely, a palpable epigastric mass or signs of metastatic disease may be evident. Risk factors include alcohol, smoking, chewing tobacco, hot drinks, obesity and reflux oesophagitis/Barrett oesophagus.

Other uncommon causes

An aortoduodenal fistula will usually present with massive haematemesis, and this should be suspected if the patient has had previous surgery for an abdominal aortic aneurysm. Angiodysplasia and congenital malformations of the vascular tree (e.g., Dieulafoy lesion) can produce major haemorrhage.

Rectal bleeding

Rectal bleeding is most commonly due to a benign cause. In acute rectal bleeding, similar to upper GI bleeding, assess bleeding severity and ensure adequate resuscitation while arranging interventions to identify and treat the bleeding source. The pattern of bleeding can inform the clinician to the likely location. Anorectal bleeding typically presents with intermittent episodes of minor, fresh, bright red bleeding during or after defecation, which is not mixed with the stool. Distal colon bleeding is darker red and may be partially mixed with stool; proximal colon bleeding is dark red and fully mixed with stool. Remember that large volume upper GI or proximal colon bleeding can present with fresh bright red bleeding (15% of patients presenting with severe PR bleeding will have an upper GI source).

Diverticular disease

Diverticulosis is the most common cause of severe acute rectal bleeding (15–42% of presentations). It typically occurs in older patients. Bleeding occurs due to erosion of a vessel in the neck of a diverticulum and is mostly fresh blood. It may result in a life-threatening bleed but stops spontaneously in 75% of patients. The long-term rebleeding rate is, however, high; up to 40% of patients who undergo conservative management of their initial bleed will rebleed at some point.

Perianal disorders

These are a common cause of rectal bleeding in all age groups. Bright red bleeding is often associated with other anorectal symptoms, such as discomfort, mucus discharge or pruritus. Causes include haemorrhoids, anal fissures, perianal Crohn's disease and anal cancer. Be aware that haemorrhoids can cause major bleeds. Always examine the anus of a patient presenting with rectal bleeding: perianal disorders are diagnosed by PR examination ± proctoscopy. Severe pain, especially during defecation, suggests anal fissure, and the patient will not tolerate PR examination. Always consider a concurrent proximal bleeding source.

Colorectal carcinoma

Colorectal carcinoma is a common cancer. The presentation is frequently insidious with minimal symptoms; be suspicious of recent weight loss, tenesmus, a change in or alternating bowel habit or colicky lower abdominal pain. Have a high degree of suspicion in older adults or those with a genetic predisposition/family history. Bleeding associated with colorectal cancer is usually low volume but recurrent. Polyps may cause rectal bleeding.

Diagnosis is made by colonic imaging (sigmoidoscopy/colonoscopy or CT colonography in patients who are unfit for endoscopic investigation.)

Inflammatory bowel disease

Colorectal inflammation may cause rectal bleeding, with this symptom being more common in ulcerative colitis than in Crohn's disease. The passage of frank blood ± mucus and tenesmus may occur in proctitis. Colitis produces bloody diarrhoea with intermittent cramping lower abdominal pain and, often, systemic upset. Endoscopy and biopsy of the colon/terminal ileum confirm the diagnosis; inflammatory markers (e.g., CRP, faecal calprotectin) provide a useful guide to disease activity. Chronicity of inflammatory bowel disease can also change the differential for PR bleeding chronic. Perianal Crohn's disease is often associated with complex perianal fistulas.

Ischaemic colitis

Ischaemic colitis (colonic ischaemia) is the most common form of ischaemic injury to the GI tract and can occur because of vascular occlusion (e.g., mesenteric artery embolism or thrombosis) or nonocclusive causes (e.g., hypoperfusion). The superior mesenteric artery supplies the ascending and transverse colon, while the inferior mesenteric artery supplies the descending and sigmoid colon. The splenic flexure and sigmoid colon are areas where the two circulations meet and are considered watershed regions where ischaemic damage is more likely in the presence of hypoperfusion. Clinical presentation varies and depends on the underlying cause. Commonly, ischaemic colitis occurs in older patients, typically resulting in severe lower abdominal pain associated with rectal bleeding. It can affect younger patients, especially those with known hypercoagulopathy. CT is often used as the initial diagnostic test, but colonoscopy is considered the gold-standard for direct visualization and confirmation of ischaemic colitis. Most cases of ischaemic colitis will improve with treatment of the underlying cause and volume replacement. A small proportion of patients (approximately 20%) will require surgery and resection of the affected bowel.

Angiodysplasia (arteriovenous malformation)

These dilated tortuous submucosal vessels are degenerative vascular malformations and are an important cause of severe lower GI bleeding, predominantly in the elderly. Typical endoscopic features may be apparent, but diagnosis is often challenging. Similar to diverticulosis, bleeding often resolves spontaneously but frequently recurs.

Other causes

GI infections (e.g., *Salmonella*, *Shigella*, *Campylobacter* and *Escherichia coli*) may cause bloody diarrhoea by causing local invasion of the mucosa, usually with systemic upset. Other small intestinal sources of rectal blood loss include Meckel's diverticulum (melaena) and intussusception ('currant jelly' bleeding) in young patients. Acute small bowel ischaemia may be associated with rectal bleeding, but the dominating feature is severe abdominal pain, and the patient is critically unwell. Small bowel tumours are rare and present with intermittent bleeding (may require capsule endoscopy).

Radiation proctocolitis should be considered in any patient with a history of pelvic radiation, such as for prostatic or gynaecological malignancy; most present within 2 years of radiotherapy.

8

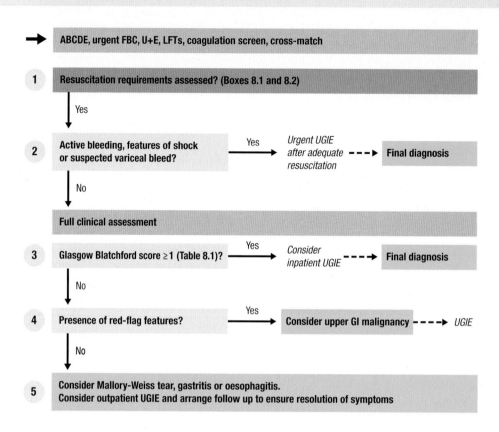

ABCDE, urgent FBC, U+E, LFTs, coagulation screen, cross-match

1 Resuscitation requirements assessed? (Boxes 8.1 and 8.2)

Yes

2 Active bleeding, features of shock or suspected variceal bleed?
→ Yes → *Urgent UGIE after adequate resuscitation* ----→ **Final diagnosis**

No

Full clinical assessment

3 Glasgow Blatchford score ≥1 (Table 8.1)?
→ Yes → *Consider inpatient UGIE* ----→ **Final diagnosis**

No

4 Presence of red-flag features?
→ Yes → **Consider upper GI malignancy** ----→ *UGIE*

No

5 Consider Mallory-Weiss tear, gastritis or oesophagitis.
Consider outpatient UGIE and arrange follow up to ensure resolution of symptoms

Box 8.1 Resuscitation in acute haemorrhage

First steps

- Recheck airway frequently, especially if ↓GCS/vomiting.
- Give high concentration O_2.
- Get help: call the medical emergency or cardiac arrest team.

Secure IV access and monitoring

- Insert 2 large-bore cannulae in antecubital veins or equivalent.
- If unable to obtain IV access quickly, consider intraosseous access early and get expert help to arrange definitive central venous access.
- Send urgent FBC, U+E, LFTs, coagulation screen, calcium, ABG/VBG and crossmatch, and inform blood bank.
- Monitor vitals and reassess peripheral perfusion every 10–15 min.
- Insert urinary catheter; monitor hourly urine output.

8

Resuscitate and reassess

Early shock features (Box 8.2) or any ongoing blood loss:

- 0.5–1 L stat of IV crystalloid
- Red cell transfusion to aim Hb >7 g/dL. Give 2 units of red cells if ongoing bleeding, haemodynamic instability, or Hb likely to drop below 7 g/dL. Target haemoglobin may be higher in patients with ischaemic heart disease or who remain unstable after initial resuscitation.

Reassess

- If advanced shock features or major blood loss (Box 8.2) on reassessment, resuscitate as per the adjacent column.
- Otherwise, continue with treatment and discuss with haematologist if any of the following:
  - Known coagulopathy/anticoagulant therapy
  - INR >1.4
  - Platelets <50 × 10^9/L
  - Fibrinogen <1 g/L
  - ≥4 L IV fluid in any form

Advance shock features (Box 8.2) or ongoing major blood loss:

- Trigger major hemorrhage protocol, or as per local procedure.
- 1–2 L stat of IV crystalloid
- Nominate person to liaise with transfusion laboratory. Give group specific red cells as soon as available.
- Consider O negative blood if significant delay in cross-matching.

Reassess

- If ongoing advanced shock features or major blood loss, administer further red cells and consider fresh-frozen plasma, platelets and cryoprecipitate, depending on the local major haemorrhage protocol, the volume of blood lost, the patient's haematological parameters and Haematology advice.
- Discuss targeted therapy for patients' medications with Haematology, such as andexanet alfa for apixaban reversal, or prothrombin complex concentrate and vitamin K for warfarin.
- Consider terlipressin and initiate broad-spectrum antibiotics if variceal bleed suspected.
- Seek specialist input, such as ICU, GI, Surgery as appropriate and discuss ongoing haemostatic support with haematologist.

Box 8.2 Clinical features of hypovolaemic shock

Early	Advanced
HR >100 bpm	Systolic BP <100 (or >40 mmHg drop from baseline)
Capillary refill time >2 secs	HR >120 bpm
Narrow pulse pressure	RR >20 breaths/min
Postural hypotension	Cold, mottled peripheries
Urine output 20–30 mL/hr	Urine output < 20 mL/hr
Pale, sweaty, anxious, thirsty	Confused, lethargic, low GCS score

1 **Resuscitation requirements assessed? (Boxes 8.1 and 8.2)**

Resuscitation is the top priority. Use Boxes 8.1 and 8.2 as a framework for evaluating resuscitation needs, but tailor your assessment to the individual. Monitoring trends of the parameters provides far more information than a single 'snapshot' assessment and is essential for evaluating response to treatment.

Do not rely exclusively on this framework. Be aware of different physiological responses to haemorrhage: young patients may compensate until blood loss is profound; heart rate may be misleading in patients on rate-limiting medications (e.g., beta blockers, calcium channel blockers) or with fixed-rate pacemakers; and compensatory vasoconstriction may not occur in patients on vasodilators.

In patients who present with fresh, red haematemesis, the subsequent vomiting of 'coffee grounds' or passage of black tarry stools may simply be a manifestation of the original bleed, but further bright red haematemesis or haematochezia implies continued active bleeding.

2 Active bleeding, features of shock or suspected variceal bleed?

All patients with haematemesis accompanied by features of shock (Box 8.2) or evidence of ongoing bleeding should have an urgent UGIE after adequate resuscitation. Variceal bleeds have a high mortality (30–50%) and require urgent endoscopic identification and treatment to arrest the bleeding following resuscitation and correction of coagulopathy. Terlipressin and broad-spectrum antibiotics should be considered pre-UGIE in patients with a suspected variceal bleed. Assume variceal bleeding in any patient with known hepatic cirrhosis or clinical and biochemical features of chronic liver disease (Box 12.5).

3 Glasgow-Blatchford score ≥1 (Table 8.1)?

In the absence of continued active bleeding or haemodynamic compromise, use the Glasgow-Blatchford Score (Table 8.1) to assess the requirement for acute endoscopic intervention. A patient with a score of ≤1 has a minimal risk of needing an intervention such as transfusion, endoscopy or surgery. These patients can be considered for an early discharge and outpatient management (see below). Any score >1 has a higher risk for needing a medical intervention such as transfusion, endoscopy, or surgery and should be admitted for further assessment. Scores of 6

Table 8.1 Glasgow-Blatchford Score

Admission risk marker	Score component value
Blood urea (mmol/L)	
6.5–8.0	2
8.0–10.0	3
10.0–25	4
>25	6
Haemoglobin (g/dL) for men	
12.0–12.9	1
10.0–11.9	3
<10.0	6
Haemoglobin (g/dL) for women	
10.0–11.9	1
<10.0	6
Systolic blood pressure (mm Hg)	
100–109	1
90–99	2
<90	3
Other markers	
Pulse ≥100/min	1
Melaena	1
Syncope	2
Hepatic disease	2
Cardiac failure	2

A score of ≤1 is associated with minimal risk of requiring an intervention such as transfusion, endoscopy or surgery. These patients can be considered for an early discharge and outpatient management. Any score >1 has an increased risk of intervention. Scores ≥6 are associated with a >50% risk of needing an intervention.

or more are associated with a >50% risk of needing an intervention.

4 Presence of red-flag features?

Request an UGIE to exclude upper GI malignancy if the patient has any of the following red-flag features:

- Weight loss
- Anorexia or early satiety
- Dysphagia
- Epigastric mass
- Lymphadenopathy
- Jaundice
- Age ≥50 years

5 Consider Mallory-Weiss tear, gastritis or oesophagitis. Consider outpatient UGIE and arrange follow up to ensure resolution of symptoms

Patients who have no red flag features, no haemodynamic compromise and a Glasgow-Blatchford score of ≤1 can safely be discharged from hospital with outpatient follow-up. A working diagnosis may be suggested by the clinical history. With a characteristic history of Mallory–Weiss tear (haematemesis preceded by forceful retching/vomiting), the diagnosis can often be made clinically, and treatment of the underlying cause may be indicated. In other cases, gastritis or oesophagitis may be the working diagnosis. Give an oral proton pump inhibitor and consider outpatient UGIE with a CLO test (for detection of *H pylori*). Arrange follow-up to ensure resolution of symptoms. If symptoms are unexplained or episodes of haematemesis are recurrent, arrange an UGIE.

8

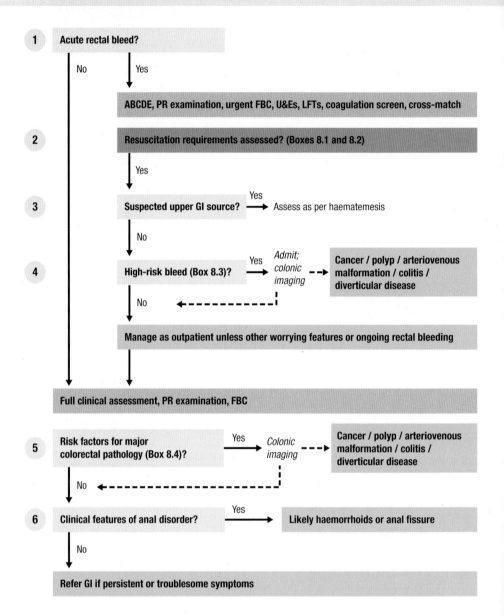

1 Acute rectal bleed?

No   Yes

ABCDE, PR examination, urgent FBC, U&Es, LFTs, coagulation screen, cross-match

2 Resuscitation requirements assessed? (Boxes 8.1 and 8.2)

Yes

3 Suspected upper GI source? → Yes → Assess as per haematemesis

No

4 High-risk bleed (Box 8.3)? → Yes → *Admit; colonic imaging* --→ Cancer / polyp / arteriovenous malformation / colitis / diverticular disease

No

Manage as outpatient unless other worrying features or ongoing rectal bleeding

Full clinical assessment, PR examination, FBC

5 Risk factors for major colorectal pathology (Box 8.4)? → Yes → *Colonic imaging* --→ Cancer / polyp / arteriovenous malformation / colitis / diverticular disease

No

6 Clinical features of anal disorder? → Yes → Likely haemorrhoids or anal fissure

No

Refer GI if persistent or troublesome symptoms

1   Acute rectal bleed?

Regard any prolonged, profuse or ongoing episode of bright red/maroon PR blood loss within the previous 24 hours as acute rectal bleeding. Assess patients with melaena in the same way as those with haematemesis (see above).

Where the predominant problem is bloody diarrhoea, evaluate as described in Chapter 9. In the absence of acute rectal bleeding, proceed to step 5.

2   Resuscitation requirements assessed? (Boxes 8.1 and 8.2)

Make adequate resuscitation your top priority. Evaluate and address resuscitation requirements as described in Boxes 8.1 and 8.2.

3   Suspected upper GI source?

Assume, initially, that melaena reflects upper GI bleeding and assess as described for haematemesis. Brisk bleeding from the upper GI tract may present with a fresh red PR blood and implies severe, life-threatening haemorrhage. The diagnosis is straightforward if there is concomitant haematemesis but otherwise a high index of suspicion is essential. Proceed with a working diagnosis of lower GI bleeding in patients without haemodynamic instability, but suspect an upper GI source in those with features of hypovolaemic shock (Box 8.2).

If shock is present, seek senior GI input and consider UGIE as the first-line investigation following resuscitation, especially if there are any recent upper GI symptoms, such as epigastric pain, or known/suspected oesophageal varices. If the source is not identified on UGIE, then CT angiography and/or colonoscopy may be considered, informed by specialist opinion.

4   High-risk bleed (Box 8.3)?

Consider early discharge (with outpatient follow-up) if the patient has no evidence of ongoing bleeding and no high-risk features (Box 8.3)—especially if there is evidence of a benign anal disorder. Do not discharge a patient without making a clear decision as to the likely cause of bleeding.

8

Box 8.3 Risk factors for adverse outcomes in acute lower GI bleeding

- Any haemodynamic instability
- Initial haematocrit <35% or need for red blood cell transfusion
- Any visualized red blood PR
- INR >1.4 or current anticoagulant use (e.g., warfarin, novel oral anticoagulants, aspirin)
- Significant comorbidity, for example, cardiorespiratory, renal, hepatic impairment or current hospital inpatient
- Low serum albumin
- Raised WCC
- Age >60 years
- A prior history of bleeding from diverticulosis or angiodysplasia

Admit any patient with risk factors for uncontrolled or recurrent bleeding (Box 8.3). Once adequately resuscitated and clinically stable, arrange colonic imaging to establish the site and cause of bleeding. Most cases of rectal bleeding settle with conservative management. Be cautious about allowing the patient to mobilize to the toilet if they need to pass stool—this may represent another bleed and they risk collapse.

Seek urgent senior surgical input in any patient with continued active bleeding, ongoing haemodynamic instability despite resuscitation or high transfusion requirements. CT angiography is the first line intervention if there is clinical evidence of ongoing bleeding despite resuscitation. Colonoscopy is the most informative investigation and the intervention of choice if the bleeding has stopped as it facilitates a final diagnosis.

5 Risk factors for major colorectal pathology?

Refer the patient for urgent lower GI investigation (usually colonoscopy) to exclude colorectal cancer if any of the criteria in Box 8.4 are present.

Also consider lower GI endoscopic assessment if the patient has:
- Systemic/extraintestinal features of inflammatory bowel disease (Box 9.3)
- A history of pelvic radiotherapy

- Recent-onset, persistent bleeding when the patient is ≥50 years or has a strong family history of colorectal cancer, such as a first-degree relative <45 years at diagnosis, or two or more first-degree relatives with the diagnosis.

Box 8.4 High-risk features for colorectal cancer in patients with rectal bleeding

- Rectal bleeding ≥4 weeks with change of bowel habit (↓ or ↑frequency or alternating bowel habit)
- Tenesmus
- Palpable rectal or abdominal mass
- Significant weight loss
- Previous excision of colorectal cancer or polyps
- History of inflammatory bowel disease
- Family history of colorectal cancer, polyps or inherited colorectal cancer syndromes
- Age >50 years without anal symptoms, such as discomfort, itching, lumps, prolapse

---

6 Clinical features of anal disorder?

Perform careful rectal examination ± proctoscopy in all patients to look for an anal disorder. Do not forget to look for anal cancer. If benign anorectal pathology is identified, provide reassurance but refer the patient for outpatient colorectal evaluation if there is diagnostic doubt or symptoms persist despite conservative management.

Arrange further GI investigation ± referral in all patients without an obvious anorectal cause in whom bleeding persists or recurs.

Diarrhoea may be defined as the passage of ≥3 loose or watery stools/day. Patients often have difficulty describing their stools. The Bristol Stool Form Scale can be helpful (Fig. 9.1).

The differential diagnosis depends on symptom duration.

- *Acute diarrhoea* (<2 weeks): usually infectious and self-limiting, e.g., norovirus or rotavirus. Less common causes include drugs, inflammatory bowel disease and ischaemic colitis. Most patients do not present to healthcare services as the symptoms are transient. However, patients may seek medical attention if their symptoms are severe, there is associated systemic upset, they are becoming dehydrated or there are concerning features such as PR bleeding. This is more likely if symptoms are due to invasive pathogens, inflammatory bowel disease, or ischaemia. The differential diagnosis and investigation of diarrhoea in immunocompromised patients is markedly different, due to the extensive range of possible pathogens and severity of the illness. These patients are best discussed with Infectious Disease (ID) specialists early in their presentation.
- *Chronic/persistent diarrhoea* (>2 weeks): As symptoms become chronic, noninfective causes become pervasive in resource-rich environments. Diarrhoea may reflect colorectal cancer or inflammatory bowel disease, but the most frequent cause is irritable bowel syndrome. In resource-limited settings, infective causes remain dominant, including mycobacterial, chronic bacterial and parasitic causes.

Infectious diarrhoea

Infectious diarrhoea is due to transmission of viruses, bacteria, bacterial toxins or parasites, usually through the faecal-oral route. Most cases are viral, self-limiting and the pathogen is rarely identified. Viruses and toxins predominantly affect the stomach and small bowel, causing large-volume, watery diarrhoea, vomiting, abdominal cramping, bloating and gas. Invasive intestinal pathogens cause inflammation of the large bowel and may cause bloody diarrhoea, often with severe abdominal cramps, passage of mucous and systemic upset (dysentery). Fever may be a feature. Pathogens include Shiga-toxin producing *Escherichia coli* (e.g., *O157*), *Shigella*, *Salmonella, Campylobacter*, enteric viruses (e.g., cytomegalovirus, adenovirus) and cytotoxic organisms such as *Clostridium difficile*. *C difficile* infection is an important cause of hospital-acquired diarrhoea, risk factors for which include broad-spectrum antibiotic therapy, immunocompromise, and advanced age. *C difficile* ranges from mild diarrhoeal illness to life-threatening pseudomembranous colitis.

Diarrhoea that persists for >10 days is unlikely to be infective, but consider protozoal infections (e.g., giardiasis, amoebiasis or *Cryptosporidium* infection) in patients who are immunocompromised or have recently travelled to the tropics.

Irritable bowel syndrome

Irritable bowel syndrome (IBS) is the most common cause of chronic diarrhoea. The predominant bowel habit may alternate between diarrhoea and constipation. Diagnosis is based on typical clinical features (Box 9.1) and the absence of apparent organic disease. Symptoms tend to follow a relapsing and remitting course, often exacerbated by psychosocial stress. There are no absolutes when considering investigations to rule out organic disease if IBS is suspected. While many female patients report cyclical features

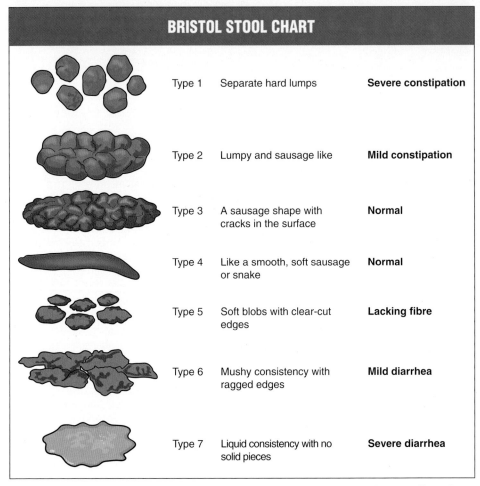

BRISTOL STOOL CHART

	Type 1	Separate hard lumps	**Severe constipation**
Type 2	Lumpy and sausage like	**Mild constipation**
Type 3	A sausage shape with cracks in the surface	**Normal**
Type 4	Like a smooth, soft sausage or snake	**Normal**
Type 5	Soft blobs with clear-cut edges	**Lacking fibre**
Type 6	Mushy consistency with ragged edges	**Mild diarrhea**
Type 7	Liquid consistency with no solid pieces	**Severe diarrhea**

Figure 9.1 Bristol stool form scale. From Arzu Ilce. Fecal incontinence: causes, management, and outcome. Chapter 2: Faecal incontinence. IntechOpen, 2014. http://dx.doi.org/10.5772/57502.

to their symptoms correlating to menstruation, it is important to rule out endometriosis as a cause for the patient's GI features. Have a low threshold for detailed investigation in patients with a known family history of ovarian or colorectal cancer.

Drugs

Many drugs, including numerous over-the-counter preparations, cause diarrhoea (Box 9.2).

Colorectal cancer

Colorectal cancer may present with diarrhoea, especially if left-sided/distal. Suggestive features include weight loss, rectal bleeding, a palpable mass or iron deficiency anaemia, but the absence of these features does not exclude malignancy. The diagnosis must be considered in any patient >45 years with new-onset, persistent diarrhoea and is usually confirmed by colonoscopy with

---

Box 9.1 Rome IV criteria for diagnosis of irritable bowel syndrome

Irritable bowel syndrome diagnostic criteria:[a]
  Recurrent abdominal pain on average at least 1 day/week in the last 3 months, associated with two or more of the following criteria:
- Related to defecation
- Associated with a change in frequency of stool
- Associated with a change in form (appearance) of stool

[a]*Criteria fulfilled for the last 3 months with symptom onset at least 6 months prior to diagnosis.*
Reprinted with permission from the Rome Foundation; all rights reserved.

Box 9.2 Drugs that frequently cause diarrhoea

- Laxatives (including occult laxative misuse)
- Antibiotics (especially macrolides)
- Alcohol (especially chronic alcohol excess)
- NSAIDs
- Metformin
- Colchicine
- Orlistat (steatorrhoea)
- Proton pump inhibitors
- SSRIs
- Nicorandil
- Digoxin
- Cytotoxic and immunosuppressive agents
- Cancer immunotherapies
- Magnesium replacement and antacids (due to magnesium content)

---

biopsy. Many countries now conduct colorectal cancer screening programmes, which has led to more cases being diagnosed at an asymptomatic stage; diagnosis following presentation with symptoms is associated with a worse prognosis.

Inflammatory bowel disease

Ulcerative colitis (UC) is an inflammatory disorder of the colonic mucosa confined to the large bowel. It typically presents with bloody diarrhoea with mucous and cramping lower abdominal pain ± tenesmus. Systemic features that occur during acute attacks include fever, anorexia and weight loss.

Crohn's disease causes transmural granulomatous inflammation affecting any part of the alimentary tract. It may present with large

---

Box 9.3 Extraintestinal features of inflammatory bowel disease

- General: fever, malaise, weight loss
- Eyes: conjunctivitis, episcleritis, iritis
- Joints: arthralgia of large joints, seronegative spondyloarthritis
- Skin: mouth ulcers, erythema nodosum, pyoderma gangrenosum
- Liver: fatty liver, gallstones, sclerosing cholangitis, cholangiocarcinoma (UC)

---

bowel symptoms, like those of UC, or with small bowel symptoms, such as watery, nonbloody diarrhoea accompanied by abdominal pain and weight loss. Both disorders are associated with a range of extraintestinal features (Box 9.3).

Microscopic colitis is an inflammatory condition affecting the musoca of the colon. It is characterized by watery, nonbloody diarrhoea, predominantly in the female population. Macroscopically, the mucosa appears normal and diagnosis is made on histological appearances. While there are a number of autoimmune disorders associated with microscopic colitis, there are no hallmark extraintestinal features.

Disorders causing malabsorption

Fat malabsorption causes pale, greasy, offensive stools that float and are difficult to flush (steatorrhoea). Other features of malabsorption include undigested foodstuffs in stool, weight loss, bloating and nutritional deficiencies. The usual underlying cause is small bowel disease, for example, coeliac disease, Crohn's disease, tropical sprue, bacterial overgrowth, lymphoma, small bowel resection or pancreatic insufficiency.

Other causes

- Diverticulitis (Chapter 7)
- Ischaemic colitis (Chapter 8)
- Hyperthyroidism, autonomic neuropathy, Addison's disease
- Carcinoid tumour, gastrinoma, VIPoma
- Amyloid
- Severe constipation with overflow

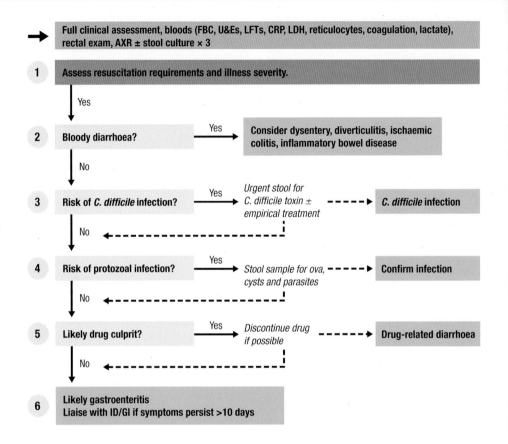

1	**Assess resuscitation requirements and illness severity**

Step 1 Are there features of shock?
Look for ↑HR, ↓BP (a late sign) or evidence of tissue hypoperfusion (Box 2.1). If present, provide IV fluid resuscitation and reassess. Although hypovolaemia from GI losses is the likeliest cause of shock, also consider intra-abdominal sepsis, and adrenal insufficiency (diarrhoea is a common feature of acute adrenal crisis).

Step 2 Is there acute kidney injury?
Hypovolaemia may result in severe 'prerenal' acute kidney injury (AKI, Chapter 29), especially if compounded by antihypertensive or nephrotoxic medication, such as diuretics, ACE inhibitors, NSAIDs. Patients with AKI require IV rehydration with close monitoring of fluid balance, urine output and U+Es. If AKI occurs in the context of bloody diarrhoea,

look for features of haemolytic uraemic syndrome, such as ↓Hb, ↓platelets, ↑bilirubin/LDH/reticulocytes. This is a hallmark and sign of disease severity in *E coli O157* infection.

Step 3 Does the patient otherwise require IV fluids/hospital admission?
Patients with clinical evidence of dehydration (thirst, dry mucous membranes, ↓skin turgor) and concomitant vomiting, or those who are unable to match oral intake to ongoing losses, require IV fluids.

Other features that may indicate a need for hospital admission include:
- Fever
- ↑WBC
- Bloody diarrhoea
- Abdominal tenderness/guarding/rigidity
- Frail, elderly or immunocompromised patient
- Significant comorbidity, such as heart/renal/hepatic failure

2 Bloody diarrhoea?

The frequent passage of bloody stools suggests either:

- Dysentery, that is, infection with invasive organisms (e.g., *Campylobacter*, *Shigella* or *Amoeba)* or cytotoxin-producing organisms (e.g., *C difficile*, *E coli O157)* OR
- Noninfectious colitis, for example, ischaemic colitis or inflammatory bowel disease

It is often difficult to differentiate dysentery from early presentations of inflammatory bowel disease: both may be accompanied by abdominal pain, tenesmus, mucus, constitutional upset and a systemic inflammatory response (Box 7.1).

- Send FBC, U+Es, LFTs, CRP, LDH, reticulocytes, venous blood gas and three stool samples in all patients, plus blood cultures if fever is present.
- Test stool for *C difficile* toxin (CDT) if the patient has risk factors (see below), severe systemic upset or ↑WBC.
- Request an abdominal X-ray to look for colonic dilatation (Fig. 7.5B).
- Liaise with the ID team and request analysis of stool for ova, cysts and parasites if recent foreign travel or immunocompromised.

If the duration of symptoms is ≤7 days, suspect an infectious cause unless there are specific pointers to an alternative diagnosis. Consider ischaemic colitis if bloody diarrhoea was preceded by sudden onset of left-sided lower abdominal pain or in any patient >50 years with known atherosclerotic disease or a source of systemic embolism, such as atrial fibrillation.

Refer any patient with known inflammatory bowel disease, extraintestinal manifestations (Box 9.3), previous similar episodes or symptoms >7 days for specialist GI evaluation.

Seek an urgent surgical review if there is evidence of peritonism or toxic megacolon, or if you suspect ischaemic colitis or diverticulitis.

3 Risk of *C difficile* infection?

Send stool for CDT in any patient who lives in an institution (e.g., nursing home), has recently been hospitalized, has received antibiotics within the last 3 months or is >65 years. In high-risk patients, send ≥3 samples before ruling out the diagnosis. If *C difficile* is confirmed, stop contributing antibiotics and proton pump inhibitors if possible, assess severity at least daily (Box 9.4) and treat as per local guidance.

4 Risk of protozoal infection?

Send three stool samples on consecutive days for ova, cysts and parasites in patients with a history of recent foreign travel or when there is known or suspected immunocompromise (e.g., chemotherapy, HIV).

5 Likely drug culprit?

Suspect drug-related diarrhoea if the onset of symptoms corresponds with initiation or ↑dose of a drug, especially those listed in Box 9.2. Seek an alternative explanation if diarrhoea does not resolve on drug discontinuation.

6 Likely gastroenteritis. Liaise with ID/GI if symptoms persist >10 days

Most cases are self-limiting viral or toxin-mediated infections and do not require further investigation or antimicrobial treatment. If symptoms persist >10 days, seek specialist advice and consider further assessment as for chronic/persistent diarrhoea.

Box 9.4 Assessing the severity of *Clostridium difficile* infection

Mild	WBC not elevated <3 episodes of loose stools/day
Moderate	↑WBC (but <15 × 10⁹/L) 3–5 loose stools/day
Severe	WBC 15 × 10⁹/L or Serum creatinine >50% above baseline or Temp >38.5°C or Evidence of severe colitis (abdominal or radiological signs)
Life-threatening	Signs of shock Partial or complete ileus Toxic megacolon or CT evidence of severe disease

Adapted from NICE 2021 (Clostridioides difficile infection: antimicrobial prescribing). Available from www.nice.org.uk/guidance/ng199. All rights reserved. Subject to Notice of rights. NICE guidance is prepared for the National Health Service in England. It is subject to regular review and updating and may be withdrawn. NICE accepts no responsibility for the use of its content in this product/publication.

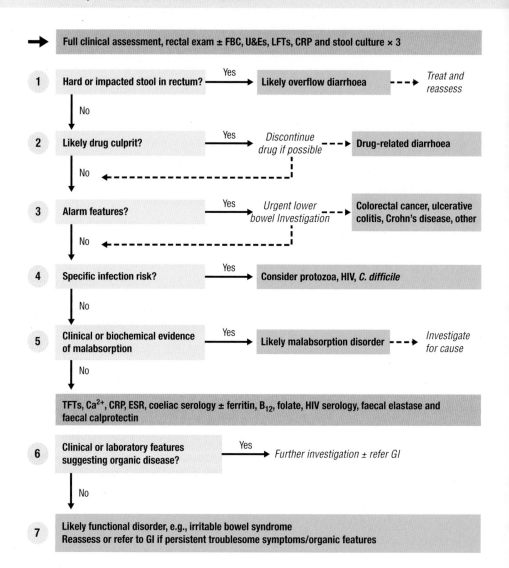

1 Hard or impacted stool in rectum?

Have a high index of suspicion for overflow diarrhoea in frail, immobile or confused elderly patients. Always do a rectal examination. If the stool is hard or impacted, treat with faecal softeners and laxatives, then reassess. If the rectal examination is normal, overflow diarrhoea is unlikely (90% of impactions are rectal) but consider an abdominal X-ray if there is strong clinical suspicion.

2 Likely drug culprit?

Look for a temporal relationship between potential drug culprits (Box 9.2) and the onset of diarrhoea. Consider trialling discontinuation where feasible, but change only one agent at any time and restart the drug if symptoms continue unaltered. Always ask about alcohol excess.

3 Alarm features?

Expedite lower bowel investigation to exclude colorectal cancer/inflammatory bowel disease if the patient has persistent diarrhoea associated with any of the following:

- Age >45 years
- Rectal bleeding or melaena
- Weight loss
- Iron-deficiency anaemia
- Pain or diarrhoea overnight
- Progressive abdominal pain
- Fever, raised inflammatory markers or other systemic symptoms
- Palpable rectal mass
- Family history of inflammatory bowel disease or colorectal cancer

Consider flexible sigmoidoscopy as a first-line investigation in patients <45 years or colonoscopy if >45 years.

4 Specific infection risk?

Exclude protozoal infection in patients with a history of travel to the tropics (e.g., giardiasis, amoebiasis) or with known HIV infection/other immunocompromise (e.g., cryptosporidiosis). Send three fresh stool samples for examination for ova, cysts and parasites. Liaise with the ID team if stool samples are negative but there is ongoing clinical suspicion of infection. Test for HIV in all patients with chronic diarrhoea.

C difficile diarrhoea may be chronic or relapsing—send stool to test for CDT in any patient with risk factors (see above).

5 Clinical or biochemical evidence of malabsorption?

Steatorrhoea signifies fat malabsorption, but its absence does not exclude a malabsorptive disorder. Screen for nutritional deficiencies (e.g., iron, B_{12}, folate, Ca^{2+}, Mg^{2+}, PO_4^{3-}, albumin) in any patient with suspected malabsorption. If steatorrhoea is present, ensure that the patient is not taking orlistat (available over the counter in the UK), and check coeliac serology and faecal elastase ($\downarrow$in pancreatic insufficiency). If $\downarrow$faecal elastase or a strong suspicion of pancreatic disease (e.g., suggestive symptoms, history of acute pancreatitis, cystic fibrosis), consider pancreatic imaging (CT/MRCP). If coeliac serology is positive, then arrange confirmatory testing for coeliac disease with endoscopy and duodenal biopsy. Note that coeliac serology and endoscopy with biopsy will detect coeliac disease only if the patient has recently been exposed to gluten; patients should continue to eat gluten-containing food during investigation.

If there is no evidence of pancreatic insufficiency or coeliac disease, but suspicion of malabsorption remains high (e.g., large-volume non-bloody stool, previous gastric/small bowel surgery or evidence of nutritional deficiencies), refer to GI for further small bowel investigation, such as duodenal biopsy or MRI.

6 Clinical or laboratory features suggesting organic disease?

Exclude inflammatory bowel disease if there is a positive family history, evidence of systemic inflammation, extra-intestinal manifestations of inflammatory bowel disease (Box 9.3) or positive faecal calprotectin. Refer to GI for further evaluation if any of the above features are present or there are other findings that suggest organic disease, such as weight loss, anorexia, painless diarrhoea, prominent nocturnal symptoms or recent onset of symptoms in a patient >45 years.

7 Likely functional disorder

If none of the above is present, a functional cause, such as irritable bowel syndrome, is likely, particularly when typical symptoms are present (Box 9.1) and baseline investigations are negative. Provide reassurance, explanation and institute a management plan.

9

10 Dysphagia

Dysphagia is the symptom of difficult or abnormal swallowing. It is an alarm ('red flag') symptom and therefore requires prompt assessment to exclude serious pathology. With the exception of acute presentations with a concomitant sore throat, oesophageal investigation is always necessary to rule out mechanical obstruction and, in particular, malignancy. History is critical to informing the differential diagnosis and can help determine whether the condition causing dysphagia is a structural or motility disorder. Structural disorders typically cause dysphagia for solids; motility disorders may cause dysphagia for solids and liquids.

Oropharyngeal dysphagia

Bulbar palsy

Lower motor neuron palsies of cranial nerves IX–XII result in weakness of the tongue and muscles of swallowing. The tongue is flaccid with fasciculation, often with a change in voice (Table 10.1). Causes include motor neuron disease (MND), Guillain-Barré syndrome, syringobulbia and brainstem tumour/infarction.

Pseudobulbar (corticobulbar) palsy

Bilateral upper motor neuron lesions of cranial nerves IX–XII cause dysphagia with a small, contracted and slowly moving tongue, weakness or paralysis of the pharyngeal muscles and a brisk jaw jerk. There may be associated speech disturbance and emotional lability (Table 10.1). It is more common than bulbar palsy, and causes include cerebrovascular disease, demyelination, MND and central pontine myelinolysis.

Myasthenia gravis

Myasthenia gravis causes fatigability of oropharyngeal muscles, resulting in increasing swallowing difficulty after the first few mouthfuls of food/fluid. Dysphagia may occur before other features of myasthenia are readily apparent.

Parkinson's disease, stroke and myopathies

These conditions frequently cause swallowing difficulty, but other features are usually more prominent.

Pharyngeal pouch

A pharyngeal pouch is formed by posterior herniation of the pharyngeal mucosa between the thyropharyngeus and cricopharyngeus muscles. It is usually found in elderly patients. In addition to dysphagia, there is classically regurgitation of undigested food, halitosis, the feeling of a lump in the neck and gurgling after swallowing liquids.

Oesophageal dysphagia (structural)

Food bolus obstruction

A food bolus obstruction causes sudden onset of complete dysphagia, often with an inability to swallow even saliva. The diagnosis is usually obvious from the history, but it may be the first manifestation of an underlying stricture.

Malignant stricture

Patients with oesophageal cancer typically present with progressive, painless dysphagia to solid foods. Weight loss may be marked, especially if presentation is delayed. Cachexia and lymphadenopathy are suggestive, but physical signs are typically absent. Risk factors include alcohol, smoking and known gastro-oesophageal reflux disease (GORD)/Barrett's oesophagus.

Benign stricture

Most commonly, benign stricture is due to gastro-oesophageal reflux, especially in elderly patients. Rarer causes include strictures weeks or months after ingestion of caustic substances,

Table 10.1 Comparison of signs in bulbar and pseudobulbar palsy

	Bulbar	Pseudobulbar
Speech	Quiet, nasal tone; difficulty forming consonants (especially 'R'); may become slurred	Slow deliberate speech
Tongue	Weak, wasted with fasciculation, folded	Small, stiff, cannot be protruded
Jaw jerk	Normal or absent	Brisk
Gag reflex	Absent	Present
Emotions	Normal	Labile (e.g., uncontrollable laughing/crying)

oesophageal webs (seen in iron deficiency), Schatzki rings (benign idiopathic strictures of the lower oesophagus), eosinophilic oesophagitis or, rarely, benign oesophageal tumours.

Hiatus hernia

Hiatus hernia with an associated intrathoracic stomach can present with dysphagia and vomiting. GORD manifests only when the lower oesophageal sphincter becomes incompetent.

Extrinsic compression

Lung cancer, thyroid goitre, mediastinal nodes, an enlarged left atrium or a thoracic aortic aneurysm may produce dysphagia by compressing the oesophagus.

Oesophageal dysphagia (dysmotility)

Achalasia

This is an uncommon disorder characterized by loss of peristalsis in the distal oesophagus and impaired relaxation of the lower oesophageal sphincter. Dysphagia is of slow onset (often years), occurs for liquids and solids and may initially be intermittent. Dysphagia for liquids is the most prominent symptom. Retrosternal discomfort and regurgitation are common.

Scleroderma

Oesophageal involvement is seen in ≈90% of cases of scleroderma; replacement of muscle with fibrous tissue results in incompetence of the lower oesophageal sphincter, impaired peristalsis and severe gastro-oesophageal reflux. Other features of scleroderma may be apparent, such as calcinosis, Raynaud's disease and telangiectasia.

Chagas disease

Chagas disease (a tropical parasitic disease caused by *Trypanosoma cruzi*) can present with achalasia; consider it in patients originating from endemic areas in Central and South America and confirm with serological testing.

Diffuse oesophageal spasm

This may cause transient episodes of dysphagia, although episodic chest pain that mimics angina is usually the predominant symptom.

Other, rarer causes

Inadequate saliva

Inadequate saliva production, which can be caused by anticholinergic side effects or connective tissue diseases such as Sjogren syndrome, may lead to problems with forming a manageable bolus and the sensation of dysphagia.

Globus

Globus is a functional disorder defined as the sensation of a lump or foreign body in the throat. It is a diagnosis of exclusion and requires that all of the Rome IV diagnostic criteria (Box 10.1) be met.

Box 10.1 Rome IV criteria for diagnosis of globus

To meet the diagnosis of globus, all of the following criteria must be fulfilled for a duration of at least 3 months, with symptom onset at least 6 months prior to diagnosis and symptom frequency of at least once per week.

1. Persistent or intermittent, nonpainful sensation of a lump or foreign body in the throat with no structural lesion identified on physical examination, laryngoscopy, or endoscopy
2. Occurrence of the sensation between meals
3. Absence of dysphagia or odynophagia
4. Absence of a gastric inlet patch in the proximal oesophagus
5. Absence of evidence that gastroesophageal reflux or eosinophilic oesophagitis is the cause of the symptom
6. Absence of major oesophageal motor disorders, such as achalasia/esophagogastric junction outflow obstruction, diffuse oesophageal spasm, jackhammer oesophagus, absent peristalsis

10

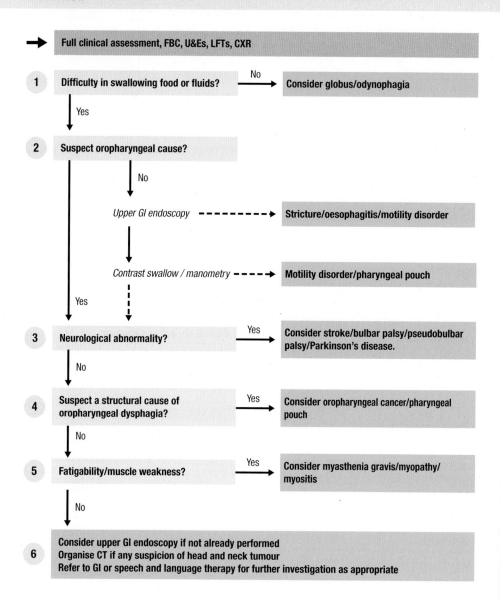

Full clinical assessment, FBC, U&Es, LFTs, CXR

1 Difficulty in swallowing food or fluids? — No → Consider globus/odynophagia

Yes

2 Suspect oropharyngeal cause?

No

Upper GI endoscopy ┈┈┈┈┈► Stricture/oesophagitis/motility disorder

Contrast swallow / manometry ┈┈┈┈► Motility disorder/pharyngeal pouch

Yes

3 Neurological abnormality? — Yes → Consider stroke/bulbar palsy/pseudobulbar palsy/Parkinson's disease.

No

4 Suspect a structural cause of oropharyngeal dysphagia? — Yes → Consider oropharyngeal cancer/pharyngeal pouch

No

5 Fatigability/muscle weakness? — Yes → Consider myasthenia gravis/myopathy/myositis

No

6 Consider upper GI endoscopy if not already performed
Organise CT if any suspicion of head and neck tumour
Refer to GI or speech and language therapy for further investigation as appropriate

1 Difficulty in swallowing foods or fluids?

Features of true dysphagia include difficulty initiating swallowing or the sensation of food 'sticking' after swallowing. Globus is the sensation of a lump in the throat; it is unrelated to swallowing and often associated with anxiety or strong emotion. Odynophagia is pain on swallowing and suggests oesophageal inflammation or ulceration.

2 Suspect oropharyngeal cause?

Suspect oropharyngeal dysphagia if the patient reports one or more of the following:
- Evidence of oral dysfunction: drooling/spillage of food from the mouth, dysarthria.
- Immediate sensation of a bolus 'catching' in the neck. Patients may identify their neck as the point of their symptoms rather than retrosternally, which is associated more with oesophageal dysphagia.
- Difficulty initiating swallow—repeated attempts are required to clear the bolus.
- Choking/coughing/aspiration on swallowing.

In patients in whom oropharyngeal dysphagia is suspected, progress to Step 3 for further investigation.

If none of these features is present, investigate for an oesophageal cause. Arrange an UGIE to look for a structural cause, especially oesophageal cancer. upper GI endoscopy (UGIE) may also reveal features of certain motility disorders (e.g., achalasia) but can be normal, especially in scleroderma or diffuse oesophageal spasm. Note that a contrast barium swallow test may be first-line investigation if the patient has a history of caustic ingestion, radiotherapy or laryngeal or oesophageal cancer—discuss with a GI specialist in the first instance.

If no cause is identified on UGIE, consult a GI specialist, as further investigation for a motility disorder (e.g., contrast swallow or oesophageal manometry) may be required. If all GI investigations are reassuring, continue to evaluate for a possible oropharyngeal cause and progress to Step 3

3 Neurological abnormality?

If the history suggests an oropharyngeal aetiology for dysphagia, neurological evaluation is essential. Although swallowing difficulty is common in stroke, Parkinson's disease and multiple sclerosis, it is very rarely the primary presenting problem. However, dysphagia may be the principal complaint in bulbar palsy and pseudobulbar palsy, so look carefully for the relevant clinical features (Table 10.1); if they are present, look for other features of MND and perform neuroimaging to exclude vascular or structural brainstem disease. Discuss with a neurologist all patients in whom there is concern about a neurological abnormality causing dysphagia.

4 Suspect structural cause of oropharyngeal dysphagia?

Exclude oropharyngeal cancer if the patient has an oropharyngeal pattern of dysphagia (Step 2) without evidence of an underlying neurological disorder. Risk factors for oropharyngeal cancer include smoking, alcohol and human papillomavirus infection. A palpable neck lump, halitosis, cough, hoarseness, sore throat, ear pain (referred pain) and weight loss are some of the clinical features that may be associated. If suspected, refer to an ENT specialist for investigation.

Investigate for a pharyngeal pouch (e.g., contrast swallow or nasoendoscopy) if there is associated regurgitation or a lump in the neck that appears after eating ± halitosis (from food lodged in the pouch), weight loss, aspiration or chronic cough.

5 Fatigability/muscle weakness?

Myasthenia gravis is rare and easily missed. The dysphagia typically presents with increasing difficulty in swallowing after the first few mouthfuls and difficulty in chewing. Ask specifically about/examine for:
- Fatigable weakness of muscles: initial strength is normal but there is a rapid decline with activity
- Weak voice with prolonged speaking
- Diplopia
- Ptosis
- Muscle fatigability (Ask the patient to count to 50 or hold the arms above the head.)

Refer to a neurologist for definitive testing if you suspect the diagnosis.

10

6 **Consider further investigation and referral to GI or speech and language therapy**

All patients should be discussed with a GI specialist. If not already done, arrange UGIE unless there is clear evidence of neurological or neuromuscular dysfunction (where referral to neurology would be essential). Request a CT if you suspect cancer of the head and neck.

Once significant pathology of the oropharynx and oesophagus has been excluded, consider referral to speech and language therapy team for a detailed swallow evaluation with video fluoroscopy. This will confirm the presence of oropharyngeal dysfunction and help to clarify the mechanism.

Nausea and vomiting 11

Nausea is the unpleasant sensation of feeling as though you will vomit. It can be associated with vomiting (the forceful expulsion of gastric contents) or dyspepsia (symptoms of indigestion). Vomiting should be differentiated from regurgitation, which is the appearance of gastric contents without any effort. Acute (≤10 days) nausea and vomiting (N&V) should be assessed separately from chronic presentations.

This chapter focuses on N&V as a principal presenting complaint. See Chapter 8 if GI bleeding is a feature.

Gastroenteritis

Gastroenteritis is the most common cause of acute N&V. The aetiology is usually viral, e.g., norovirus, rotavirus, adenovirus. It may affect any age group but has a higher incidence and associated harm in children and the elderly. Gastroenteritis may also be caused by bacteria or parasites. The sudden onset of N&V is likely due to the ingestion of a toxin such as *Staphylococcus aureus* enterotoxin or *Bacillus cereus* emetic toxin; vomiting tends to develop within 1–6 hours of ingestion of poorly prepared/cooked foodstuffs. Enteric viruses (e.g., norovirus, rotavirus) are transmitted via the faeco-oral route and manifest slightly later. Parasitic infections causing GI upset include nematodes and are associated with ingestion of raw fish.

A detailed history may reveal known contacts with similar symptoms or a history of travel, eating out or eating unusual foods recently. Accompanying features may include fever, abdominal cramping and diarrhoea.

GI obstruction

Mechanical obstruction of the GI tract (e.g., due to a tumour, adhesions or incarcerated hernia) may cause vomiting, usually accompanied by colicky abdominal pain (Chapter 7)

and absolute constipation (absence of flatus) ± abdominal distension. The characteristics of the vomitus may suggest the location of obstruction: gastric juices—gastric outlet obstruction; bilious material—small bowel obstruction; feculent material—distal obstruction (or coloenteric/cologastric fistula).

Gastroparesis

Gastroparesis is a disorder which causes delayed gastric emptying and N&V as a result of reduced peristalsis of the stomach. It is frequently associated with autonomic neuropathy and so is common in patients with diabetes. It can also be associated with other conditions such as scleroderma and can occur in patients who have had previous gastric surgery. In a significant proportion of patients, it is idiopathic.

Functional nausea and vomiting disorders

Functional nausea and vomiting disorders are diagnoses of exclusion, but there are symptoms to be alert for. Cyclical vomiting syndrome is characterized by repeated, sudden-onset, severe N&V with no identified cause; discrete episodes of N&V typically last <1 week. Patients with cannabinoid hyperemesis syndrome may report symptoms similar to cyclical vomiting. The syndrome is associated with prolonged cannabis use; symptoms may be alleviated by prolonged warm baths and showers. Functional nausea and vomiting disorders have specific criteria that must be met for at least 3 months, with symptom onset at least 6 months before diagnosis.

Other GI tract disease

Peptic ulcer disease may present with N&V, typically associated with epigastric discomfort or a history of dyspeptic symptoms. N&V may

Box 11.1 Common toxic/therapeutic causes of nausea and vomiting

Alcohol	Colchicine
Antiarrhythmics	Digoxin
Anticonvulsants	NSAIDs/Aspirin
Antibiotics (especially erythromycin and tetracyclines)	Oestrogen and progestogen-containing drugs
Anti-Parkinsonian treatments	Opioids
Cannabinoids	Psychotropic medications
Chemotherapy agents	Theophylline

Box 11.2 Clinical/biochemical features often present in patients with adrenal insufficiency

Symptoms (often insidious)

- Lethargy, fatigue, low mood
- Anorexia, weight loss
- Nausea and vomiting
- Postural hypotension
- Abdominal pain
- Diarrhoea/constipation

Physical signs

- Pigmentation (palmar creases, mucous membranes)
- Vitiligo
- Postural hypotension
- In Addisonian crisis: shock (low BP, reduced tissue perfusion), pyrexia, coma

Blood

- Hyponatraemia
- Hyperkalaemia
- Hypoglycaemia (fasting or spontaneous)
- Hypercalcaemia
- Anaemia
- Normal anion gap metabolic acidosis (mild)

Other

- History of other autoimmune disorders

be a prominent feature of acute inflammatory abdominal pathology (e.g., acute pancreatitis/appendicitis/cholecystitis) but abdominal pain is almost always the principal complaint (Chapter 7). Severe constipation may lead to N&V, particularly in frail elderly patients.

Medications

Numerous medications or toxins can result in N&V; some of the more common are listed in Box 11.1. Alcohol misuse is a very frequent cause of both acute and chronic N&V.

Hypercalcaemia

N&V may be the main presenting symptom in hypercalcaemia, especially since other features tend to be nonspecific, e.g., fatigue, depression, constipation, abdominal pain, anorexia. Confusion and renal impairment may complicate severe hypercalcaemia. Patients presenting with hypercalcaemia require investigations to identify the underlying cause, which may be life-threatening. The main diagnoses to consider are malignancy (myeloma, bone metastases, ectopic secretion of parathyroid hormone–related peptide from tumour) and primary hyperparathyroidism. Rarer causes include sarcoidosis, adrenal insufficiency, lithium toxicity and tertiary hyperparathyroidism.

Other metabolic disturbance

Chronic renal failure with uraemia tends to present nonspecifically, and nausea ± vomiting is often a prominent feature. Conversely, severe N&V is an important cause of acute kidney injury due to hypovolaemia. The assessment of acute kidney injury is discussed in Chapter 29.

Diabetic ketoacidosis and, to a lesser extent, hyperosmolar hyperglycaemic state (HHS), may present with N&V. Suggestive features include a history of polyuria and/or polydipsia and a background of diabetes (particularly type 1).

GI upset, including N&V, is also common in adrenal insufficiency, including acute adrenal crisis. Hypotension and illness severity are usually disproportionate to the degree of vomiting. Other suggestive features are shown in Box 11.2.

CNS causes

Raised intracranial pressure (ICP) may produce vomiting, often without nausea. The vomiting can be profound. When raised ICP is chronic (e.g., space-occupying lesion), vomiting classically occurs shortly after wakening in the morning and is associated with headache (worse on lying, bending or straining) and, possibly, papilloedema. In acute causes (e.g., intracerebral haemorrhage), there may be sudden-onset headache with vomiting followed by progressive neurological symptoms, including reduced consciousness level. Nausea, with or without vomiting, occurs during episodes of migraine in ≈80% of patients and is often severe; however, headache ±aura is usually the dominant symptom (Chapter 13).

N&V accompanied by vertigo suggests vestibular or brainstem pathology (Chapter 17). Vomiting may also occur in CNS infection (e.g., meningitis, encephalitis) but usually not as the main presenting feature.

Other causes

Always consider pregnancy in women of child-bearing age with new-onset nausea ±vomiting. Symptoms are not always confined to morning and may occur at any time of the day.

In bulimia nervosa, recurrent vomiting may be concealed by the patient. There is frequently a history of psychiatric disorder, deliberate self-harm, laxative misuse or evidence of altered body image.

Infections other than gastroenteritis (e.g., urinary tract infection, meningitis, hepatitis or otitis media) may present with vomiting in association with other symptoms, particularly in more vulnerable groups such as children and the elderly.

Myocardial infarction may present with N&V as the predominant symptoms. Historically, this was associated more frequently with inferior infarcts, but recent work suggests it is more likely related to infarct size.

11

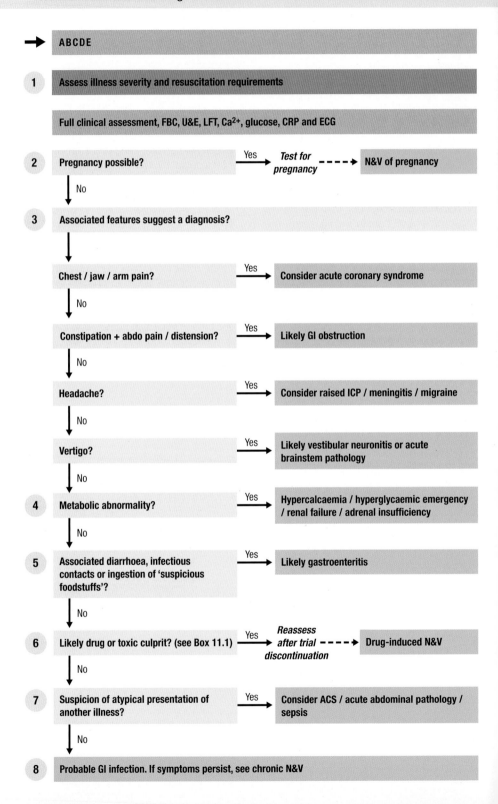

ABCDE

1 Assess illness severity and resuscitation requirements

Full clinical assessment, FBC, U&E, LFT, Ca^{2+}, glucose, CRP and ECG

2 Pregnancy possible? — Yes → *Test for pregnancy* ----→ N&V of pregnancy

No

3 Associated features suggest a diagnosis?

Chest / jaw / arm pain? — Yes → Consider acute coronary syndrome

No

Constipation + abdo pain / distension? — Yes → Likely GI obstruction

No

Headache? — Yes → Consider raised ICP / meningitis / migraine

No

Vertigo? — Yes → Likely vestibular neuronitis or acute brainstem pathology

No

4 Metabolic abnormality? — Yes → Hypercalcaemia / hyperglycaemic emergency / renal failure / adrenal insufficiency

No

5 Associated diarrhoea, infectious contacts or ingestion of 'suspicious foodstuffs'? — Yes → Likely gastroenteritis

No

6 Likely drug or toxic culprit? (see Box 11.1) — Yes → *Reassess after trial discontinuation* ----→ Drug-induced N&V

No

7 Suspicion of atypical presentation of another illness? — Yes → Consider ACS / acute abdominal pathology / sepsis

No

8 Probable GI infection. If symptoms persist, see chronic N&V

1 Assess illness severity and resuscitation requirements

Step 1 Are there features of shock?

Look for ↑HR, ↓BP (a late sign) or evidence of tissue hypoperfusion (Box 2.1). If present, reassess following IV fluid resuscitation and monitor urine output (consider urinary catheterization if necessary). Exclude diabetic ketoacidosis if ↑capillary blood glucose. Suspect adrenal insufficiency in patients with a history of Addison disease (or other autoimmune disease), chronic corticosteroid use or suggestive clinical features (Box 11.2); also consider whenever the severity of shock appears disproportionate to fluid losses: take blood for random cortisol levels and treat immediately with IV hydrocortisone.

Step 2 Is there acute renal impairment?

Hypovolaemia may result in severe 'prerenal' acute kidney injury (AKI), especially if compounded by antihypertensive or nephrotoxic medication, such as diuretics, ACE inhibitors, NSAIDs. Patients with AKI due to volume depletion require IV rehydration with close monitoring of fluid balance, urine output and electrolytes, particularly potassium. Consider other potential drivers of both AKI and N&V (e.g., sepsis, drug toxicity) in patients without clinical evidence of hypovolaemia. Consider renal failure as the cause of N&V in patients with severe impairment. See Chapter 29 for further assessment of acute kidney injury.

Step 3 Does the patient otherwise require IV fluids/hospital admission?

Patients with clinical evidence of dehydration (thirst, dry mucous membranes, ↓skin turgor) and ongoing vomiting, require IV hydration.

Other features that may indicate a need for hospital admission include:

- Evidence of sepsis (Chapter 26)
- Acute kidney injury (Chapter 29)
- Frail, elderly or immunocompromised patient
- Significant comorbidity, such as heart/renal/hepatic failure

2 Pregnancy possible?

Ascertain gynaecological history and test for pregnancy in any women of reproductive age presenting with N&V.

3 Associated features suggest a diagnosis?

Perform an AXR if N&V is accompanied by absent bowel movements and abdominal pain or distension. Consider gastritis, peptic ulcer disease or acute pancreatitis if there is severe upper abdominal pain and assess as per Chapter 7.

Headache may occur secondary to dehydration in acute vomiting, but consider the possibility of serious CNS pathology. Assess as per Chapter 13 if headache is a prominent feature, especially if the onset is acute.

Acute onset of N&V accompanied by vertigo (dizziness with an illusion of movement, e.g., spinning) is likely to represent either vestibular neuronitis or acute brainstem pathology, such as infarction or haemorrhage; assess as per Chapter 17.

Suspect ACS and assess as per Chapter 3 if N&V occurs with chest/jaw/neck/arm pain and ECG changes.

11

4 Metabolic abnormality?

Test for diabetes and exclude ketoacidosis in any patient without a preexisting diagnosis who has ↑capillary blood glucose (see Table 25.2). Consider HHS in older patients with markedly ↑ glucose, dehydration, biochemical derangement (↑urea, ↑osmolality) and confusion.

Assess patients with acute kidney injury as described in Chapter 29.

Hypercalcaemia more commonly presents with chronic N&V and is discussed below but may present for the first time with apparent acute N&V. Reassess symptoms after rehydration and other corrective treatment. Investigate the cause of the hypercalcaemia as it may reflect serious underlying disease, such as malignancy.

Consider adrenal insufficiency in patients with ↓Na+/↑K+ or ↓blood glucose, especially when there are suggestive clinical features (Box 11.2). If suspected, check a morning cortisol level ± ACTH stimulation test ('short synacthen test').

5 Associated diarrhoea, infectious contacts or ingestion of 'suspicious foodstuffs'?

Suspect acute gastroenteritis if any of these features are present. Most cases are self-limiting viral or toxin-mediated infections and do not require further investigation or antimicrobial treatment. Investigate appropriately if there are concerning features, such as bloody diarrhoea (Chapter 9), abdominal pain (Chapter 7) or an excessive systemic inflammatory response (Box 7.1). Warn patients that they may require further investigation if symptoms persist >10 days (see assessment of chronic N&V below).

6 Likely drug or toxic culprit? (Box 11.1)

Always ask about recent changes to medications or dosages—including over-the-counter medicines. Enquire about alcohol and recreational drug use, particularly cannabis and opiates. In drugs with a narrow therapeutic window (e.g., digoxin, lithium, some anticonvulsants), check serum levels to exclude toxicity. Resolution of symptoms with drug discontinuation (where possible) confirms the diagnosis.

7 Suspicion of atypical presentation of another illness?

Consider nonspecific presentation of major pathology in patients who appear seriously unwell (e.g., autonomic upset, physiological derangement). Be mindful of atypical presentations in frail elderly patients or those with cognitive impairment, immunocompromise (including chronic corticosteroid treatment) or longstanding diabetes. Perform an ECG to look for evidence of ACS. Undertake a septic screen (see Chapter 26) if there is fever or ↑inflammatory markers. Have a low threshold for erect CXR, AXR ± further abdominal imaging, such as CT or USS. Severe constipation may lead to N&V in immobile, frail or elderly patients, so enquire about bowel movements and consider PR exam ± AXR.

8 Probable GI infection

In the absence of alternative pathology, GI infection is the most likely cause of acute N&V; it is almost always self-limiting, so further investigation is usually not required. Reevaluate if the patient is unwell or deteriorating. Proceed to assessment of chronic N&V symptoms persist for >10 days.

11

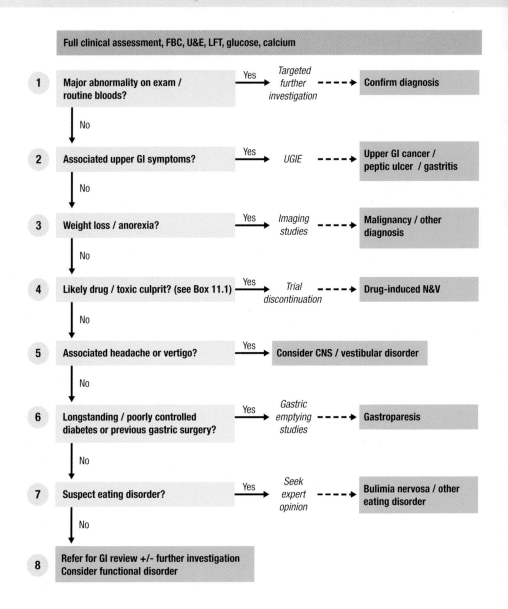

	Full clinical assessment, FBC, U&E, LFT, glucose, calcium

1. **Major abnormality on exam / routine bloods?** — Yes → *Targeted further investigation* ----→ **Confirm diagnosis**
   - No ↓

2. **Associated upper GI symptoms?** — Yes → *UGIE* ----→ **Upper GI cancer / peptic ulcer / gastritis**
   - No ↓

3. **Weight loss / anorexia?** — Yes → *Imaging studies* ----→ **Malignancy / other diagnosis**
   - No ↓

4. **Likely drug / toxic culprit? (see Box 11.1)** — Yes → *Trial discontinuation* ----→ **Drug-induced N&V**
   - No ↓

5. **Associated headache or vertigo?** — Yes → **Consider CNS / vestibular disorder**
   - No ↓

6. **Longstanding / poorly controlled diabetes or previous gastric surgery?** — Yes → *Gastric emptying studies* ----→ **Gastroparesis**
   - No ↓

7. **Suspect eating disorder?** — Yes → *Seek expert opinion* ----→ **Bulimia nervosa / other eating disorder**
   - No ↓

8. **Refer for GI review +/- further investigation. Consider functional disorder**

1 Major abnormality on examination/routine blood tests?

Screen patients with persistent or recurrent N&V for the following abnormalities to narrow the differential diagnosis.

Deranged LFTs ± jaundice

Arrange an urgent abdominal USS, review alcohol intake/all recent medications and assess further, as described in Chapter 12. Continue to look for alternative causes of N&V if only minor LFT derangement without jaundice.

Renal failure

Severe renal failure frequently presents non-specifically with nausea ± vomiting, lethargy and anorexia. Distinguish this from 'prerenal'

AKI due to protracted vomiting and assess for an underlying aetiology (Chapter 29).

Palpable abdominal or pelvic mass

Arrange urgent imaging to exclude underlying malignancy. Consider USS initially, particularly for young patients. Arrange CT abdomen/pelvis if no cause is found (or to further characterize/stage abnormalities).

Anaemia

Arrange urgent upper GI endoscopy in any patient with persistent N&V and evidence of iron-deficiency anaemia to rule out gastric malignancy. In patients without iron deficiency, continue anaemia work-up (Chapter 25) but consider other causes of N&V if no clear explanation is identified.

Hypercalcaemia

The critical steps in the management of hypercalcaemia are correcting the calcium and addressing the underlying cause. Check a parathyroid hormone (PTH) level to narrow the differential diagnosis. If PTH is elevated in the context of hypercalcaemia, the likely cause is primary hyperparathyroidism. If the PTH is low (suppressed), then investigate for malignancy (e.g., bone metastasis, myeloma, tumour secretion of PTH-related peptide). To treat hypercalcaemia, rehydrate with IV fluid, and consider a bisphosphonate if the patient remains hypercalaemic despite fluids. Refer to the appropriate specialty to treat the underlying cause. If mildly ↑ Ca^{2+}, continue to evaluate for other causes of N&V as small calcium elevations are seen in dehydration.

2   Associated upper GI symptoms?

Associated symptoms of dysphagia, early satiety, epigastric discomfort or dyspepsia suggest upper GI tract pathology such as oesophageal/gastric cancer, peptic ulcer disease or gastritis. Ask about NSAID use/alcohol intake and arrange an UGIE if any of these are present or if vomiting persists for >4 weeks (urgently if weight loss, dysphagia or new onset symptoms in patient aged ≥50 years). Refer for formal GI review if persistent symptoms with no cause identified on endoscopy.

3   Weight loss/anorexia?

Investigate for underlying malignancy if N&V is accompanied by significant weight loss (e.g., ≥5% of body weight in ≤12 months) ± anorexia, especially in patients with relatively recent onset of symptoms. Arrange an UGIE if not already performed and, if normal, request CT chest/abdomen/pelvis. If no cause identified, continue to assess as below. Consider chronic presentation of adrenal insufficiency if there are other suggestive clinical features (Box 11.2).

4   Likely drug/toxic culprit?

Take a detailed medication history (including over-the-counter medications, Box 11.1). Establish alcohol intake and ask specifically about cannabis and/or opiate use. Suspect a toxic aetiology if there is a clear temporal relationship between starting the drug and symptom onset. Reassess after trial discontinuation (if safe to do so) and look for alternative causes if symptoms persist. Check serum levels to exclude toxicity in drugs with a narrow therapeutic window, such as digoxin, lithium, theophylline.

5   Associated headache or neurological symptoms?

Consider ↑ intracranial pressure if vomiting is associated with recurrent headache that is most prominent on waking from sleep; aggravated by bending, straining or lying; or accompanied by papilloedema—arrange urgent CT of the brain (Chapter 13).

See Chapter 17 for assessment of patients with concomitant vertigo.

6   Longstanding/poorly controlled diabetes or previous gastric surgery?

Suspect gastroparesis in diabetic patients with longstanding poor control and/or significant microvascular complications or in patients with previous gastric surgery (including weight reduction surgery). Consider prokinetic (i.e. metoclopramide) if no evidence of obstruction/contraindication and refer to GI. Nuclear scintigraphy scan confirms the diagnosis.

11

7 Suspect eating disorder?

Consider an eating disorder in patients with persistent/recurrent vomiting despite reassuring GI investigations and in the presence of low mood/self-esteem concerning features of body dysmorphia or where family members raise concern. Typically, vomiting occurs after eating and is not directly witnessed. Explore the issue sensitively and, if suspected, seek expert input at an early stage.

8 Refer for GI review/further investigation

Arrange an UGIE (if not already performed) and refer for GI evaluation if symptoms persist without a clear cause. Investigate for chronic pancreatitis if there is associated epigastric discomfort, a history of chronic alcohol excess and/or steatorrhoea; check faecal elastase and arrange abdominal CT. Consider functional vomiting if investigations are consistently reassuring, but be vigilant for underlying eating disorder.

Jaundice 12

Jaundice describes the yellow pigmentation of skin, sclerae and mucous membranes that results from accumulation of bilirubin (hyperbilirubinaemia). It is often classified according to the anatomical location of the pathology:

- Prehepatic—haemolysis
- Hepatic—hepatocellular dysfunction and/or intrahepatic bile duct obstruction
- Posthepatic—extrahepatic bile duct obstruction

It is important to remember that patients may have more than one aetiology (e.g., alcoholic hepatitis on a background of cirrhosis due to chronic hepatitis C infection).

Prehepatic

Haemolytic disorders cause accumulation of unconjugated bilirubin in plasma due to ↑ red cell destruction. LFTs are otherwise normal, but there may be anaemia with evidence of haemolysis on blood tests and film. Clinical features of prehepatic jaundice include normal coloured urine and dark stools. Biochemically there is unconjugated hyperbilirubinaemia. See Clinical Tool: Further assessment of anaemia (Chapter 25) for further information on the causes and investigation of haemolysis.

Hepatic

Problems with conjugation

Gilbert syndrome is a benign, congenital condition affecting 2–5% of the population. Decreased glucuronyl transferase activity limits bilirubin conjugation and therefore excretion into the bile, causing mild jaundice during periods of fasting or intercurrent illness. There are no other clinical/biochemical features of liver disease.

Acute liver injury

A broad range of liver insults may lead to acute liver injury, such as toxic, infective, autoimmune, metabolic and vascular. Jaundice results from impaired bilirubin uptake and conjugation by hepatocytes. There may also be obstruction of biliary canaliculi due to inflammation and/or oedema. There is typically a disproportionate increase in ALT and AST relative to ALP and GGT. Extensive liver injury may cause acute liver failure, characterized by encephalopathy (Table 12.1) and failure of synthetic function (i.e., coagulopathy; typically, INR >1.5) in the absence of preexisting liver disease. Causes of acute liver failure are shown in Box 12.1. Potential causes of acute drug-induced liver injury are listed in Box 12.2. LFTs may take months to normalize after drug cessation, especially with cholestatic injury.

In acute viral hepatitis, jaundice is usually preceded by a 1–2-week prodrome of malaise, arthralgia, headache and anorexia. Hepatitis A–E viruses are responsible for most cases; less common causes include cytomegalovirus (CMV), Epstein–Barr virus (EBV) and herpes simplex. Diagnosis is confirmed by serology. Recovery occurs over 3–6 weeks in most cases, but chronic infection develops in up to 10% of patients with hepatitis B and 80% with hepatitis C.

Autoimmune hepatitis most often presents with established cirrhosis, but 25% of cases manifest as an acute hepatitis with jaundice and constitutional symptoms. It is more common in females (ratio 3:1), and there is an association with other autoimmune conditions. Serum immunoglobulin (IgG) levels are raised, and serum autoantibodies may be present.

Wilson disease, an inherited disorder of copper metabolism, can present with acute hepatitis and occasionally causes acute liver failure. A ↓serum caeruloplasmin level is highly suggestive.

Hepatic vein thrombosis (Budd–Chiari syndrome) typically presents with upper abdominal pain, hepatomegaly and marked ascites due to liver outflow venous congestion.

Ischaemic hepatitis ('shocked liver') may result from impaired hepatic perfusion in a

Table 12.1 West Haven grading of hepatic encephalopathy

Stage	Alteration of consciousness
0	No change in personality or behaviour No asterixis
1	Impaired concentration and attention span Sleep disturbance, slurred speech Euphoria or depression Asterixis present
2	Lethargy, drowsiness, apathy or aggression Disorientation, inappropriate behaviour, slurred speech
3	Confusion and disorientation, bizarre behaviour Drowsiness or stupor Asterixis usually absent
4	Comatose with no response to voice commands Minimal or absent response to painful stimuli

Box 12.1 Causes of acute liver failure

Drugs/toxins

- Paracetamol overdose[a]
- Anti-tuberculous drugs
- Ecstasy
- Halothane
- *Amanita phalloides*
- Carbon tetrachloride

Infection

- Acute viral hepatitis (A, B, E)[a]
- Cytomegalovirus (CMV), Epstein–Barr virus (EBV), herpes simplex

Vascular

- Shocked liver/ischaemic hepatitis
- Budd–Chiari syndrome

Other

- Wilson disease
- Autoimmune hepatitis
- Acute fatty liver of pregnancy
- Extensive malignant infiltration

[a]Denotes common cause.

Box 12.2 Drugs causing acute hepatotoxicity

Acute hepatitis

- Paracetamol (in overdose)
- Cocaine, ecstasy
- Aspirin, NSAIDs
- Halothane
- Anti-tuberculous therapy: pyrazinamide, isoniazid, rifampicin
- Antifungals: ketoconazole
- Antihypertensives: methyldopa, hydralazine, dronedarone

Cholestasis/cholestatic hepatitis

- Antibiotics: penicillins, such as flucloxacillin, co-amoxiclav, ciprofloxacin, macrolides, such as erythromycin
- Chlorpromazine
- Azathioprine
- Oestrogens (including the oral contraceptive pill)
- Amitriptyline
- Carbamazepine
- ACE inhibitors
- Cimetidine/ranitidine
- Sulphonamides

Acute alcoholic hepatitis may occur in individuals without chronic liver disease following intensive binge drinking and presents with jaundice, malaise, tender hepatomegaly and fever. The Glasgow Alcoholic Hepatitis Score can be used to predict mortality and guide pharmacological treatment (Table 12.2).

Table 12.2 Glasgow Alcoholic Hepatitis Score (GAHS)

	Score given		
	1	2	3
Age (years)	<50	≥50	—
WCC (10^9/L)	<15	≥15	—
Urea (mmol/L)	<5	≥5	—
PT ratio or INR	<1.5	1.5–2.0	>2.0
Bilirubin (µmol/L)	<125	125–250	>250

A score of 9 or more identify patients most at risk of death. A score of 9 or more can be used either on day 1 (admission day) or day 6–9.

patient with shock; the ALT is usually markedly raised. Cardiac failure may cause hepatic injury due to vascular congestion, with resultant jaundice and ↑ALT.

Cirrhosis

Chronic liver injury results in extensive hepatocellular loss, fibrosis and disturbance of the normal hepatic architecture. Hepatocellular insufficiency leads to jaundice, coagulopathy and ↓albumin. Architecture disturbance causes portal hypertension; consequent portosystemic shunting of blood results in oesophageal varices and hepatic encephalopathy (Table 12.1). Portal hypertension, ↓albumin and generalized salt and water retention, due to haemodynamic and endocrine abnormalities, lead to ascites. There may be characteristic 'stigmata' on examination

Box 12.3 **Stigmata of chronic liver disease**

- Spider naevi
- Digital clubbing
- Palmar erythema
- Loss of axillary/pubic hair
- Parotid swelling
- Gynaecomastia
- Testicular atrophy

(Box 12.3). Causes of chronic liver injury are listed in Box 12.4.

Hepatic tumours

Malignant infiltration by primary or, more commonly, metastatic tumours may cause jaundice due to intrahepatic duct obstruction or extensive replacement of liver parenchyma. Common associated features include cachexia, malaise, hepatomegaly and RUQ pain (secondary to stretching of the liver capsule).

Post-hepatic/biliary causes of jaundice

Jaundice due to biliary obstruction is associated with a pronounced rise in ALP and GGT (produced in the biliary epithelium). Clinical features may include pale stools, dark urine and intractable itch. A raised prothrombin time (PT) may occur due to vitamin K malabsorption from the GI tract.

Gallstones

Obstructing gallstones are the most common cause of extrahepatic cholestasis; the onset of jaundice is relatively rapid, may be intermittent and is typically accompanied by epigastric/RUQ pain. Cholecystitis is diagnosed on abdominal USS by the appearance of an inflamed gallbladder (thick-walled) containing gallstones. A dilated common bile duct on USS implies extrahepatic biliary obstruction and may be due to gallstones lodged in the common bile duct (choledocholithiasis). The presence of RUQ pain, fever and rigors suggests bacterial infection proximal to the obstruction (ascending cholangitis) and requires prompt antibiotics and decompression (ERCP). More information about gallstones is detailed in Abdominal Pain (Chapter 7).

Benign strictures

Benign strictures may result from trauma, particularly during biliary surgery or as a

Box 12.4 **Causes of cirrhosis**

- Chronic alcohol excess
- Chronic viral hepatitis (hepatitis B or C)
- Nonalcoholic fatty liver disease
- Autoimmune hepatitis
- Cholestatic
  - Primary sclerosing cholangitis
  - Primary biliary cholangitis
  - Secondary biliary cholangitis
- Metabolic
  - Hereditary haemochromatosis
  - Wilson disease
  - Alpha1-antitrypsin deficiency
  - Cystic fibrosis
- Venous obstruction
  - Cardiac failure
  - Budd–Chiari syndrome
- Drugs, such as methotrexate
- Cryptogenic

12

consequence of inflammation within the biliary tree, such as recurrent cholangitis, pancreatitis.

Autoimmune

In primary biliary cholangitis (previously referred to as primary biliary cirrhosis), there is progressive destruction of the intrahepatic bile ducts. Ninety percent of patients are female. Pruritus usually precedes jaundice. The presence of antimitochondrial antibodies is diagnostic. Primary sclerosing cholangitis causes inflammation, fibrosis and strictures of the intrahepatic and extrahepatic biliary tree. It is more common in men and has a strong association with ulcerative colitis.

Malignancy

Painless jaundice may represent a malignant cause of obstructive jaundice. Cancer of the head of the pancreas typically presents with insidious, progressive jaundice due to extrinsic compression of the common bile duct, often with marked weight loss, nausea and anorexia. Pain may be absent in the early stages.

Cholangiocarcinoma is a malignant tumour of the intrahepatic or extrahepatic biliary tree that most commonly presents with painless jaundice, often with pruritus.

Other important causes of malignant extrinsic biliary compression include duodenal ampullary tumours and enlarged lymph nodes at the porta hepatis.

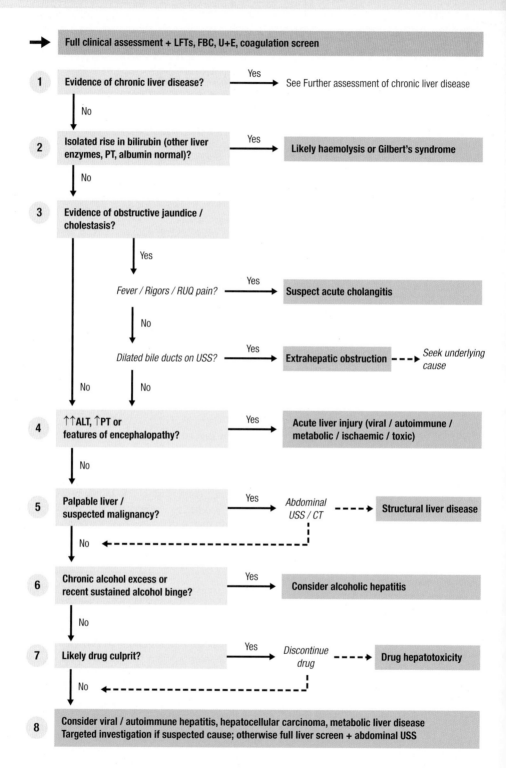

Full clinical assessment + LFTs, FBC, U+E, coagulation screen

1 Evidence of chronic liver disease? — Yes → See Further assessment of chronic liver disease

No

2 Isolated rise in bilirubin (other liver enzymes, PT, albumin normal)? — Yes → **Likely haemolysis or Gilbert's syndrome**

No

3 Evidence of obstructive jaundice / cholestasis?

Yes

Fever / Rigors / RUQ pain? — Yes → **Suspect acute cholangitis**

No

Dilated bile ducts on USS? — Yes → **Extrahepatic obstruction** - - - → *Seek underlying cause*

No   No

4 ↑↑ALT, ↑PT or features of encephalopathy? — Yes → **Acute liver injury (viral / autoimmune / metabolic / ischaemic / toxic)**

No

5 Palpable liver / suspected malignancy? — Yes → *Abdominal USS / CT* - - - → **Structural liver disease**

No

6 Chronic alcohol excess or recent sustained alcohol binge? — Yes → **Consider alcoholic hepatitis**

No

7 Likely drug culprit? — Yes → *Discontinue drug* - - - → **Drug hepatotoxicity**

No

8 Consider viral / autoimmune hepatitis, hepatocellular carcinoma, metabolic liver disease
Targeted investigation if suspected cause; otherwise full liver screen + abdominal USS

1   Evidence of chronic liver disease?

In the absence of an established diagnosis, look for signs of chronic liver disease, particularly physical stigmata (Box 12.3) and evidence of complications of cirrhosis, such as portal hypertension.

- Multiple spider naevi, in the absence of pregnancy/pro-oestrogenic drugs, strongly suggest chronic liver disease. The other stigmata lack specificity individually but are helpful in combination.
- Ascites is a useful pointer to portal hypertension but may have other causes in jaundiced patients, e.g., intra-abdominal malignancy or right heart failure with hepatic congestion. The rapid onset of ascites, jaundice, hepatomegaly and abdominal pain suggests acute thrombotic complication, that is, Budd–Chiari syndrome.
- Hepatic encephalopathy (Table 12.1) and synthetic dysfunction (see below) may occur in acute liver failure but are highly suggestive of chronic liver disease when they occur against a background of previous clinical/biochemical evidence of liver disturbance.
- Abdominal USS can demonstrate morphologic features of cirrhosis (e.g., coarse echotexture, ↑nodularity) and provide supportive evidence of portal hypertension (splenomegaly, reversed flow in the portal vein).

Evaluate any patient with jaundice and a background of established or suspected cirrhosis as described in Further assessment of chronic liver disease below.

2   Isolated rise in bilirubin (other liver enzymes, PT, albumin normal)?

Consider haemolysis if features of liver disease are absent and blood results suggest ↑red cell breakdown (e.g., ↓Hb, ↑LDH, ↓haptoglobin, red cell fragments on blood film) ± evidence of ↑red cell production (e.g., ↑reticulocytes, polychromasia).

If there are no features of haemolysis or chronic liver disease, jaundice is mild (bilirubin <100 μmol/L) and LFTs are otherwise normal, the likely diagnosis is Gilbert syndrome.

3   Evidence of obstructive jaundice/cholestasis?

A rise in ALP/GGT out of proportion to ALT/AST suggests that jaundice is due to impaired biliary excretion. If there are features of sepsis, take blood cultures, give IV antibiotics, arrange urgent abdominal USS and discuss with the surgical team. Otherwise, perform USS to look for bile duct dilatation (indicating extrahepatic obstruction) and an underlying cause, such as gallstones.

If USS does not show dilated bile ducts, proceed to step 4.

If USS shows dilated bile ducts but does not reveal the underlying cause, arrange further imaging. MRCP is the gold standard modality for biliary tree imaging—request this if you suspect gallstones (acute or recurrent RUQ pain) or if there is a history of biliary pathology. CT allows better visualization of the pancreas—arrange if pancreatic cancer is suspected, e.g., jaundice is painless with an insidious, progressive onset, especially in the elderly.

4   ↑↑ALT, ↑PT or features of encephalopathy?

Identify patients with acute liver failure

Look for features of acute liver failure in all jaundiced patients without preexisting liver disease or extrahepatic biliary obstruction, especially if there is evidence of extensive hepatocellular injury (↑↑ALT).

Hepatic encephalopathy (Table 12.1) may be subtle; look closely for ↓concentration/alertness, mild disorientation, behavioural changes and reversal of the sleep/wake cycle. Test specifically for constructional apraxia (e.g., ask the patient to draw a five-pointed star or clock face) and asterixis. Seek collateral history if possible and exclude hypoglycaemia and other metabolic abnormalities. Consider CT brain to exclude intracranial pathology, especially if there are focal neurological abnormalities.

12

An ↑PT (in the absence of anticoagulation, preexisting coagulopathy or extensive cholestasis) indicates ↓hepatic synthetic function. If ↑, do not correct acutely unless there is major haemorrhage.

Seek cause of acute liver injury

Enquire about alcohol and paracetamol intake, all recent drugs (prescribed or otherwise) and possible exposure to environmental/occupational toxins, e.g., carbon tetrachloride. Check viral serology (IgM antibodies to hepatitis B core antigen [HBc], hepatitis A virus [HAV], hepatitis E virus [HEV], CMV and EBV), serum caeruloplasmin, autoantibodies (ANA, ASMA, LKM) and gamma-globulins, and paracetamol level (on admission blood draws). Arrange abdominal USS to exclude Budd–Chiari syndrome and extensive malignant infiltration.

Repeatedly monitor and reassess patients with acute liver failure

Monitor closely in ICU or a high-dependency unit (HDU) for complications, including:
- Hypoglycaemia
- Hyperkalaemia
- Metabolic acidosis
- Renal failure (develops in >50%, often necessitating haemofiltration)
- Cerebral oedema with ↑intracranial pressure
- Bacterial or fungal infection

Use the King's College Hospital criteria (Box 12.5) to identify patients who may require transplantation. Liaise early with a specialist liver unit to enable timely transfer if necessary.

5 Palpable liver/suspected malignancy?

Consider abdominal USS or CT to exclude malignant or other structural liver disease if the patient has:
- Clinical evidence of hepatomegaly
- Known malignancy with metastatic potential
- A palpable abdominal/rectal mass or lymphadenopathy
- Ascites in the absence of chronic liver disease
- Insidious constitutional upset, such as unexplained weight loss/anorexia/cachexia.

> ### Box 12.5 King's College Hospital criteria for liver transplantation in acute liver failure
>
> **Paracetamol overdose**
> - pH <7.25 at or beyond 24 hours following the overdose
>
>   *or*
> - Serum creatinine >300 µmol/L or anuria *plus* PT >100 seconds (INR > 6.5) *plus* encephalopathy grade 3 or 4
>
> **Nonparacetamol cases**
> **Severe encephalopathy and**
> - PT >100 seconds (INR >6.5)
>
>   *or*
> - Any three of the following:
>   - Jaundice to severe encephalopathy time >7 days
>   - Age <10 or >40 years
>   - Indeterminate (non-A, non-B hepatitis) or drug-induced causes
>   - Bilirubin >300 µmol/L
>   - PT >50 seconds (INR >3.5)
>
> Creatinine of 300 µmol/L ≅ 3.38 mg/dL. Bilirubin of 300 µmol/L ≅ 17.6 mg/dL.
>
> *Modified from O'Grady JG, Alexander GJ, Hayllar KM, Williams R. Early indicators of prognosis in fulminant hepatic failure. Gastroenterology. 1989;97(2):439–445.*

6 Chronic alcohol excess or recent sustained alcohol binge?

Establish alcohol intake in all jaundiced patients. A tactical approach is to ask a general enquiry, before quantifying typical weekly intake. In addition to the weekly total number of drinks, consider the alcohol content and, for spirits, the measure per drink. Seek a collateral history from relatives and friends and observe closely for features of alcohol withdrawal if you suspect covert alcohol abuse.

Suspect alcoholic hepatitis in any patient with longstanding excessive consumption, e.g., >40 units/week or recent binge drinking (e.g., >100 units/week), or who develops severe withdrawal symptoms after 24–48 hours in hospital. Helpful supporting features for alcoholic hepatitis include tender hepatomegaly and an AST:ALT ratio of >1. Once the diagnosis is made, calculate the Glasgow alcoholic hepatitis score to assess prognosis and guide treatment (Table 12.2).

7 Likely drug culprit?

Enquire about all drugs taken within the preceding 6 weeks, including those which are prescribed, recreational and over-the-counter, such as NSAIDs, paracetamol and herbal remedies. Box 12.2 contains some common causes of hepatotoxicity, but there are many others; consult with a pharmacist or review the literature if uncertain. Wherever possible, discontinue any suspected drug culprit and observe the effect on bilirubin and LFTs. If paracetamol toxicity is suspected, immediate treatment with acetylcysteine may be required; treat as per a poison information resource such as TOXBASE® (www.toxbase.org).

Liver biochemistry may take months to normalize in drug-induced liver injury, so consider further investigations (see below) in the interim unless clinical suspicion of drug toxicity is very high, for example, the patient recently started co-amoxiclav or anti-tuberculous therapy.

8 Consider other causes. Targeted investigation or full liver screen

If the cause remains uncertain, conduct a basic liver screen for viral, autoimmune, hereditary and metabolic conditions (Box 12.6), arrange an abdominal USS if not already performed and confirm alcohol intake. If there is fever, purpura, ↓platelets, conjunctival congestion or recent exposure to potentially contaminated water (e.g., freshwater sports, sewage worker), send blood and urine samples for leptospiral culture, serology ± PCR (liaise with the Microbiology laboratory) and consider empirical antibiotic treatment. Liver biopsy may be required if jaundice persists without a clear cause and potential drug culprits have been removed.

Box 12.6 Screening investigations in jaundice/suspected liver disease

Serology
- Hepatitis B surface antigen (HBsAg), hepatitis C antibodies HCV Ab (+ IgM antibodies to HBc, HAV, HEV, CMV and EBV if acute)

Metabolic
- Ferritin, alpha-1 antitrypsin level, caeruloplasmin

Autoimmune
- AMA, ASMA, ANA, LKM, immunoglobulins

Other
- Abdominal USS, alpha-fetoprotein, paracetamol level, toxicology screen

---

12

Further assessment of chronic liver disease

Step 1 Establish the underlying cause

Determine the underlying aetiology in all new presentations of cirrhosis. Assess alcohol intake and perform screening investigations as listed in Box 12.6. Exclude causes with specific interventions (e.g., Wilson disease, hepatitis virus B and C, haemochromatosis). Consider referral for liver biopsy if the cause remains uncertain.

Step 2 Look for evidence of complications/decompensation

Evaluate for hepatic encephalopathy, portal hypertension and other complications of liver disease; examine for confusion, ascites, oedema, jaundice and malnutrition. Measure albumin and PT to assess hepatic synthetic function, as well as bilirubin, U+Es (hyponatraemia, hepatorenal syndrome) and FBC (anaemia, thrombocytopenia). Consider investigation for pulmonary complications such as pleural effusion, hepatopulmonary syndrome and pulmonary hypertension in patients with breathlessness, cyanosis or $\downarrow$SpO$_2$. If not already done, screen for oesophageal varices with UGIE and for hepatocellular carcinoma with 6–12 monthly abdominal USS; USS will also detect small-volume ascites and splenomegaly.

Step 3 Seek precipitants of decompensation

Patients with cirrhosis have limited metabolic reserve, so many factors can precipitate acute decompensation, including spontaneous bacterial peritonitis, other intercurrent infection, surgery, alcohol excess, hepatotoxic drugs, constipation and hepatocellular carcinoma.

In a decompensated cirrhotic patient (i.e., acute worsening of jaundice, coagulopathy or encephalopathy):

- Perform a full sepsis screen including an ascitic tap for microscopy and culture if ascites is present.
- Review all drugs and alcohol intake.
- Ensure that an abdominal USS has been performed within the last 6 months.

Additionally, in patients with encephalopathy:

- Seek evidence of upper GI bleeding (stool evaluation, $\downarrow$Hb, $\uparrow$urea).
- Look for and correct constipation (PR examination, stool chart)/dehydration/electrolyte disturbance.
- Minimize use of opioids/other sedative drugs or drugs that may precipitate constipation.

In cases of worsening ascites, evaluate salt and water intake and compliance with diuretics, exclude spontaneous bacterial peritonitis, and consider Budd–Chiari syndrome.

Step 4 Assess prognosis

Use the Child–Pugh classification (Table 12.3) to assess prognosis in patients with cirrhosis. Other poor prognostic factors include $\uparrow$creatinine and $\downarrow$Na$^+$, a small liver, and variceal haemorrhage. Consider referral to a transplant centre for patients with Child–Pugh grade B or C. Absolute contraindications to transplantation include severe extrahepatic disease with a predicted mortality of >50% at 5 years, severe irreversible pulmonary disease, active malignancy (excluding specific neuroendocrine malignancies), and active alcohol/illicit drug abuse. Ongoing extrahepatic sepsis and untreated HIV are also absolute contraindications, but discussion with a Liver Transplant unit would be merited given their possible temporary nature.

Table 12.3 Child–Pugh classification of cirrhosis

Score	1	2	3
Bilirubin (µmol/L)	<34	34–51	>51
Albumin (g/L)	>35	28–35	<28
Ascites	None	Mild	Marked
Encephalopathy (Table 12.1)	None	Grade 1-2	Grade 3-4
Prolongation of PT (seconds)	<4	4–6	>6

Child A = Score <7: 2-year survival 85%
Child B = Score 7–9: 2-year survival 60%
Child C = Score >9: 2-year survival 35%

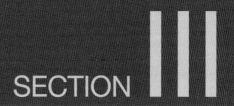
Neurological System

13 Headache

Headache is an extremely common symptom and the vast majority of headaches are benign in origin. Detailed history is central to identifying the small minority of patients with serious underlying pathology and those with disorders that respond to specific treatments. Headache may be the result of a primary headache syndrome (e.g., migraine, cluster headache, thunderclap headache) or be associated with a more serious underlying pathology in secondary headache syndromes (e.g., subarachnoid haemorrhage [SAH], dissection of the carotid/vertebrobasilar arteries, cerebral venous sinus thrombosis). Assessment should focus first on identifying any serious or life-threatening underlying condition causing the headache before considering a primary headache syndrome.

Acute headache

Subarachnoid haemorrhage (SAH)

A SAH is most commonly caused by rupture of an intracranial saccular aneurysm. It is associated with a classic 'thunderclap' headache, which is a sudden, severe occipital headache, reaching maximal intensity within 1–5 minutes. Headache in SAH varies in the abruptness of onset but almost always reaches maximal intensity within 5 minutes and rarely resolves in <1 hour. Distress and photophobia are common, but neck stiffness may take hours to develop. Associated complications may include transient loss of consciousness, reduced GCS score, seizures or focal neurological signs, but neurological examination can often be normal. A SAH should reliably be detected on a noncontrast CT head scan by a skilled radiologist if performed within 6 hours of the onset of the headache (diagnostic accuracy, 95–100%). Beyond 6 hours, the accuracy of CT is reduced to around 85–90%. Therefore,

in the event of a negative CT, an LP should be considered given the morbidity and mortality associated with SAH. An LP is performed to detect xanthochromia—elevated bilirubin as a result of metabolized red blood cells in the CSF. It is important to wait for at least 12 hours from the onset of the headache before performing the LP to allow sufficient time for bilirubin to be reliably detected in the CSF.

Other vascular causes of acute headache

Intracerebral/intraventricular haemorrhage or ischaemic stroke may present with headache, but there will be associated focal neurological deficit ± ↓GCS score to alert the clinician to a more serious underlying cause. Intracerebellar haemorrhage typically presents with acute-onset headache, nausea, vomiting, dizziness and ataxia ±↓GCS score. Any patient with focal neurological deficits should immediately undergo radiological imaging to identify the underlying pathology.

In 85% of patients with cerebral venous sinus thrombosis (CVST), headache is the presenting symptom, but this may be described in a variety of ways, including 'thunderclap', throbbing, and 'band-like'. Frequently the headache is associated with signs and symptoms of increased ICP (e.g., nausea, vomiting, seizures, cranial nerve palsies, ataxia and ↓GCS). Risk factors have been identified which should alert the clinician to this rare but serious condition (e.g., oral contraceptive pill, pregnancy, cancer, coagulopathies, antiphospholipid syndrome, perimeningeal infections, such as sinusitis, otitis media), but in a proportion of patients, no underlying aetiology can be found. CT venogram is the first-line diagnostic investigation with 95% sensitivity, but CT angiography may be required in cases of diagnostic uncertainty.

Dissection of the carotid or vertebrobasilar arteries may present with an acute headache, neck pain or facial pain. Symptoms can be variable, but carotid artery dissection can result in ipsilateral headache, facial pain, neck pain and Horner syndrome. While neurological features may be absent, contralateral motor and sensory disturbance may develop. Vertebrobasilar artery dissection typically results in acute-onset occipital/posterior neck pain with brainstem signs and symptoms, including vomiting.

Meningoencephalitis

Meningoencephalitis is a critical diagnosis that requires a high degree of suspicion so that appropriate treatment can be administered at the earliest opportunity. Patients present with headache, fever and meningism. While the headache may be acute, typically it develops in a more subacute manner over several hours. Bacterial meningitis is life-threatening, and presenting features may include ↓GCS, signs of shock (Box 2.1), purpuric rash (Fig. 27.12) and focal neurological signs. Encephalitis may present with altered mental status, seizures and/or coma. Performing an LP (Clinical tool) is essential in the diagnosis but should not delay initiation of treatment. Viral meningitis is a milder form of the condition and usually self-limiting, with headache the most prominent clinical feature.

Migraine

Migraine is a type of headache characterized by recurrent severe attacks lasting several hours to a few days. Patients typically describe a pulsating throbbing on one side of their head, which may be accompanied by photophobia, hyperacusis and nausea ± vomiting. There are two types of migraine:

- Migraine with aura: Patients can describe a range of symptoms (Box 13.1) which typically occur for up to 60 minutes before the onset of headache.
- Migraine without aura: This is the more common form of migraine that occurs without warning, usually on one side of the head with associated symptoms as described above.

The patient usually prefers to lie in a quiet, darkened room. Possible triggers include cheese, chocolate, alcohol and oral

> ### Box 13.1 What constitutes a migraine aura?
>
> Auras are focal neurological phenomena that precede or accompany a migrainous headache. They occur in 20–30% of patients, usually developing gradually over 5–20 minutes and lasting <60 minutes. Most are visual but they may also be sensory or motor. Common examples include:
> - 'Fortification spectra': shimmering zigzag lines that move across the visual field
> - Flashing lights or spots
> - Temporary loss of vision
> - Numbness/dysaesthesia on one side of the body
> - Expressive dysphasia

contraceptives. A first attack aged >40 years is uncommon. In patients who have a history of migraine with recurrent similar attacks, the diagnosis is more straightforward. However, if there is diagnostic uncertainty, particularly in patients who are presenting with a first headache or abrupt change in migraine symptoms, it is important to maintain an open mind with respect to the diagnostic process.

Benign headache syndromes

Benign headache syndromes describe thunderclap, exertional or coital headache where there is no underlying serious pathology and intracranial causes have been excluded. A significant proportion of patients who experience benign headache syndromes have a history of migraine or will develop it. However, it is important to remember that this is a diagnosis of exclusion as these diagnoses share many features with life-threatening causes of headache, such as coital headache and subarachnoid haemorrhage.

Subacute headache

Acute angle-closure glaucoma

Acute angle-closure glaucoma occurs due to a sudden increase in intraocular pressure and represents an ophthalmological emergency due to potential sight loss. The typical patient is long-sighted, middle-aged or elderly, and presents with periorbital pain (± frontal headache), nausea and vomiting, blurred vision with

13

halos around lights and conjunctival injection. Urgent ophthalmology referral is mandatory (Chapter 16).

Giant cell arteritis (GCA)

A large-vessel vasculitis, closely associated with polymyalgia rheumatica, more commonly diagnosed in women and unusual in patients <50 years. Clinical features may include localized headache (temporal/occipital), scalp tenderness, jaw claudication, visual loss, constitutional upset (malaise, night sweats, pyrexia, weight loss) and an abnormal temporal artery (inflamed, tender, nonpulsatile). ESR/CRP are almost always raised. Untreated GCA can lead to rapid-onset irreversible visual loss, and clinical features suggesting impending visual loss necessitate immediate treatment with steroids (Chapter 16). Temporal artery ultrasound/biopsy may confirm the diagnosis but should not delay steroid treatment.

Raised intracranial pressure

Subacute presentations of raised intracranial pressure may occur as a primary disorder (idiopathic intracranial hypertension [IIH]) or secondary to an intracranial space-occupying lesion. IIH is a rare condition, and risk factors include females aged 20–50 years, obesity and the oral contraceptive pill. Intracranial hypertension secondary to a space-occupying lesion may be associated with focal neurological signs, seizures, or change in personality and mood. The headache tends to be worse in the morning and has a strong positional element, that is, exacerbated by lying flat, coughing or straining. There may be associated vomiting, often without nausea, and papilloedema on fundoscopy. CT ± LP is required to establish the underlying diagnosis.

Chronic subdural haematoma

Patients may present insidiously with headache ± confusion and/or balance problems. The headache may be exacerbated by straining, bending or exercise. At least one quarter of patients have no clear history of head trauma, so have a high index of suspicion, particularly in older patients or those taking anticoagulants. Diagnosis is confirmed by CT imaging.

Sinusitis

Sinusitis causes a dull, throbbing headache associated with facial pain over the sinuses. It tends to be worse on bending forward. There are invariably associated nasal symptoms (e.g., congestion or discharge) which help to make the diagnosis. Persistent sinusitis lasting >12 weeks requires CT to confirm the diagnosis and rule out other causes or complications.

Hypertensive crisis

Hypertensive crisis (malignant hypertension) refers to patients with severely elevated blood pressure >180/120 mmHg and evidence of evolving organ damage secondary to capillary bed dysfunction. End-organ damage can be cardiac (e.g., myocardial ischaemia/infarction, heart failure), vascular (e.g., aortic dissection), neurological (e.g., intracranial haemorrhage or ischaemia, hypertensive encephalopathy) or renal (e.g., AKI). Headache is a common symptom, with other clinical features correlating to organ damage, such as nausea and vomiting and visual disturbances in encephalopathy, chest pain and dyspnoea as symptoms of myocardial infarction. While management should clearly focus on gaining control of the blood pressure, further investigations are required to identify any underlying cause and specific management of end-organ damage.

Recurrent/chronic headache

Cluster headache

This refers to severe, unilateral, retro-orbital headache with restlessness, agitation and ipsilateral lacrimation, conjunctival injection and rhinorrhoea. The pain associated with cluster headache is usually reported to be more severe than other causes of headache; they are generally considered one of the most painful medical conditions and are associated with suicidal ideation. Attacks are short-lived (15–90 minutes) but occur frequently and repeatedly (often at the same time each day) in 'clusters' lasting days to weeks; these are separated by months without symptoms. The male-to-female ratio is 5:1 with a strong family propensity.

Tension headache

The headache is usually bilateral (often generalized or frontal) and described as 'dull', 'tight' or 'pressing' in nature. Unlike migraine, nausea and photophobia are uncommon and the patient can often continue with normal activities.

Medication overuse headache

A common cause of chronic frequent headache (often daily) caused by excessive use of analgesics (e.g., codeine) or triptans.

Treatment of choice is withdrawal of the overused medication, though this is often difficult to achieve.

Other causes

- Cervicogenic headache
- Carbon monoxide poisoning
- Hypercapnia
- Drugs: vasodilators, such as nitrates, 'recreational' drugs, such as solvents
- Trigeminal neuralgia (brief, repetitive episodes of intense shooting/stabbing/'electric shock'-like pain in II and III divisions of trigeminal nerve)
- Trauma: extradural haemorrhage, subdural haemorrhage, concussion

13

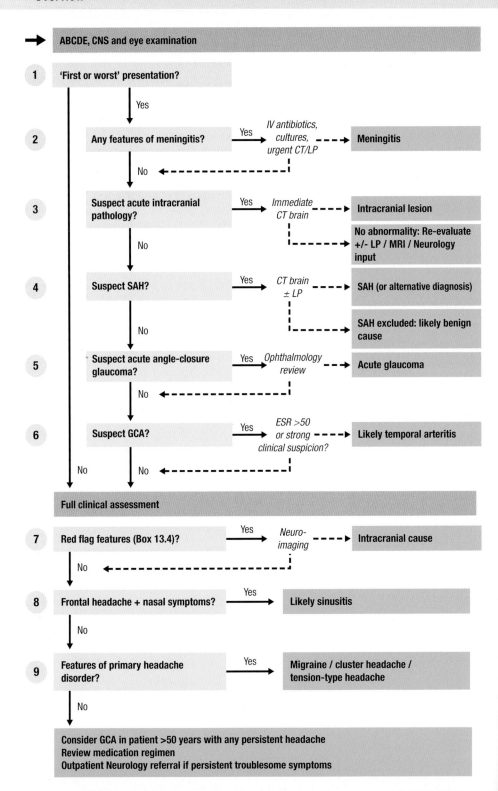

1 'First or worst' presentation?

Acute severe pathology is less likely in patients with recurrence of a longstanding problem than in patients with a first presentation of headache. However, patients with a preexisting headache disorder (e.g., migraine) may also present acutely with another diagnosis, such as SAH. If a patient with chronic headaches presents with a new headache that is markedly different in severity or character to normal, assess it as new-onset headache.

2 Any features of meningitis?

Identifying patients with bacterial meningitis is the top priority to allow rapid, potentially life-saving, antibiotic treatment. Patients may lack classical features but, in almost all cases, there will be at least one of:
- Fever (≥38°C)
- Rash (not always petechial)
- Signs of shock (Box 2.1)

- Headache, which may be acute, or more commonly subacute over a period of hours with meningism (Box 13.2).

SAH may also present with severe headache and meningism but is less likely if the headache onset was not sudden (see below).

If you suspect meningitis, take blood cultures and throat swabs. If there is evidence of severe sepsis, a rapidly progressing rash, or there will be a delay of >1 hour to perform an LP, give IV antibiotics immediately as per the local policy. Otherwise, provided there are no contraindications, perform an LP prior to giving antibiotics to maximize the diagnostic yield of the CSF sample. A CT head is required before an LP only if there is evidence of raised intracranial pressure (see Clinical tool). It is difficult to distinguish viral from early bacterial meningitis clinically, so manage as bacterial meningitis pending CSF analysis.

13

Box 13.2 Meningism?

Meningism (neck stiffness, photophobia, positive Kernig sign) denotes irritation of the meninges. To test for neck stiffness, lie the patient supine with no pillow, place your fingers behind their head and gently attempt to flex the head until the chin touches the chest (Fig. 13.1A); firm resistance to passive flexion and rigidity in the neck muscles indicate neck stiffness. To test for Kernig sign, flex one of the patient's legs at the hip and knee with your left hand placed over the medial hamstrings. Extend the knee with your right hand, maintaining the hip in flexion (Fig. 13.1B). Resistance to extension by spasm in the hamstrings ± flexion of the other leg indicates a positive test.

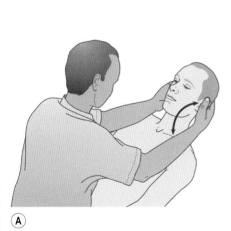

(A)

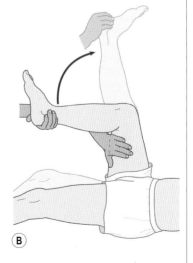

(B)

Fig. 13.1 Testing for meningeal irritation.

Clinical tool
LP and CSF interpretation

Contraindications to LP

- Radiological evidence of raised intracranial pressure.
- Clinical suspicion of raised intracranial pressure: ↓GCS, focal neurological signs, papilloedema, new seizures, vomiting
- Coagulopathy or platelets <50 × 10⁹/L
- Severe agitation and restlessness
- Infected skin over the needle entry site

CSF interpretation

Routine interpretation of CSF results includes (Table 13.1):
- Opening pressure (supine position)
- Protein
- Glucose (always compare with blood glucose)
- Cell count

Additional tests, such as culture, PCR, oligoclonal bands, may be required in some circumstances.

Additional points to consider

- Early bacterial meningitis may be mistaken for viral meningitis as there is a predominance of lymphocytes in the CSF. If there is any possibility of bacterial meningitis, treat the patient with antibiotics pending further investigation, such as blood/CSF culture.
- If there is a ↑lymphocyte count, send CSF for viral PCR, including herpes and enterovirus.
- Symptoms and signs in tuberculous meningitis are often mild or obscure—consider it if the patient is immunocompromised or is from an endemic TB region, especially if the CSF results suggest the diagnosis (Table 13.1). If suspected, send CSF for acid-fast bacilli and mycobacterial PCR and culture.
- Rarely, non-infective disorders can produce a lymphocytic picture, including lupus, sarcoidosis and malignant meningitis.
- A difficult procedure may result in a 'traumatic tap', that is, red cells in the CSF. This can complicate interpretation of the WBC. A rule of thumb is that 1 white cell per 1000 red cells is normal. However, if the CSF picture is unclear, then the clinical history must be taken into account.

13

Table 13.1 Interpretation of CSF results

Condition	Opening pressure	CSF protein (mg/L)	CSF glucose (mmol/L)	Lymphocytes (× 10⁶/L)	Neutrophils (× 10⁶/L)	Red cells (× 10⁶/L)
Normal	5–18 cm H₂O	200–450	>60% of blood glucose 3–5	<5	0	0
Bacterial meningitis	↑ or normal	↑	<50% of blood glucose	↑: usually <neutrophils but may be predominant cell type in early stages	Usually >100 ≥1 is +ve May be 0 in very early stages	0
Viral meningitis	↑ or normal	↑ or normal	>60% of blood glucose 3–5	Usually >50 >5 is +ve	0	0
TB meningitis	↑	↑↑: may be >1,000	<30% of blood glucose	100% >50	0	0
Subarachnoid haemorrhage	↑	↑	>60% of blood glucose	0; if ↑red cells, then 1 white cell per 1,000 red cells is normal	0	↑: often in thousands
Late subarachnoid haemorrhage	↑ or normal	↑	>60% blood glucose	0	0	0 but +ve for xanthochromia (haem breakdown product)

3 Suspect acute intracranial pathology?

Arrange immediate neuroimaging to exclude life-threatening intracranial pathology (e.g., haemorrhage or space-occupying lesion with mass effect) if any of the following is present:

- ↓GCS
- Focal neurological signs
- New-onset seizures
- History of recent head injury
- Anticoagulation or coagulopathy

LP may be required to exclude meningitis or SAH if CT does not yield a diagnosis and no alternative cause is apparent, such as toxicity, metabolic derangement. Further imaging with MRI/CT venogram may be appropriate depending on clinical features. Seek urgent Neurology input if the cause remains unclear.

4 Suspect SAH?

Exclude SAH in any patient with a severe 'first or worst' headache that reaches peak intensity within 5 minutes of onset and persists for >1 hour. No clinical features can reliably rule out the diagnosis, so neuroimaging ± CSF analysis is mandatory. If a CT head performed within 6 hours of onset of the headache is negative, SAH can be excluded. Beyond 6 hours, if the CT is normal, then LP, at least 12 hours from the onset of headache, must be performed to look for xanthochromia; its absence effectively excludes SAH. The major differential diagnosis is benign thunderclap headache; however, all sudden-onset severe headaches should, ideally, be discussed with Neurology.

5 Suspect acute angle-closure glaucoma?

Acute angle-closure glaucoma is sight-threatening. Request urgent Ophthalmology review if the patient has acute-onset headache (especially frontal or periorbital) accompanied by any of the following features:

- Conjunctival injection
- Clouding of the cornea
- Irregular/nonreactive pupil

Box 13.3 Features suggesting GCA

- Pain localized to temporal or occipital region
- Inflamed, thickened, pulseless or tender temporal artery
- Scalp tenderness
- Jaw claudication
- Visual loss (may be temporary initially)
- Constitutional symptoms: fever, malaise, fatigue, night sweats, weight loss
- Symptoms of polymyalgia rheumatica (proximal pain, stiffness)

- ↓visual acuity or blurred vision
- Coloured 'halos' around lights

6 Suspect Giant Cell Arteritis? (Box 13.3)?

Suspect GCA in patients >50 years with new-onset headache and any features shown in Box 13.3. Check ESR and CRP urgently; normal inflammatory markers make the diagnosis highly unlikely. Clinical features that suggest impeding visual loss are jaw claudication and transient visual disturbances. If either of these features are present, start 60mg of prednisolone once a day immediately. Refer any patient with suspected GCA and visual disturbance urgently to Ophthalmology. Discuss all other patients urgently with Rheumatology. Seek advice on steroid initiation and arrange plans for follow-up investigation with temporal artery US or biopsy. A prompt response to steroids is supportive of the diagnosis, but further testing is necessary to ensure that those patients who do not have GCA do not receive a prolonged course of steroids.

7 Red flag features (Box 13.4)?

Regardless of headache duration, you must exclude serious underlying intracranial pathology if any features in Box 13.4 are present. Arrange CT brain ± MRI and, if normal, seek input from Neurology. Consider idiopathic intracranial hypertension in patients with features of ↑intracranial pressure but no mass on neuroimaging. An LP is required to confirm the diagnosis in such circumstances.

Box 13.4 Red flag features

- New-onset headache/change in headache in patients over 50 years.
- Focal CNS signs, ataxia or new cognitive or behavioural disturbance.
- Persistent visual disturbance.
- Headache that changes with posture or wakes the patient up.
- Headache brought on by physical exertion.
- Papilloedema.
- New-onset headache in a patient with HIV, active malignancy or immunocompromised.

Box 13.5 Green flag features

- The current headache has already been present during childhood.
- The headache occurs in temporal relationship with the menstrual cycle.
- The patient has headache-free days.
- Close family members have the same headache "phenotype".
- Headache occurred or stopped more than one week ago.

From H. Pohl, Do TP, García-Azorin D, et al. Green flags and headache: a concept study using the Delphi method. Headache. 2021;61(2): 300-309.

---

8   Frontal headache + nasal symptoms?

Whilst frontal headache may raise the suspicion of sinusitis, the diagnosis should be made only when there are associated nasal symptoms. Look for at least two of:

- Nasal blockage/congestion
- Rhinorrhoea/discharge
- Loss of smell
- Facial pressure or tenderness

Further investigation is not necessary in acute sinusitis, but refer the patient to ENT if there are chronic symptoms.

9   Features of primary headache disorder?

Primary headache disorders (e.g., cluster headache, tension headache, migraine) are responsible for most headaches. Diagnosis relies on associated features and patterns of presentation (see above). By definition, they cannot be diagnosed on the basis of a single episode. However, where the presentation is typical, it may be reasonable to class a case as a likely first presentation of a primary headache disorder. Following exclusion of 'red flag' symptoms (Box 13.4), 'green flags' may be used to suggest a primary headache disorder (Box 13.5). Where a recurrent headache does not fit neatly into a diagnostic category or in any area of uncertainty, refer to Neurology.

13

14 Limb weakness

Limb weakness may be a result of focal or generalized pathology. Diagnosis relies on careful clinical assessment, complemented, in most cases, by appropriate brain or spinal imaging. Current stroke management mandates urgent evaluation of unilateral limb weakness. Focal limb weakness can also be caused by many nonstroke pathologies, and these should not be overlooked during the acute assessment.

When describing patterns of limb weakness, it is useful to characterize between upper motor neuron and lower motor neuron patterns of weakness. Upper motor neuron (UMN) weakness is caused by lesions in the central nerve system above the level of the anterior horn cells in the spinal cord. They typically cause increased tone, spasticity, hyperreflexia, an upgoing plantar reflex and clonus. Lower motor neuron (LMN) weakness is caused by lesions of the peripheral nervous system, beyond the anterior horn cells of the spinal cord. They typically cause reduced tone, diminished reflexes, muscle atrophy and fasciculation.

Stroke

Stroke is the most common cause of unilateral limb weakness; infarction or bleeding presents with sudden-onset focal neurological symptoms correlating to the affected brain territory. Patients typically have sudden-onset weakness of the arm, leg and/or facial muscles. Symptoms persist for >3 hours and often do not resolve. There may be associated signs of cortical dysfunction (Box 14.1) or other sensory, visual or coordination problems. Aside from rare examples, such as those affecting certain areas of the brainstem, symptoms and signs are consistently unilateral. An initial flaccid paresis progresses to stereotypical UMN weakness days later.

Transient ischaemic attack (TIA)

TIAs are temporary, focal, ischaemic insults to the brain. Comparable to ischaemic strokes in their acute presentations, symptoms and signs usually last for at least 10 minutes but resolve entirely without permanent neurological sequelae. The traditional definition of TIA describes a syndrome lasting less than a day, but this does not correlate with modern knowledge of stroke—symptoms >3 hours are likely to show permanent ischaemic damage on advanced brain imaging. With rare exceptions, TIAs do not cause loss of consciousness. One in 12 patients will go on to have a stroke within a week if treatment is not initiated.

Space-occupying lesions

Space-occupying lesions (e.g., tumour, abscess, chronic subdural haematoma) can cause symptoms and signs mimicking stroke, but the onset is typically more gradual and progressive. There may be features of raised ICP (Box 15.1). Raised ICP may produce vomiting (classically occurs shortly after wakening), headache (worse on lying, bending or straining) and possibly papilloedema. In acute causes of raised ICP (e.g., intracerebral haemorrhage), there may initially be a sudden onset headache followed by progressive neurological symptoms, including a decline in GCS. Assessment of patients with space-occupying lesions should include screening for potential underlying pathology (e.g., malignancy) or a source of septic emboli, such as infective endocarditis.

Spinal cord lesions

Transverse spinal cord lesions produce bilateral UMN limb weakness (para-/tetraparesis), with loss of all sensory modalities below the affected cord level and disturbance of sphincter function. Unilateral lesions (Brown–Séquard

Box 14.1 Signs of cortical dysfunction

- Visual field defect
- Dysphasia
- Dyspraxia
- Sensory/visual or motor neglect including inattention

syndrome) cause ipsilateral UMN weakness and loss of proprioception below the cord level, with contralateral loss of pain and temperature sensation.

Causes may be compressive lesions (e.g., intervertebral disc prolapse, trauma, vertebral metastases) or intrinsic pathology (e.g., transverse myelitis, glioma, spinal infarct, vitamin B_{12} deficiency). Circumferential pain that crosses dermatomes or sensory loss below a thoracic or lumbar dermatome suggest cord compression but are not always present—the level should correlate with neurological examination of the lower limbs.

Cauda equina syndrome

Cauda equina syndrome describes compression of the lumbosacral nerve roots below the termination of the spinal cord. The most common cause is intervertebral disc herniation into the spinal canal. Clinical features include saddle anaesthesia, bowel/bladder disturbance, back pain and bilateral leg weakness and pain. Features of bladder and bowel disturbance can include urgency, difficulty initiating urination, urinary retention, overflow incontinence, reduced anal tone and faecal incontinence. Unlike lesions of the spinal cord, the weakness in cauda equina syndrome will have a LMN pattern.

Peripheral nerve lesions

LMN weakness may result from generalized disease of peripheral nerves (peripheral neuropathy) or from lesions affecting a plexus (plexopathy), spinal root (radiculopathy) or single nerve (mononeuropathy). In peripheral neuropathy, the longest nerves tend to be affected first, leading to a 'glove-and-stocking' pattern of weakness and sensory loss; in the other lesions, weakness and sensory loss reflect the muscles/skin regions innervated by the affected nerve(s) or nerve root.

Motor neuron disease

Motor neuron disease (amyotrophic lateral sclerosis) describes a chronic degenerative condition that presents with gradual, progressive weakness and a combination of UMN and LMN signs. There may be bulbar involvement, but sensory features are absent.

Other causes

Encephalitis may cause limb weakness as part of a constellation of central neurological symptoms, including confusion, seizures and altered consciousness. Multiple sclerosis can present with almost any pattern of UMN limb weakness, though paraparesis secondary to transverse myelitis is most typical. Transient focal limb weakness can occur immediately after an epileptic seizure (Todd paresis). Myasthenia gravis causes 'fatigability' of limb muscles. Migraine occasionally causes limb weakness (hemiplegic migraine), but this is a diagnosis of exclusion.

Generalized muscle weakness may result from congenital/inflammatory myopathy (e.g., polymyositis, muscular dystrophy), endocrine or metabolic disturbance (e.g., Cushing syndrome, hypokalaemia) or drugs/toxins (e.g., corticosteroids, alcohol); it is also a common, nonspecific presentation of acute illness in frail, elderly patients.

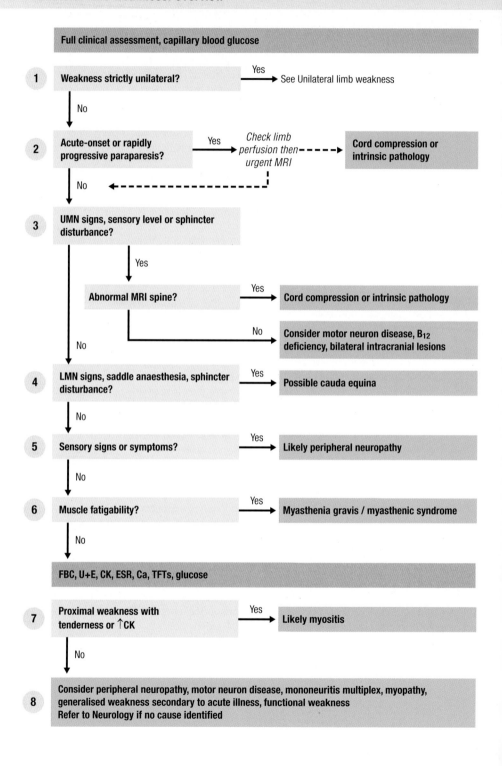

1   Weakness strictly unilateral?

Assess power in all four limbs and grade according to the MRC scale (Table 14.1). Ask about any preexisting limb weakness that predates the current presentation (e.g., old stroke) and whether it has changed. In any rapid-onset weakness, perform a CBG test; if <4.0 mmol/L, send blood for lab glucose measurement, but treat immediately with IV dextrose and then reassess.

If the current presentation of limb weakness is confined to one side of the body, assess as per unilateral limb weakness (this includes patients with contralateral facial weakness). Otherwise, continue on the current diagnostic pathway, even if signs are markedly asymmetrical.

2   Acute-onset or rapidly progressive paraparesis?

In any patient with sudden-onset or rapidly progressive paraparesis or tetraparesis:
- Immobilize the cervical spine pending imaging if there is suspicion of recent trauma.
- Discuss immediately with a vascular surgeon if weakness is accompanied by features of acute limb ischaemia, such as pain; cold/pale/mottled skin; absent pulses.
- Otherwise, arrange urgent spinal imaging, usually MRI, to exclude cord compression or traumatic injury.

If MRI confirms a compressive lesion, discuss with Neurosurgery or Oncology, depending on the clinical context and likely cause.

Table 14.1 Medical Research Council (MRC) power rating

Grade	Findings on examination
1	No movement, not even muscle flicker
2	Flicker of muscle contraction only
3	Movement possible only when action of gravity is removed and against no resistance
4	Can move against gravity but not completely against full active resistance
5	Normal power against full active resistance

If MRI excludes cord compression (and does not yield a definitive alternative diagnosis), consider spinal stroke if the onset of weakness was very sudden, especially when accompanied by severe back pain. Examine for sparing of proprioception and vibration sense and look specifically for MRI changes of spinal infarction. Otherwise, seek urgent neurological review and continue to assess as described below.

3   UMN signs, sensory level or sphincter disturbance?

- Bilateral weakness associated with UMN signs, a sensory level (Fig. 14.1) and/or bladder/bowel dysfunction suggests a spinal cord lesion (i.e., a myelopathy). Arrange an MRI spine to exclude cord compression and structural intrinsic spinal disease, e.g., syringomyelia, glioma, abscess.
- If neither is present, check whether the patient has had previous radiotherapy (postradiation myelopathy), and measure plasma vitamin B_{12} levels to exclude subacute combined degeneration of the cord.
- Suspect transverse myelitis if the MRI shows evidence of inflammatory change and the time from first onset of symptoms to maximal weakness was between 4 hours and 21 days—refer to Neurology for further evaluation, such as CSF analysis, autoimmune and infective screen.
- Suspect motor neuron disease if weakness is slowly progressive and sensory features are absent, especially when there are associated LMN signs or bulbar involvement.

Consider brain imaging to exclude bilateral intracranial lesions (e.g., cerebral emboli/metastases, venous stroke, demyelination) in any patient with bilateral UMN limb weakness and:
- No evidence of myelopathy (i.e., normal MRI spine, no sensory level/sphincter disturbance) or
- Associated cortical signs (Box 14.1), features of ↑ICP (Box 15.1), cranial nerve lesions or cerebellar involvement.

14

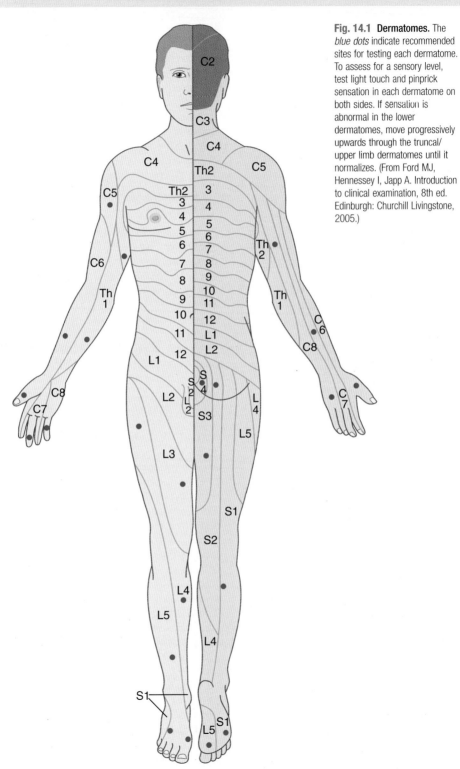

Fig. 14.1 Dermatomes. The *blue dots* indicate recommended sites for testing each dermatome. To assess for a sensory level, test light touch and pinprick sensation in each dermatome on both sides. If sensation is abnormal in the lower dermatomes, move progressively upwards through the truncal/upper limb dermatomes until it normalizes. (From Ford MJ, Hennessey I, Japp A. Introduction to clinical examination, 8th ed. Edinburgh: Churchill Livingstone, 2005.)

Discuss with Neurology and consider CT angiography of the Circle of Willis to exclude basilar artery thrombosis in patients with a normal CT brain but bilateral and asymmetrical neurology associated with drowsiness and change in behaviour. Obtain specialist neurological input in any suspected case of motor neuron disease or multiple sclerosis, or if the cause remains unclear.

4   LMN signs, saddle anaesthesia, sphincter disturbance

Suspect cauda equina syndrome in any patient with bilateral LMN weakness with associated bowel/bladder disturbance or saddle anaesthesia. Supportive features include back pain, bilateral leg pain or sensory disturbance in the lumbosacral nerve root dermatomes. Cauda equina syndrome is a surgical emergency; urgent MRI of the spine and consultation with Neurosurgery must be organized if it is suspected.

5   Sensory signs or symptoms?

In the absence of clinical features of a spinal cord lesion or cauda equina syndrome, the combination of bilateral or generalized limb weakness with sensory disturbance is usually due to peripheral neuropathy.

Consider Guillain–Barré syndrome if distal lower limb numbness or tingling is followed by rapidly ascending weakness and absent tendon reflexes (Table 14.2).

- Confirm the diagnosis with nerve conduction studies and a LP (↑CSF protein with normal cell count and glucose).
- Check and monitor vital capacity for evidence of respiratory depression.
- Refer early to Neurology for further evaluation.

Slowly progressive limb weakness that is more marked distally with a 'glove-and-stocking' pattern of sensory loss strongly suggests a sensorimotor peripheral neuropathy, such as chronic inflammatory demyelinating polyneuropathy, hereditary sensorimotor neuropathy.

- Arrange nerve conduction studies to confirm peripheral nerve disease, and

Table 14.2 Clinical features of Guillain–Barré syndrome

Remember these as the five 'A's:

Acute course:	Time from onset to maximal weakness = hours to 4 weeks.
Ascending weakness:	Initially in legs, progressing to arms ± respiratory/bulbar/facial muscles. At presentation 60% have weakness in all four limbs; 50% have facial weakness.
Areflexia:	Absence of tendon reflexes helps to distinguish Guillain–Barré syndrome from myelopathy.
Associated sensory symptoms:	Distal numbness, tingling or pain often precedes weakness. Loss of proprioception more common than pain and temperature.
Autonomic involvement:	Sinus tachycardia, postural hypotension, impaired sweating often present. Urinary retention and constipation are later features.

differentiate demyelination from axonal degeneration.
- Investigate for an underlying cause, e.g., blood glucose/HbA1c, vitamin B_{12}, ESR, serum protein electrophoresis, HIV test, urinary porphyrins, and syphilis serology.

Consider spinal imaging to exclude bilateral radiculopathy if sensory loss and motor signs follow a nerve root distribution (Table 14.4).

6   Muscle fatigability?

Consider myasthenia gravis if the history or examination findings suggest fatigable muscle weakness: initially normal muscle power that rapidly weakens with sustained or repeated activity. Ocular and bulbar muscles tend to be affected before limb muscles.

Ask about the effect of exercise and other activities on weakness.

- Enquire specifically about diplopia during reading, weakening of the voice when speaking, and difficulty in chewing/swallowing after the first few mouthfuls of food.
- Examine for ptosis.

14

- Observe patients as they hold their arms above their head for a sustained period.
- Listen while the patient counts to 50.

In suspected cases, consult Neurology and consider a Tensilon test if rapid confirmation is required, e.g., myasthenic crisis or severe global weakness; otherwise, check for anti-acetylcholine receptor antibodies, arrange a thoracic CT to exclude thymoma and seek expert neurological input. Avoid medications which may provoke crisis, such as beta blockers, gentamicin, tetracyclines, and opiates.

7 Proximal weakness with tenderness or ↑CK

Suspect myositis if symmetrical proximal muscle weakness is accompanied by ↑CK. Assess for signs of connective tissue disease such as fever, rash, raised inflammatory markers, and joint pain. If the patient is taking statins, reassess after a period of discontinuation. Otherwise, send an autoantibody screen, including anti-synthetase antibodies (e.g., anti-Jo-1 — associated with polymyositis); exclude other toxic causes (e.g., cocaine); and arrange muscle biopsy.

Even if the CK is normal, consider further investigation with muscle biopsy in any patient with symmetrical proximal muscle weakness associated with aching, tenderness, pyrexia or ↑ESR.

8 Consider other causes

Advanced myopathy may cause a degree of muscle wasting and diminished tendon reflexes, but suspect a LMN lesion if there is flaccidity, absent reflexes and/or fasciculation.

- Suspect lumbosacral plexopathy if there is severe pain and progressive weakness/wasting of quadriceps with absent knee reflexes—arrange imaging to exclude malignant infiltration of the plexus and check fasting blood glucose to exclude diabetes mellitus (diabetic amyotrophy).
- Exclude other causes of motor neuropathy—check serum lead levels and urinary porphyrins and arrange nerve conduction studies.
- If nerve conduction studies are normal, the most likely diagnosis is motor neuron disease (progressive muscular atrophy)—arrange electromyography and refer the patient to a Neurologist.

In patients with a 'patchy' pattern of weakness, examine to exclude multiple discrete peripheral nerve lesions (Fig. 14.2), that is, mononeuritis multiplex; if suspected, arrange

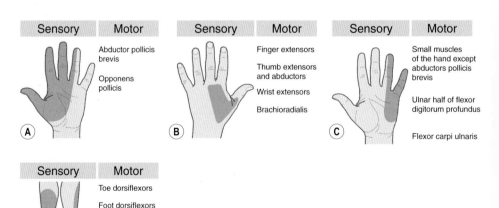

Fig. 14.2 Clinical signs in peripheral nerve lesions. (A) Median nerve. (B) Radial nerve. (C) Ulnar nerve. (D) Common peroneal nerve. (From Douglas G, Nicol F, Robertson C. Macleod's clinical examination, 12th ed. Edinburgh: Churchill Livingstone, 2009.)

neurophysiological assessment and investigate for an underlying malignant, vasculitic or infiltrative disorder.

In patients with proximal muscle weakness ± wasting and no associated neurological abnormality, screen for underlying metabolic, nutritional, endocrine, genetic and drug-related causes.

Enquire about alcohol intake.

- Consider trial discontinuation of any potentially causative medication, such as statin, fibrate.
- Check for an underlying biochemical disorder, such as $\downarrow K^+$, $\uparrow Ca^{2+}$.
- Look for clinical/biochemical features of diabetes, Cushing's syndrome, Addison's disease, thyroid disorders and acromegaly.
- Consider osteomalacia. Check 25(OH) cholecalciferol alongside serum calcium, ALP and parathyroid hormone. At-risk groups include the elderly, patients with cirrhosis, malnourished patients and ethnic minority groups, but this is overall a more common problem than is recognized. Consider a genetic myopathy, e.g., limb girdle muscular dystrophy. Enquire about a family history of muscle weakness.
- Assess frail, elderly patients with generalized weakness as described in Chapter 22.

Refer for specialist neurological evaluation if the cause remains unclear. Consider a functional aetiology if there are no objective features of organic disease and the severity or pattern of weakness is inconsistent, especially when the patient has a background of other functional disorders.

14

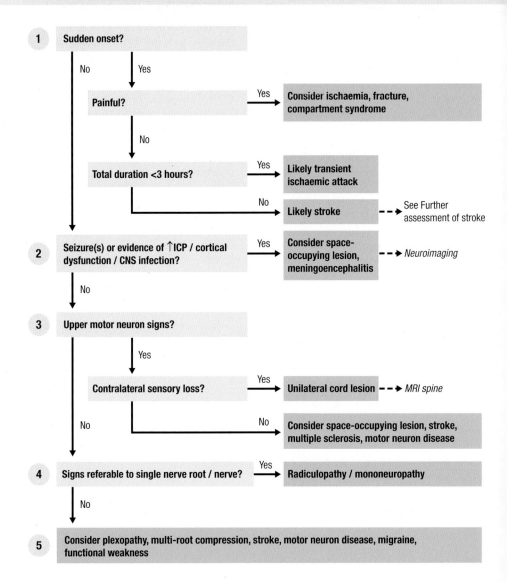

1 Sudden onset?

Evaluate weakness as 'sudden-onset' if it reaches maximal intensity within a few minutes from the first appearance of symptoms.

If there is painful weakness of a single limb, consider vascular and orthopaedic causes:

- Compare pulses, colour, temperature and capillary refill with the unaffected limb — seek immediate Vascular review if there is any suspicion of acute limb ischaemia.
- Request an X-ray of the limb if there is any history of trauma.
- Measure CK and request an urgent Orthopaedic review if there are features of compartment syndrome (Box 20.3).

Consider postictal weakness (Todd paresis) if the history suggests seizure activity immediately prior to the onset of weakness — arrange rapid neuroimaging unless the patient has known epilepsy and the patient's typical postictal phase is known to include limb weakness and the weakness is improving.

Acute non-neurological illness or hypotension may exacerbate established limb weakness from an old stroke — suspect this if the current weakness is confined to the same territory as a previously documented persistent neurological deficit and there are other clinical/laboratory features to suggest acute systemic illness. Maintain a low threshold for further neuroimaging.

In the absence of the above causes, sudden-onset unilateral weakness is highly likely to represent a stroke or TIA. Proceed to Further assessment of stroke.

Diagnose TIA if symptoms have resolved completely and lasted <3 hours.

- Evaluate for risk factors and sources of embolism as described under Further assessment of stroke.
- Assess the risk of impending stroke using the ABCD2 score (Table 14.3).
- Admit or arrange next-day specialist referral for any patient with >1 TIA in a week or an ABCD2 score ≥4 for urgent control of risk factors and carotid Doppler USS.
- Otherwise, consider discharge with appropriate secondary prevention and specialist follow-up within a week.

Table 14.3 ABCD2 score in TIA

	1	2
Age	≥60 years	—
Blood pressure	Systolic ≥140 or diastolic ≥90 mmHg	—
Clinical features	Speech disturbance, no weakness	Unilateral weakness
Duration of attack	10–59 minutes	≥60 minutes
Diabetes	Yes	—

- Arrange neuroimaging prior to discharge in any patient taking warfarin/direct oral anticoagulation (DOAC).

2 Seizure activity or evidence of ↑intracranial pressure/cortical dysfunction/CNS infection?

New-onset seizures, signs of cortical dysfunction (Box 14.1) or evidence of ↑ICP (Box 15.1) suggest underlying brain pathology.

- Arrange prompt neuroimaging (usually CT brain) to identify the cause. Seek anaesthetic review prior to scanning if GCS score <8 or signs of airway compromise.
- See Chapter 24 for further assessment of seizures.
- In all cases, seek expert Neurological advice, and consider further investigation with LP ± MRI if CT fails to reveal an underlying cause.

Consider meningoencephalitis if there is onset of limb weakness over hours accompanied by fever, meningism (Box 13.2), purpuric rash or features of shock (Box 2.1). If meningoencephalitis is suspected, manage as described in Chapter 13.

3 UMN signs?

A progressive onset of UMN pattern weakness suggests a space-occupying lesion, whilst rapid onset favours a vascular or inflammatory cause.

Exclude a unilateral cord lesion if there is dissociated sensory loss (ipsilateral proprioception/vibration; contralateral pain/temperature) or a clear sensory level. Otherwise, arrange brain imaging; CT is the usual first-line modality, but consider MRI if CT is inconclusive,

14

especially when there are brainstem features, such as contralateral cranial nerve palsies or cerebellar signs.

Consider an atypical presentation of motor neuron disease (usually bilateral) if neuroimaging fails to reveal a cause and sensory features are absent, especially when there are associated LMN signs.

4   Signs referable to single nerve root/nerve?

In the absence of UMN signs, suspect a radiculopathy if clinical signs are correlated to a single nerve root (Table 14.4), and consider spinal MRI urgently if the weakness is progressive. Investigate for mononeuropathy if they correspond to a single peripheral nerve (Fig. 14.2).

5   Consider other causes

Perform CT and/or MRI in any patient presenting with hemiparesis, even if there are no obvious UMN features; if results are normal, consider hemiplegic migraine.

If weakness is confined to a single limb, consider multilevel root compression (Table 14.4) or plexopathy, e.g., lumbosacral plexopathy (see above) or brachial plexopathy.

Otherwise, consider mononeuritis multiplex (see above), an atypical presentation of motor neuron disease (usually bilateral) or functional weakness.

Seek expert Neurological input in any case where the diagnosis remains unclear.

Table 14.4 Clinical signs of nerve root compression			
Root	Weakness	Sensory loss (Fig. 14.1)	Reflex loss
C5	Elbow flexion (biceps), arm and shoulder abduction (deltoid)	Upper lateral arm	Biceps
C6	Elbow flexion (brachioradialis)	Lower lateral arm, thumb, index finger	Supinator
C7	Elbow (triceps), wrist and finger extensors	Middle finger	Triceps
L4	Inversion of foot	Inner calf	Knee
L5	Dorsiflexion of hallux/toes	Outer calf and dorsum of foot	
S1	Plantar flexion	Sole and lateral foot	Ankle

Further assessment of stroke

Step 1 – Maintain physiological stability

- Monitor and protect the airway (if necessary). Ensure nil by mouth unless acute management complete.
- Ensure capillary blood glucose remains >4.
- Measure blood pressure. Do not treat hypertension unless clinical evidence of hypertensive emergency and/or as directed by a Stroke physician. If thrombolysis is indicated, emergency antihypertensive therapy may be necessary but should only be initiated by specialists—lowering blood pressure acutely may reduce cerebral perfusion.

Step 1 Assess eligibility for thrombolysis/mechanical clot retrieval

If facilities are available, refer immediately to the Stroke team for consideration of thrombolysis/mechanical clot retrieval in any patient with a potentially disabling stroke whose first onset of symptoms occurred within the last 4.5 hours (potentially longer time frame if mechanical clot retrieval available). Where the time of onset is uncertain (e.g., symptoms present on awakening), define it as the last time the patient was known to be well, but note that this is a poor surrogate marker for when the stroke occurred, and advanced imaging techniques can be used in some centres to ascertain how recently the stroke has occurred and whether thrombolysis/mechanical thrombectomy may be beneficial. Assess rapidly for contraindications (Box 14.2) and ascertain stroke severity score, e.g., National Institutes of Health Stroke Scale (NIHSS), in conjunction with the on-call Stroke team. In patients who meet clinical eligibility criteria, arrange immediate CT brain to exclude haemorrhagic stroke.

Step 2 Classify stroke according to clinical and radiological findings

Arrange urgent neuroimaging (CT brain usually) to differentiate haemorrhagic stroke from ischaemic stroke and to exclude nonstroke pathology, such as space-occupying lesion. Perform a CT brain urgently if:

- The patient is eligible for thrombolysis (see above)

Box 14.2 Contraindications to thrombolysis[a]

- Seizure at stroke onset
- Symptoms suggestive of subarachnoid haemorrhage
- Prior intracranial haemorrhage
- Intracranial tumour
- Stroke or serious head trauma within last 3 months
- Arterial puncture at a noncompressible site or LP within 1 week
- GI or urinary bleeding in last 21 days
- Severe liver disease (cirrhosis, varices, hepatic failure)
- Active haemorrhage
- Suspected bacterial pericarditis/endocarditis or aortic dissection
- Systolic BP >185 mmHg or diastolic BP >110 mmHg
- INR >1.7, thrombocytopenia or bleeding disorder
- Pregnancy

[a]Most are relative contraindications—seek guidance from the on-call stroke team if the patient is otherwise eligible.

- Coagulation is impaired (including receiving anticoagulant therapy)
- ↓GCS score
- Symptoms include a severe headache
- There is a rapidly progressive neurological deficit
- Cerebellar haemorrhage is suspected (to exclude obstructive hydrocephalus).

Otherwise, perform CT within 12 hours of presentation. Irrespective of CT findings, use the Bamford classification (Box 14.3) to categorize stroke.

Step 3 Evaluate for risk factors/underlying cause

In any patient with ischaemic stroke, identify modifiable risk factors for vascular disease, including hypertension, hypercholesterolaemia, smoking and diabetes; arrange Doppler USS to determine the presence and severity of carotid stenosis unless the affected territory is within the posterior circulation or the patient is unfit for vascular surgery.

Suspect a cardiac source of cerebral embolism if the patient has

- Current or previous evidence of atrial fibrillation
- A recent MI
- Clinical features suggesting endocarditis, such as fever and new murmur

14

Box 14.3 Bamford classification of stroke

This separates stroke into four clinical presentations that relate to the affected vascular territory and correlate with prognosis.

TACS (total anterior circulation stroke)

- All three of:
  1. Weakness/sensory deficit affecting 2 out of 3 of face/arm/leg
  2. Homonymous hemianopia
  3. Cortical dysfunction, such as dysphasia, apraxia

PACS (partial anterior circulation stroke)

- Two out of three of the TACS criteria, or cortical dysfunction alone

LacS (lacunar stroke)

- Causes limited motor/sensory deficits with *no* cortical dysfunction

PoCS (posterior circulation stroke)

- Causes a variety of clinical syndromes, including homonymous hemianopia, cerebellar dysfunction and the brainstem syndromes

- ≥2 cerebral infarcts (especially in different territories)
- Other systemic embolic events, such as lower limb ischaemia

Consider further investigation with transthoracic and, in selected cases, transoesophageal echocardiography.

Investigate for an unusual cause of stroke in younger patients without vascular risk factors.

- Perform a vasculitis and thrombophilia screen.
- Request a bubble-contrast echocardiography to detect a right-to-left shunt, e.g., patent foramen ovale that would permit 'paradoxical embolism' from the venous circulation.
- Consider MRA to exclude carotid/vertebral artery dissection.

Coma and altered consciousness 15

Coma and reduced consciousness are generally considered states of impaired responsiveness and/or lack of wakefulness. A reduction in consciousness requires prompt investigation to preserve brain function and prevent loss of life.

Consciousness is a poorly defined, ill-understood term. 'Normal' consciousness requires:

- An intact ascending reticular activating system (located in the brainstem and responsible for wakefulness) and,
- Normal function of the cerebral cortex, thalamus and their connections (responsible for cognition).

Altered consciousness results if either malfunctions. Minor defects (e.g., memory impairment, disorientation or slow cerebration) can be subtle and difficult to detect/describe, especially if there are coexistent language, visual or speech problems. Altered consciousness is often multifactorial at the time of presentation, such as a patient who has taken alcohol falls in the street, sustaining a head injury, lying for hours and becoming hypothermic.

The Glasgow Coma Scale (GCS; Table 15.1) was developed to assess and prognosticate head injury and is commonly used to record consciousness level. It is not validated as a prognostic indicator in nontraumatic conditions (e.g., sedative toxidromes) but can be used to capture fluctuating consciousness during the course of an admission. A GCS score <15/15 indicates altered consciousness. 'Coma' denotes a patient with no eye response and a GCS ≤8/15. Do not use terms such as semiconscious, stuporous, or obtunded as they lack clarity, especially when monitoring a patient's altered consciousness during the course of an admission.

The assessment pathway in this chapter is appropriate for patients with a GCS <15 and:

- Known or suspected head injury
- A clinical picture not suggestive of delirium (Chapter 21)

As the patient is unlikely to be able to give a clear history, it is essential to obtain a history from witnesses, relatives or the ambulance crew.

Ask about:

- Situation: the circumstances in which the patient was found, for example, exposure to temperature extremes or poisons.
- Preceding symptoms: A history of headache and vomiting would be suggestive of raised intracranial pressure; a preceding temperature or flu-like illness would be consistent with intracranial infection.
- Progression: the speed and nature of deterioration. Sudden-onset altered consciousness may suggest subarachnoid haemorrhage, seizure or trauma; gradual onset could be due to an expanding intracranial lesion or metabolic conditions; fluctuating consciousness could represent recurrent seizures.
- Trauma: e.g., road traffic accident, falls, assault.
- Drugs: previous/known alcohol and recreational drug use. Inquire about a history of overdose or suicidal ideation. Appraise current known medications (prescribed and over-the-counter).
- Medical history:

Table 15.1 **Glasgow Coma Scale**	
Criterion	Score
Eye opening	
Spontaneous	4
To speech	3
To pain	2
No response	1
Verbal response	
Orientated	5
Confused: talks in sentences but disorientated	4
Verbalizes: words not sentences	3
Vocalizes: sounds (groans or grunts) not words	2
No vocalization	1
Motor response	
Obeys commands	6
Localizes to pain, such as brings hand up beyond chin to supraorbital pain	5
Flexion withdrawal to pain: no localization to supraorbital pain but flexes elbow to nail bed pressure	4
Abnormal flexion to pain	3
Extension to pain: extends elbow to nail bed pressure	2
No response	1
Record the GCS score as a total and its three separate components, that is, GCS 9/15: E3, V2, M4	

Important causes to consider are listed below.

CNS causes

- Trauma: intracranial bleeding (extradural, subdural, intracerebral, subarachnoid), diffuse axonal injury. Note that patients taking anticoagulants or with bleeding disorders may have intracranial bleeding following minor, unrecognized trauma.
- Infection: meningitis, encephalitis, cerebral abscess, cerebral malaria
- Stroke: cortex or brainstem
- Subarachnoid haemorrhage
- Epilepsy including nonconvulsive status epilepticus (NCSE)
- Intracranial space-occupying lesion such as primary or secondary tumour
- Hypertensive encephalopathy

Metabolic causes

- Hypo-/hyperglycaemia
- Hypo-/hyperthermia
- Hypo-/hypernatraemia
- Hypothyroidism
- Metabolic acidosis

Drugs/toxins

- Alcohol
- Pharmaceuticals: opioids, benzodiazepines, tricyclic antidepressants, barbiturates
- 'Recreational' drugs, such as gamma hydroxybutyrate/gamma-butyrolactone (GHB/GBL), ketamine, heroin

- Carbon monoxide/other cellular toxins, such as cyanide

Organ failure

- Shock
- Respiratory failure (hypoxia and/or hypercapnia)
- Renal failure (uraemic encephalopathy)
- Liver failure (hepatic encephalopathy)

Other

- Psychogenic

15

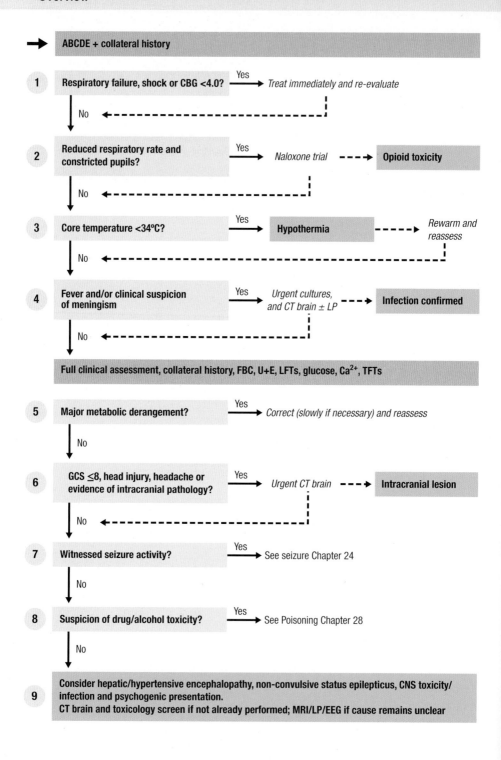

1 Respiratory failure, shock or CBG <4.0?

Ensure a patent airway and provide cervical spine control if trauma is suspected. If the GCS score is ≤8, then definitive airway management may be required. Look for and treat rapidly reversible causes of reduced GCS as per the ABCDE assessment:

- Assess oxygenation and ventilation by blood gas analysis. Treat hypoxia and hypercapnia urgently.
- Check carboxyhaemoglobin (COHb) and methaemoglobin concentration on the blood gas. Clinical features of CO poisoning are nonspecific, so the diagnosis may be missed unless specifically considered. Nonsmokers typically have a COHb concentration of 1–2%, while in smokers this baseline may be 5–10%. In the presence of methaemoglobinaemia (normal level <1.5%) patients usually appear cyanosed due to reduced oxygen-carrying capacity (Chapter 28).
- Check a capillary blood glucose (CBG); if <4.0 mmol/L, treat immediately with IV dextrose or IV/IM glucagon. Send blood for formal laboratory glucose measurement.
- Look for evidence of shock (Box 2.1); if present, assess and treat as per (Chapter 2).

2 Reduced respiratory rate and constricted pupils?

Consider opioid toxicity in any patient who has clinical features of opioid toxidrome (Table 28.2). Look for additional clues in the history (e.g., medication history, use of recreational drugs) and examination findings (e.g., presence of needle marks, fentanyl patch). Give a therapeutic/diagnostic dose of naloxone if opioid

toxicity is suspected. A rapid improvement in consciousness level and oxygenation supports the diagnosis and indicates that opioids are, at least in part, contributing to the clinical state. The half-life of naloxone is shorter than that of most opioids, and so ongoing monitoring and repeated naloxone doses ± an infusion may be required.

If a drug cause is suspected and a sedative toxidrome is not fully reversed by naloxone (e.g., improved respiratory rate but GCS score remains low), then consider mixed overdose with other sedative agents and proceed as per the sedated poisoned patient flow chart (Chapter 28).

3 Core temperature <34°C?

Suspect a contribution to altered consciousness from hypothermia if the core temperature is <34°C. Rewarm and reassess whilst searching for additional causes. Check TFTs and consider treatment with IV tri-iodothyronine (T3) or IV levothyroxine (T4) (preceded by IV corticosteroid) if there is any suspicion of myxoedema coma.

4 Fever and/or clinical suspicion of meningism

Patients presenting with fever, features of meningism (Box 13.2) and/or purpuric rash should be considered to have meningoencephalitis until definitively excluded. If suspected, take blood cultures, give empiric antibiotics/antivirals, arrange CT scanning and conduct LP for culture for further analysis (unless it is contraindicated).

5 Major metabolic derangement?

Altered consciousness is common in hypo- and hypernatraemia. It tends to reflect the rate of sodium alteration rather than absolute values. If the disturbance is known to be acute, correct promptly then reassess; otherwise, correct cautiously, at a slow rate, with frequent remeasurement to avoid excessive neuronal fluid shifts, which may cause cerebral oedema or central pontine myelinolysis. There may be a lag between correction of the metabolic derangement and return of normal consciousness level.

15

Box 15.1 Symptoms and signs suggestive of raised intracranial pressure

- Severe headache
- Reduced GCS
- CN VI nerve palsy and unilateral pupillary dilation
- Vomiting
- Bradycardia/systolic hypertension
- Papilloedema

Altered consciousness is a common feature of diabetic emergencies. Hypoglycaemia should be excluded in all presentations during the initial assessment. Suspect DKA if the patient has type 1 diabetes mellitus; confirm the diagnosis by identifying metabolic acidosis on VBG and raised capillary blood ketones. Suspect hyperosmolar hyperglycaemic state (HHS) rather than DKA if there is marked hyperglycaemia and hyperosmolarity in the absence of ketoacidosis (Box 25.2).

Suspect a contribution to altered consciousness from uraemia only if derangement is severe. Similarly, hypercalcaemia may alter consciousness when profoundly elevated (Chapter 11).

6   GCS score ≤8, head injury, headache or evidence of intracranial pathology?

Once you have identified and initiated treatment of major physiological derangement and medically reversible causes of ↓GCS score, it is vital to investigate for intracranial causes of altered consciousness. In general, immediate brain CT is required in patients with any of:

- GCS score ≤8
- A history of headache, focal neurological symptoms, lateralizing neurological signs (e.g., unilateral pupillary abnormality, absence of limb movement or extensor plantar response), or signs of ↑ICP (Box 15.1)
- Known or suspected head injury
- CSF shunt in situ

Seek senior advice prior to scanning if GCS score ≤8 or evidence of airway compromise as advanced airway/breathing support with intubation and controlled ventilation may be needed.

If CT brain fails to reveal underlying cause, discuss with Neurology and consider further investigation, such as MRI, LP.

7   Witnessed seizure activity?

↓GCS score is common in postictal patients, but seizures can be precipitated by a wide spectrum of conditions, including hypoglycaemia, head injury ± intracranial haematoma, alcohol withdrawal, and recreational or prescribed drug use. Therefore, it is essential to consider the potential precipitants for seizure activity. A clear, detailed history from an eyewitness is crucial. Consider atypical seizure activity in any patients with a fluctuating GCS score with a normal CT brain.

In status epilepticus, associated hypoxia/hypercapnia aggravates any preexisting cerebral injury. Mortality is ≈10%, so urgent intervention is required. Assess further as described Chapter 24.

8   Suspicion of drug/alcohol toxicity?

Even in patients with a history or features of acute or chronic alcohol intake, never assume that altered consciousness is due to alcohol alone. The correlation between breath or blood alcohol levels and consciousness level is poor, so beyond confirming that alcohol is present, these values are of limited help and can be potentially misleading. Look for (and treat) alcohol-related hypoglycaemia, occult head injury, intracranial bleeding and recreational drug use or overdose.

Examine for characteristic clinical sedative 'toxidromes' and manage accordingly (Chapter 28).

9   Consider further investigation if no clear cause identified

If the cause remains unclear, arrange CT brain if not already performed. Consider hepatic encephalopathy if the patient has known or suspected liver disease, or hypertensive encephalopathy if BP is consistently >180/120 mmHg with capillary bed dysfunction (i.e., retinopathy or proteinuria/AKI). Otherwise, seek neurological and/or critical care input and consider MRI, EE and LP.

Psychogenic unresponsiveness is a diagnosis of exclusion but consider it if comprehensive investigation fails to reveal an underlying cause and there are suggestive signs, e.g., response to tickling, resistance to passive eye opening and gaze deviating towards the floor in any position.

Accurate sight requires light to be able to enter the eye, the retina to detect that light, transmission of neural impulses from the retina to the visual processing centres, and accurate processing of those impulses. Pathology that interrupts any stage of this pathway can result in visual loss.

Acute visual loss can be complete monocular visual loss, an acute reduction in visual acuity, or loss of part of the visual field. It is important to be able to diagnose the cause of visual loss in a timely manner to allow urgent intervention of sight-threatening conditions (e.g., acute open-angle glaucoma) or diagnose an underlying systemic disease (e.g., vitreous haemorrhage and diabetic proliferative retinopathy). In all patients with visual symptoms, check visual acuity (VA; with corrective lenses if necessary), pupillary responses, visual fields, and eye movements and perform fundoscopy.

Keratitis

Keratitis is an inflammation/ulceration of the cornea causing an intensely painful red eye with associated photophobia and watering. VA may be reduced and the eyelids swollen. Keratitis is usually infective, but other causes include autoimmune conditions, radiation, and eye dryness due to incomplete eyelid closure. Infectious agents can be bacterial, viral (herpes simplex infection can produce corneal ulcers with a characteristic dendritic branching pattern), fungal or protozoal. The main risk factor for developing infectious keratitis is contact lens use. Keratitis, if untreated or severe, can lead to sight-threatening complications.

Scleritis

Scleritis is a serious, localized inflammation of the sclera (Fig. 16.1). It presents with pain (worse on eye movement and often severe enough to disturb sleep), redness, photophobia, and lacrimation. Scleral injection may affect only one quadrant of the eye or be diffuse. Visual loss is possible but is not present in all cases. In its most severe form, scleritis can cause perforation of the globe. Cases may be idiopathic, infective, or associated with systemic diseases, which include seronegative spondyloarthropathies, rheumatoid arthritis, systemic vasculitis, and connective tissue disease.

Uveitis

The uvea is the middle of the three layers of the eye, lying between the inner retina and the outer sclera and cornea. It includes the choroid, the ciliary body, and the iris (Fig. 16.2). Inflammation of the uvea, known as uveitis, is classified based on acuity and the structures which are inflamed. Acute uveitis is characterized by onset within hours to days and a duration of <3 months.

Anterior uveitis, where inflammation affects the iris and ciliary body, is the most common form of acute uveitis. Anterior uveitis is associated with systemic disease, including human leukocyte antigen (HLA)-B27–associated disorders (e.g., seronegative spondyloarthropathies, inflammatory bowel disease), sarcoidosis, and Behçet disease. Other causes include infection (particularly with herpes viruses), trauma and idiopathic causes. It presents with ocular pain (exacerbated by pupillary constriction), redness, photophobia, ↓ VA and lacrimation. Redness is typically ciliary or limbal (at the junction of the cornea and sclera (Fig. 16.3). Symptoms are usually unilateral but can be bilateral in patients with systemic disease.

Posterior uveitis is less common, has a more insidious onset, and presents with floaters and visual loss.

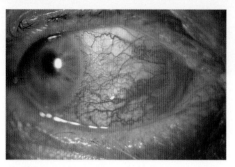

Fig.16.1 Scleritis

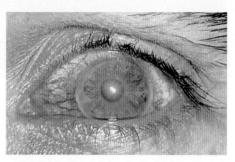

Fig. 16.3 Anterior uveitis. Note the distribution of inflammation at the junction between the cornea and the sclera.

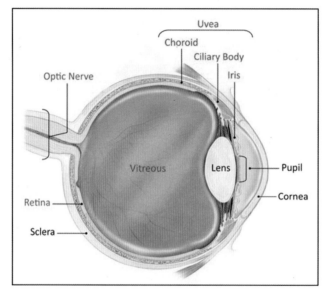

Fig. 16.2 Anatomy of the eye. Uvea consists of the iris, ciliary body, and the choroid. (From https://www.nei.nih.gov/learn-about-eye-health/eye-conditions-and-diseases/uveitis.)

Acute angle-closure glaucoma

Acute angle-closure glaucoma is a sight-threatening ophthalmic emergency caused by sudden blockage of the drainage of aqueous humour leading to ↑↑↑intraocular pressure. Middle-aged/elderly, long-sighted patients with shallow anterior chambers are at particular risk. Pupil dilation can precipitate the condition, so the onset may be more common in the evening and be precipitated by sympathomimetic, anticholinergic, and other drugs. Presentation is with acute, usually unilateral, severe eye pain with redness, ↓VA, seeing halos around lights, a cloudy cornea and a fixed, mid-dilated, often oval-shaped, pupil (Fig. 16.4). Headache, abdominal pain, nausea and vomiting may also be evident. The globe feels hard on gentle palpation through the eyelid.

Vitreous haemorrhage

Vitreous haemorrhage is a result of bleeding into the vitreous humour. This is most commonly secondary to diabetic proliferative retinopathy, where neovascularization results in extension of fragile blood vessels into the vitreous humour. Other causes include retinal

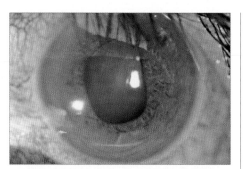

Fig. 16.4 Acute angle-closure glaucoma. The pupil is oval-shaped, and there is corneal haziness. (From Ophthalmology, 6th ed. Philadelphia: Elsevier; 2023.)

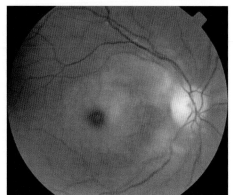

Fig. 16.6 Central retinal artery occlusion. Note the cherry-red spot at the fovea with the surrounding pallor due to retinal oedema. (From Anthony Schapira. Neurology and clinical neuroscience, 1st ed. Philadelphia: Elsevier; 2007.)

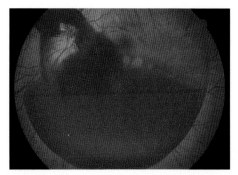

Fig. 16.5 Vitreous haemorrhage. (From Eye essentials for every doctor. Chatswood, NSW, Australia: Elsevier Australia; 2013.)

tears, hypertensive retinopathy, neovascularization due to sickle cell disease or previous retinal vein occlusion, subarachnoid haemorrhage, and trauma. Presentation is with floaters or cobwebs followed by painless visual loss. Vision may have a red hue. The degree of visual loss will vary according to the severity of the haemorrhage. Vitreous haemorrhage may obscure the retina on fundoscopy (Fig. 16.5).

Central retinal artery occlusion

Occlusion of the central retinal artery leads to retinal ischaemia, resulting in sudden onset, severe, unilateral, painless visual loss. The occlusion can be temporary or permanent, with a permanent occlusion leading to retinal infarction and irreversible visual loss. Permanent central retinal

artery occlusion is equivalent to an ocular stroke, with a temporary occlusion being equivalent to a TIA. Transient monocular visual loss secondary to temporary occlusion of the central retinal artery is often called amaurosis fugax and typically lasts up to several minutes. Most cases of central retinal artery occlusion are caused by thromboembolism, commonly from carotid artery atherosclerosis. On fundoscopy, the retina appears pale, with a cherry-red spot at the fovea (Fig. 16.6), and an embolism may be visible. The pupil is poorly responsive.

16

Central retinal vein occlusion

Occlusion of the central retinal vein by thrombus results in sudden, unilateral, painless loss of vision. Thrombus develops due to venous obstruction, usually secondary to compression from adjacent atherosclerotic arteries, or due to raised intraocular pressure. Risk increases with advancing age, with other risk factors including hypertension, diabetes, atherosclerotic disease, and glaucoma. Occlusion of the venous system results in venous tortuosity, retinal haemorrhage, and retinal oedema, all of which can be seen on fundoscopic examination (Fig. 16.7). Occlusion of a branch retinal vein results in a visual field defect, and the retinal changes localized to one quadrant.

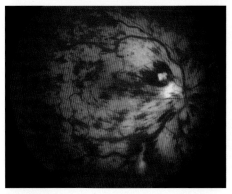

Fig. 16.7 Central retinal vein occlusion. (From Goldman-Cecil medicine, 27th ed. Philadelphia: Elsevier; 2024.)

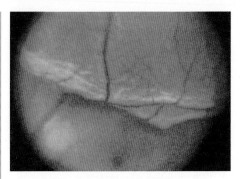

Fig. 16.8 Retinal detachment. (From The ophthalmic assistant: a text for allied and associated ophthalmic personnel, 11th ed. Philadelphia: Elsevier; 2023.)

Retinal detachment

Retinal detachment is the separation of the neural retina from the retinal pigment epithelium. It is most commonly caused by a retinal tear. Risk factors include advancing age, ocular trauma, previous cataract surgery and myopia. It presents with a painless loss of vision either centrally or in the peripheral visual fields. Patients may describe this is a curtain or veil moving over their field of vision. The visual loss may be preceded by floaters or flashes of light. Diagnosis is confirmed based on examination findings (Fig. 16.8). Retinal detachments may be missed on handheld fundoscopy and frequently require indirect fundoscopy or slit lamp examination performed by an ophthalmologist to be diagnosed.

Optic neuritis

Optic neuritis is inflammation of the optic nerve. It presents with eye pain, which is typically worse on movement, with associated visual loss. Symptoms develop over 1 to 2 days, are at their worst after roughly 2 weeks, and then improve. The degree of visual loss is variable, but can range from mild ↓VA, to scotomata, to complete blindness. Colour vision is frequently affected. On examination, a relative afferent pupillary defect is present. Fundoscopy appearances may be normal if inflammation lies behind the optic disc or may demonstrate swelling of the optic disc

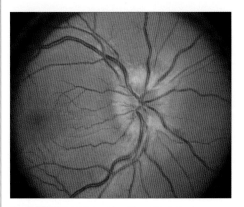

Fig. 16.9 Optic disc swelling. (From Ophthalmology, 6th ed. Philadelphia: Elsevier; 2023.)

(Fig. 16.9). Most cases of optic neuritis are caused by demyelination. Demyelination can occur in isolation (idiopathic optic neuritis) or be a manifestation of multiple sclerosis (MS). Risk factors are the same as those for MS, with optic neuritis being more common in females between the ages of 20 and 50.

Giant cell arteritis

Giant cell arteritis (GCA) is a medium to large vessel vasculitis that preferentially affects the extracranial branches of the carotid artery. It can present with headaches, fatigue, fevers, jaw claudication, temporal artery tenderness, proximal muscle stiffness and pain and raised CRP/ESR in patients over 50 years of age. Profound, irreversible visual loss due to central retinal artery occlusion or ischaemic optic neuropathy can develop if branches of the ophthalmic artery are involved. Irreversible visual loss may be preceded by transient monocular visual loss, flashing lights or diplopia. Sometimes, visual loss may be the only presenting symptom of GCA, making it hard to identify. Patients with suspected GCA and visual symptoms require urgent treatment to prevent permanent visual loss.

The most common ocular manifestation of GCA is ischaemic optic neuropathy due to infarction of the optic disc. Ischaemic optic neuropathy presents with severe visual loss without eye pain. Ophthalmic examination may reveal swelling of the optic disc (Fig. 16.9) and a relative afferent pupillary defect. Nonarteritic ischaemic optic neuropathy (i.e., not related to GCA) can occur and is more common than arteritic ischaemic optic neuropathy. It occurs in patients over 50 and is associated with cardiovascular risk factors. Visual loss tends to be less severe than in the arteritic form.

Stroke

Cerebral ischaemia can present with a range of visual field defects depending on which part of the visual pathway has been affected. The most common visual field defect associated with stroke is a homonymous hemianopia, but other potential defects include quadrantinopias, scotomata, bitemporal hemianopia, and cortical blindness secondary to bilateral infarcts of the primary visual cortex in the occipital lobe (Fig. 16.10). Visual changes may happen in isolation or in combination with other neurological symptoms (Chapter 14). A stroke may be preceded by transient monocular visual loss or other symptoms of TIA.

Migraine

Migraine aura can cause temporary visual loss with or without headache. Other visual symptoms can include photophobia, flashing lights and scotomata. For further details, see Chapter 13.

16

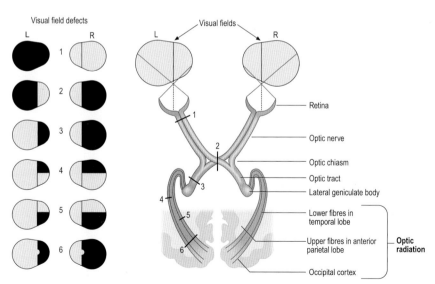

Fig. 16.10 Visual field defects. (1) Total loss of vision in one eye because of a lesion of the optic nerve. (2) Bitemporal hemianopia due to a lesion at the optic chiasm. (3) Right homonymous hemianopia from a lesion of the optic tract. (4) Upper right quadrantanopia from a lesion of the lower fibres of the optic radiation in the temporal lobe. (5) Lower quadrantanopia from a lesion of the upper fibres of the optic radiation in the anterior part of the parietal lobe. (6) Right homonymous hemianopia with sparing of the macula due to a lesion of the optic radiation in the occipital lobe. (From Macleod's clinical examination, 15th ed. Philadelphia: Elsevier; 2024.)

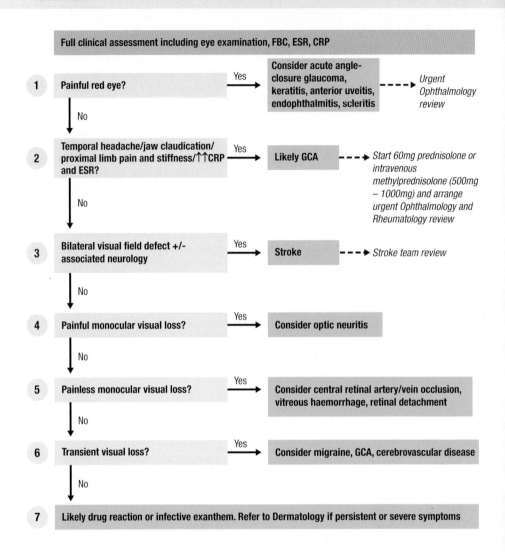

1 Painful red eye?

In patients with a combination of acute visual loss and a painful red eye, refer urgently to Ophthalmology. Conditions presenting in this way are sight-threatening if untreated, and accurately determining the cause of the presentation requires detailed examination by an Ophthalmologist.

Some specific clinical features may suggest a causative diagnosis in advance of ophthalmological assessment. Suspect acute angle-closure glaucoma if there are associated symptoms of nausea, vomiting, abdominal pain and headache, and examination findings of corneal haziness and a fixed, mid-dilated pupil. Prolonged contact lens use may suggest keratitis, while a history or symptoms of autoimmune disease may suggest anterior uveitis or scleritis. Inflammation localized to one quadrant of the eye would suggest scleritis (Fig. 16.1), while limbal inflammation would suggest anterior uveitis (Fig. 16.3).

| 2 | Temporal headache/jaw claudication/proximal limb pain and stiffness/↑↑CRP and ESR? |

Strongly suspect GCA in patients with symptoms of visual loss with associated symptoms of temporal headache, jaw claudication, fever, fatigue, and proximal muscle pains and stiffness. Examine for temporal artery thickness, tenderness, nodularity, and loss of arterial pulses. Check ESR/CRP if not done already. Symptoms of jaw claudication, diplopia, flashing lights, and transient monocular visual loss all suggest imminent progression to permanent visual loss and require urgent treatment with steroids. In patients who have already suffered permanent monocular visual loss, the loss is irreversible, but treatment is required urgently to prevent ischaemic changes in the other eye. Give 60 mg of prednisolone daily and refer urgently to Ophthalmology for further evaluation.

| 3 | Bilateral visual field defect/associated unilateral neurology? |

Consider stroke in patients with homonymous hemianopia, particularly when there is associated unilateral neurology. Note that though homonymous hemianopia is the most common visual field defect, other patterns of visual loss are possible (Fig. 16.10). Assess as described in Chapter 14.

| 4 | Painful monocular visual loss? |

Suspect optic neuritis in patients with visual loss associated with eye pain (which is worse on eye movement) and loss of colour vision, without eye redness. Fundoscopy may reveal optic disc swelling (Fig. 16.9). Take a detailed history with the aim of identifying any previous episodes of transient neurology, including transient visual loss, or ongoing symptoms of weakness, numbness, balance disorders or bladder dysfunction. Perform a full neurological examination. Refer patients with suspected optic neuritis to both Ophthalmology and

Neurology and consider administering high-dose IV steroids.

| 5 | Painless, monocular visual loss? |

Painless, monocular visual loss is likely to represent a primary eye pathology. Symptoms preceding visual loss (e.g., floaters, flashes of light, red hue to vision), or risk factors for the conditions causing painless visual loss, might suggest the cause, but the diagnosis can be confirmed only on examination. Perform fundoscopy looking for features of retinal artery occlusion (Fig. 16.6), retinal vein occlusion (Fig. 16.7), vitreous haemorrhage (Fig. 16.5) or retinal detachment (Fig. 16.8). Refer to Ophthalmology for more detailed examination and management.

| 6 | Transient visual loss? |

Transient visual loss can either be benign (e.g., migraine) or an indicator of more severe underlying pathology (e.g., GCA, cerebrovascular disease). In patients where visual symptoms are followed by a typical migraine headache, or transient visual loss is accompanied by positive visual symptoms such as flashing lights or zigzag lines, no further action is required. Otherwise, assess for features of GCA, and if present, start treatment with 60 mg prednisolone urgently. In the absence of features of GCA, inquire about other transient neurological symptoms associated with visual changes, and refer to the Stroke team for further evaluation.

| 7 | Consider chronic vision loss presenting acutely |

It is possible that patients with a more chronic, progressive visual loss may present acutely when it is noticed for the first time. Establish whether there have been progressive changes and consider risk factors for chronic visual loss (e.g., hypertension/diabetes). Refer all patients with unexplained visual loss for further assessment by Ophthalmology.

16

The key to assessing dizziness lies in establishing the exact nature of the patient's symptoms. Dizziness is a subjective symptom; occasional, transient alteration of consciousness or focal neurological deficit may be described as a 'dizzy turn'. Most patients reporting dizziness have vertigo, light-headedness/presyncope or a sensation of unsteadiness.

Disorders causing vertigo

Vestibular neuronitis

This is inflammation of the vestibular nerve, usually due to viral infection. There is abrupt onset of severe vertigo, associated with nausea and vomiting. Labyrinthine involvement (labyrinthitis) causes tinnitus and/or hearing impairment.

Benign paroxysmal positional vertigo (BPPV)

BPPV is caused by particles in the semicircular canals which alter endolymph flow. Brief episodes of vertigo, typically lasting 10–60 seconds, are provoked by changes in head position. BPPV does not cause prolonged vertigo, tinnitus, hearing loss or neurological abnormalities. If any of these features are present then an alternative diagnosis should be sought.

Ménière's disease

Recurrent attacks of a triad of vertigo, fluctuating low-frequency hearing loss and tinnitus are caused by increased volume of endolymph in the semicircular canals. A sense of aural fullness is also often described.

Acoustic neuroma

This cerebellopontine angle tumour usually presents with unilateral sensorineural hearing loss. Vertigo may occur but is rarely the predominant problem.

Brainstem/cerebellar pathology

Vertigo may be due to infarction, haemorrhage, demyelination or a space-occupying lesion in the brainstem or cerebellum. There may be associated features of brainstem dysfunction, such as diplopia, dysarthria or cranial nerve palsies. Vertigo, vomiting (with the absence of nausea), and nystagmus tend to be constant and protracted. Vertebrobasilar transient ischaemic attacks (TIAs) may cause recurrent, transient episodes of vertigo.

Other causes

These include migraine-associated vertigo, ototoxicity (e.g., gentamicin, furosemide, cisplatin), herpes zoster oticus (Ramsay Hunt syndrome) and perilymphatic fistula.

Disorders causing presyncope/light-headedness

Reflex presyncope (vasovagal episode)

Reflex vasodilatation and/or bradycardia occur in response to a 'trigger' such as intense emotion or noxious stimuli, such as venesection. There is a prodrome of nausea, sweating and 'greying-out' of vision/loss of peripheral vision. Syncope often ensues but may be averted by lying down.

Orthostatic hypotension

Orthostatic hypotension may result from antihypertensive medication, hypovolaemia (dehydration, blood loss) or autonomic dysfunction, especially in older patients or people with diabetes.

Arrhythmia

Brady- and tachyarrhythmia can reduce cardiac output and thereby compromise cerebral perfusion. There may be associated palpitation, ECG abnormalities or a known cardiac history.

Structural cardiac disease

Severe left ventricular outflow tract obstruction (e.g., aortic stenosis or hypertrophic obstructive cardiomyopathy) can result in light-headedness by reducing cardiac output. Episodes may be provoked by exertion. There will usually be abnormalities on examination (e.g., systolic murmur) and ECG (e.g., left ventricular hypertrophy.)

Disorders causing unsteadiness

Ataxia

Lack of coordination of muscle movements may cause profound unsteadiness and difficulty walking; it is most commonly due to cerebellar pathology.

Multisensory impairment

Balance requires input from multiple sensory modalities (visual, vestibular, touch, proprioceptive);

reduced function in more than one of these modalities, even if relatively minor, may cause unsteadiness. This is most often seen in the elderly.

Weakness

Lesions anywhere in the motor tract (cerebral cortex, upper motor neuron, lower motor neuron, motor endplate or muscle) can result in unsteadiness due to weakness.

Other causes

Joint pathology, Parkinson's disease, gait dyspraxia and loss of confidence may all cause unsteadiness.

Other disorders causing dizziness

Many other conditions can cause dizziness, including hypoglycaemia, focal (temporal lobe) seizure, migraine variants, normal pressure hydrocephalus, hyperventilation and anxiety.

17

DIZZINESS

Initial assessment: overview

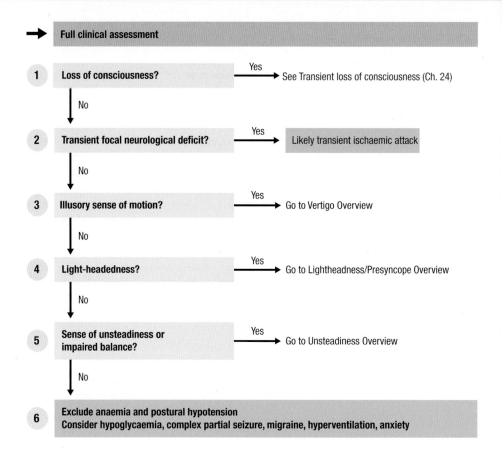

Full clinical assessment

1   **Loss of consciousness?** — Yes → See Transient loss of consciousness (Ch. 24)

No ↓

2   **Transient focal neurological deficit?** — Yes → Likely transient ischaemic attack

No ↓

3   **Illusory sense of motion?** — Yes → Go to Vertigo Overview

No ↓

4   **Light-headedness?** — Yes → Go to Lightheadness/Presyncope Overview

No ↓

5   **Sense of unsteadiness or impaired balance?** — Yes → Go to Unsteadiness Overview

No ↓

6   **Exclude anaemia and postural hypotension**
Consider hypoglycaemia, complex partial seizure, migraine, hyperventilation, anxiety

1 Loss of consciousness?

Establish whether there has been loss of consciousness first, as this requires a different diagnostic approach (see Chapter 24). If possible, obtain an eyewitness account of the episode; otherwise, suspect transient loss of consciousness if there is a history of 'coming to' on the ground or if facial injuries were sustained.

2 Transient focal neurological deficit?

A TIA is often described by the patient as a 'funny turn', and careful questioning may be required to elicit a history of transient focal neurological disturbance. The most common presentations include hemiparesis, hemisensory disturbance, facial droop, speech disturbance, diplopia and monocular visual loss (amaurosis fugax). Vertigo may occur with a vertebrobasilar TIA, usually accompanied by other brainstem features.

3 Illusory sense of motion?

Vertigo is an illusory sensation of rotational motion. The rotational aspect differentiates vertigo from unsteadiness. When present, it is invariably aggravated by movement. If the nature of the dizziness is not apparent from the patient's own account, then ask: 'When you have dizzy spells, do you simply feel light-headed or do you see the world spin around you as if you had just got off a playground roundabout?' The latter indicates vertigo (overview below).

4 Light-headedness?

Consider presyncope in patients who describe a feeling of light-headedness, 'as if I might faint or pass out', or one that is akin to the familiar transient sensation experienced after standing up quickly. If any of the episodes has been associated with blackout, assess as described for transient loss of consciousness (Chapter 24); otherwise. continue diagnostic process for lightheadness/presyncope (overview below).

5 Sense of unsteadiness or impaired balance?

In some patients with dizziness, the principal problem is an impaired sense of balance associated with falls or the feeling that one might fall. This usually occurs while standing and is aggravated by walking. The patient may need to hold onto furniture or other people. Examination of the gait (Chapter 22) may be revealing. The underlying problem is often impaired central processing of the body's position in space (e.g., cerebellar disorders, impaired proprioception, peripheral neuropathy, visual loss, poorly compensated vestibular disorders), which may be exacerbated by reduced muscle strength or confidence, particularly in the elderly. Continue diagnostic process for unsteadniness (overview below).

6 Consider other causes

If the description of dizziness is unclear, ask for more details: 'Imagine you are having one of your dizzy turns now. Talk me through exactly what happens and what you feel.' If the account is not consistent with any of the above categories, consider alternative causes. If there are episodes of amnesia, altered consciousness or unusual behaviour, then seek advice from Neurology.

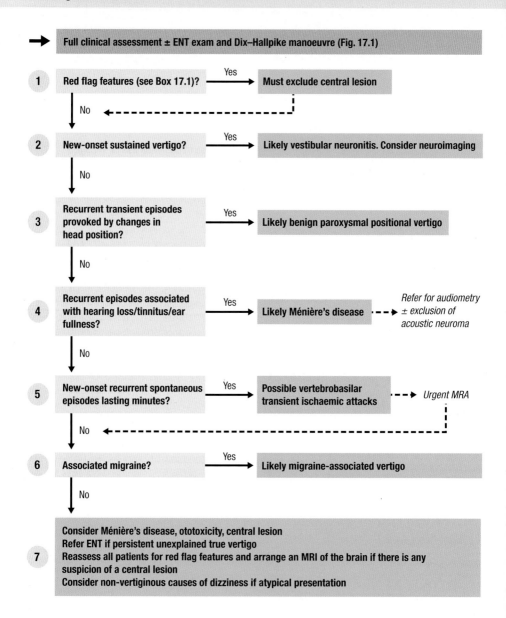

Full clinical assessment ± ENT exam and Dix–Hallpike manoeuvre (Fig. 17.1)

1 Red flag features (see Box 17.1)? — Yes → Must exclude central lesion

No

2 New-onset sustained vertigo? — Yes → Likely vestibular neuronitis. Consider neuroimaging

No

3 Recurrent transient episodes provoked by changes in head position? — Yes → Likely benign paroxysmal positional vertigo

No

4 Recurrent episodes associated with hearing loss/tinnitus/ear fullness? — Yes → Likely Ménière's disease ···→ *Refer for audiometry ± exclusion of acoustic neuroma*

No

5 New-onset recurrent spontaneous episodes lasting minutes? — Yes → Possible vertebrobasilar transient ischaemic attacks ···→ *Urgent MRA*

No

6 Associated migraine? — Yes → Likely migraine-associated vertigo

No

7 Consider Ménière's disease, ototoxicity, central lesion
Refer ENT if persistent unexplained true vertigo
Reassess all patients for red flag features and arrange an MRI of the brain if there is any suspicion of a central lesion
Consider non-vertiginous causes of dizziness if atypical presentation

1   Red flag features (Box 17.1)?

The presence of any of the features in Box 17.1 and/or a positive HINTS (head impulse, nystagmus and test of skew) assessment (Box 17.2) raises the possibility of serious intracranial pathology (i.e. 'central vertigo').

If the presentation is sudden, consider acute haemorrhagic or ischaemic stroke and arrange urgent neuroimaging. Where less acute, the main concern is to exclude an intracranial mass lesion.

CT is usually the initial imaging modality, but MRI offers superior visualization of the posterior fossa. All patients with progressive sensorineural hearing loss require an MRI to exclude acoustic neuroma.

2   New-onset sustained vertigo?

In the absence of red flag features, new-onset sustained vertigo is most likely due to vestibular neuronitis. The usual story is of abrupt-onset severe vertigo with nausea and vomiting but without hearing loss or tinnitus. The patient has difficulty walking but can usually stand unsupported. There is unilateral nystagmus enhanced by asking the patient to look to the side or by blocking visual fixation (place a blank piece of paper a few inches in front of the eyes and inspect from the side). A positive head impulse test (Box 17.2) confirms the diagnosis.

Consider neuroimaging (preferably MRI) to exclude acute cerebellar stroke if the patient has a negative head impulse test, is unable to stand without support or has a history of vascular disease.

Box 17.1 Red flag features in vertigo

- Focal neurological symptoms or signs: dysarthria, diplopia, facial weakness, swallowing difficulties, dysdiadochokinesis or focal limb weakness
- Papilloedema, drowsiness or ↓GCS
- Inability to stand or walk
- Atypical nystagmus (down-beating, bidirectional gaze evoked, pure torsional, not suppressed with fixation on object)
- New-onset headache: sudden onset and severe or worse in morning/lying down
- Progressive unilateral hearing loss

In vestibular neuronitis, severe vertigo typically persists for several days with recovery in 3–4 weeks; reassess if symptoms persist beyond this period.

3   Recurrent transient episodes provoked by changes in head position?

A history of repeated, brief episodes of vertigo provoked by changes in head position (e.g., turning over in bed or looking up) strongly suggests BPPV. Episodes may occur in bouts lasting several weeks interspersed

Box 17.2 The HINTS examination

The HINTS examination is composed of three tests that can be used in combination to assess whether vertigo is likely to be caused by a peripheral vestibular or intracranial pathology. It is composed of the head impulse test, an assessment of nystagmus and a test of skew.

- Head impulse test—Stand in front of the patient, grasp his/her head in your hands and instruct him/her to focus on your nose. Turn the head as rapidly as possible to one side by 15° (do not perform in patients with known or suspected neck pathology) and observe eye movements. Failure to maintain fixation on the target is evidenced by the need for a voluntary, corrective eye movement back towards the target. This indicates peripheral vestibular dysfunction on the side to which the head was turned. Perform the test in both directions. Unilateral impairment of the vestibulo-ocular reflex is seen in vestibular neuronitis and excludes a central cause for vertigo. See the video at the website of the *Journal of Neurology, Neurosurgery, and Psychiatry*: http://jnnp.bmj.com/content/suppl/2007/09/13/jnnp.2006.109512.DC1/78101113webonlymedia.mpg
- Assessment of nystagmus—Assess eye movements through their full range. Bidirectional nystagmus, where the fast phase of nystagmus changes direction to the side towards which the patient is looking, vertical nystagmus or rotatory nystagmus are all suggestive of a central cause of vertigo.
- Test of skew—Alternate between covering each of the patient's eyes with your hand while they focus on your nose. In cases of central vertigo, as each eye is alternately uncovered, a vertical deviation of the pupil will be seen. If there is no deviation, the test is negative.

A central cause for vertigo is suggested by a negative head impulse test, characteristic nystagmus and a positive test of skew.

17

with periods of remission. A positive Dix–Hallpike test (Fig. 17.1) confirms the diagnosis but, even if negative, BPPV remains the likely diagnosis.

4 Recurrent episodes associated with hearing loss/tinnitus/ear fullness?

Diagnosis of Ménière's disease requires the following criteria:

- Recurrent attacks of vertigo lasting minutes to hours (± nausea and vomiting)
- Fluctuating sensorineural hearing loss, especially for low frequencies (audiometry is usually required to detect this.)
- Tinnitus or a sense of pressure/fullness in the ear

Consider acoustic neuroma for any patient with unilateral hearing loss and vertigo, especially if the presentation is recent in onset or atypical for Ménière's disease. Refer the patient to ENT.

5 New-onset recurrent spontaneous episodes lasting minutes?

Vertebrobasilar TIAs are normally associated with other neurological features (e.g., diplopia, dysarthria, facial numbness) but occasionally present with episodes of vertigo as the only symptom. Patients with a crescendo pattern of symptoms may have impending thrombosis and require prompt referral for imaging of the posterior circulation, such as MRA.

6 Associated migraine?

Enquire about possible migrainous symptoms in all patients with episodic vertigo. Those who have typical migrainous symptoms and have episodic vertigo with no other obvious cause have probable migraine-associated vertigo; definitive diagnosis requires a temporal association between vertigo and migraine headache or aura.

7 Consider other causes/ENT referral

Reassess all patients for red flag features and arrange an MRI of the brain if there is any suspicion of a central lesion.

In Ménière's disease, the patient is often unaware of low-frequency hearing loss or tinnitus during attacks, and hearing may have returned to normal by the time of audiometry. In these circumstances, recurrent attacks of spontaneous vertigo may be the only presenting feature.

Suspect ototoxicity in any patient with new-onset vertigo or other balance/hearing disturbance if gentamicin, furosemide or cisplatin has recently been prescribed. Persistent symptoms despite drug cessation may indicate irreversible vestibulocochlear dysfunction.

Patients with dizziness who present constantly over weeks or whose dizziness is not improved by remaining still are unlikely to have true vertigo. If symptoms are consistent with vertigo but the cause is unclear, refer to ENT for further evaluation.

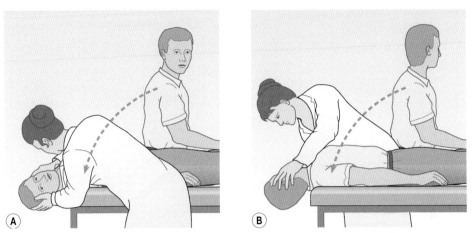

Fig. 17.1 The Dix–Hallpike test. Start with the patient sitting upright on the couch. Explain what you are going to do. (A) Rapidly lay the patient supine with the head (supported by your hands) extended over the end of the couch and turned to the right. Maintain this position for at least 30 seconds, asking the patient to report any symptoms whilst observing for nystagmus. (B) Repeat with the head turned to the left. The test is positive if the patient develops symptoms of vertigo and nystagmus. (From Boon NA, Colledge NR, Walker BR. Davidson's principles and practice of medicine, 20th ed. Edinburgh: Churchill Livingstone, 2006.)

17

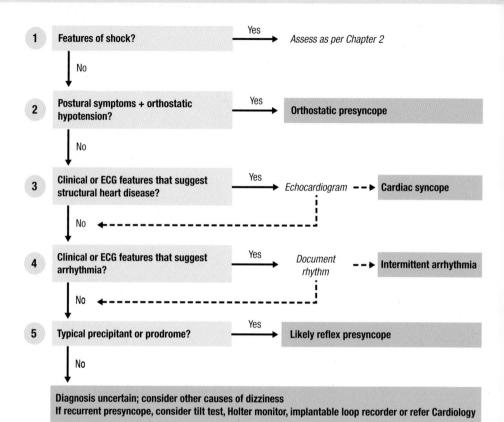

1. **Features of shock?** — Yes → *Assess as per Chapter 2*

   No ↓

2. **Postural symptoms + orthostatic hypotension?** — Yes → **Orthostatic presyncope**

   No ↓

3. **Clinical or ECG features that suggest structural heart disease?** — Yes → *Echocardiogram* --▶ **Cardiac syncope**

   No ↓

4. **Clinical or ECG features that suggest arrhythmia?** — Yes → *Document rhythm* --▶ **Intermittent arrhythmia**

   No ↓

5. **Typical precipitant or prodrome?** — Yes → **Likely reflex presyncope**

   No ↓

Diagnosis uncertain; consider other causes of dizziness
If recurrent presyncope, consider tilt test, Holter monitor, implantable loop recorder or refer Cardiology

1 Features of shock?

Acute light-headedness may signify haemodynamic instability. Look for shock (Box 2.1), including early features, such as ↑HR, narrow pulse pressure, pallor or postural ↓BP. If present, assess as described in Chapter 2.

2 Postural symptoms + orthostatic hypotension?

In all patients with orthostatic symptoms, measure erect and supine BP and perform a FBC to exclude anaemia. A secure diagnosis of orthostatic presyncope requires:

- A clear temporal relationship between light-headedness and standing up
- Demonstration of a significant postural BP drop (≥20 mmHg in systolic BP or ≥10 mmHg in diastolic BP within 3 minutes of changing from a lying to a standing position)

If orthostatic presyncope is detected, search for underlying causes, for example, antihypertensive medication, dehydration, autonomic neuropathy (e.g., diabetes mellitus).

3 Clinical or ECG features that suggest structural heart disease?

Consider echocardiography to exclude structural heart disease in patients with:

- Exertional presyncope
- A family history of sudden unexplained death
- A history or clinical signs of aortic stenosis/hypertrophic cardiomyopathy
- Clinical features of cardiac failure
- Relevant ECG abnormalities, such as severe left ventricular hypertrophy, right heart strain, deep anterior T-wave inversion

4 Clinical or ECG features that suggest arrhythmia?

Suspect an arrhythmic aetiology if episodes of light-headedness are associated with palpitation, occur whilst supine, are associated with significant ECG abnormalities (Box 3.2), or if the patient has a history of MI.

The key to clinching the diagnosis is to document the rhythm during a typical episode. If episodes are relatively frequent, arrange ambulatory monitoring (see Chapter 5 for more detail).

5 Typical precipitant or prodrome?

Consider whether episodes of light-headedness occurred while the patient was standing and had a clear precipitating trigger (e.g., intense emotion, venepuncture or prolonged standing) and/or were accompanied by other 'prodromal' features such as nausea, sweating and disturbance of vision. A tilt test may help to clinch the diagnosis of reflex presyncope.

17

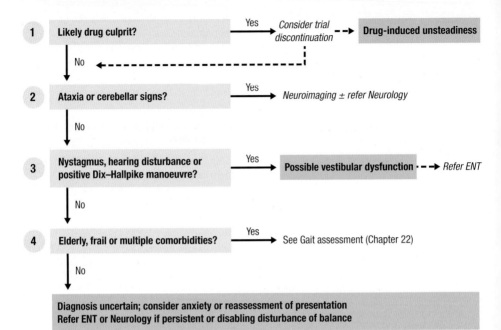

1 Likely drug culprit? — Yes → *Consider trial discontinuation* - - → **Drug-induced unsteadiness**

No ↓

2 Ataxia or cerebellar signs? — Yes → *Neuroimaging ± refer Neurology*

No ↓

3 Nystagmus, hearing disturbance or positive Dix–Hallpike manoeuvre? — Yes → **Possible vestibular dysfunction** · - → *Refer ENT*

No ↓

4 Elderly, frail or multiple comorbidities? — Yes → See Gait assessment (Chapter 22)

No ↓

**Diagnosis uncertain; consider anxiety or reassessment of presentation
Refer ENT or Neurology if persistent or disabling disturbance of balance**

1 Likely drug culprit?

Drug causes of unsteadiness are numerous and common but close attention should be paid to the following agents:
- Alcohol
- Antihypertensives
- Sedatives, such as benzodiazepines
- Antipsychotics, such as haloperidol
- Antidepressants with anticholinergic properties, such as amitriptyline
- Anticonvulsants, such as carbamazepine

If safe to do so, discontinue potential drug culprits and reassess.

2 Ataxia or cerebellar signs?

Suspect cerebellar dysfunction if there is ataxia (broad-based, unsteady gait; inability to heel–toe walk) or other typical clinical features, e.g., intention tremor, dysdiadochokinesis, past-pointing, dysarthria or nystagmus. If any of these is present, enquire about current and previous alcohol intake and consider an MRI of the brain and/or Neurology referral.

3 Nystagmus, hearing disturbance or positive Dix–Hallpike manoeuvre?

Even if the patient's account of dizziness is not suggestive of vertigo, the presence of nystagmus, hearing disturbance or a positive Dix–Hallpike manoeuvre suggests vestibular dysfunction (see Vertigo Overview, above). Consider referral to ENT.

4 Elderly, frail or multiple comorbidities?

Multiple factors may contribute to unsteadiness, particularly in the elderly, including limb weakness, sensory neuropathy, impaired proprioception, joint disease, impaired visual acuity and loss of confidence. Several factors commonly coexist. If the patient has evidence of more than one of these, is frail/elderly or exhibits unsteadiness during walking, assess as described for mobility problems (Chapter 22).

17

SECTION IV

Musculoskeletal System

Joint swelling 18

This chapter relates primarily to the acute swelling of a single large joint, such as the knee, elbow, shoulder, wrist, or ankle. Swelling may arise from the joint itself or from periarticular structures (e.g., bursae, tendons, ligaments, muscles). Conditions affecting the joint usually cause diffuse swelling, warmth, tenderness and both active and passive restriction in all planes of motion. In contrast, bursitis/tendinopathies cause localized tenderness and swelling over the inflamed structure. Pain and restricted motion are limited to certain planes of movement, and pain is generally worse with active rather than passive movement.

Septic arthritis

Septic arthritis has a high associated mortality and can lead to irreversible joint destruction, so should be identified early in the diagnostic process. Haematogenous spread or direct inoculation into the joint from local infection or trauma are the usual routes of infection. Common organisms are *Staphylococcus aureus, Staphylococcus epidermidis* and *Streptococcus* species. *Neisseria gonorrhoeae* is more common in young adults and can be associated with polyarthralgia, malaise and cutaneous manifestations. Gram-negative species are more common in patients who are elderly, immunosuppressed, or use IV drugs. Risk factors include a history of inflammatory arthritis, a prosthetic joint, skin infection, joint surgery,

diabetes mellitus, increasing age, immunocompromise and IV drug use. Pain, swelling, tenderness, erythema and restricted joint movement are typical presenting features. The joint is often held in a fixed position with the patient extremely reluctant to move it. Fever and ↑WBC/CRP may be present but are unreliable features, particularly in patients taking steroids or NSAIDs and in the immunosuppressed.

Trauma and haemarthrosis

Trauma may result in haemarthrosis if there is an injury to a vascular structure within the joint (a fracture or ligamentous injury). A traumatic effusion may cause joint swelling following an injury, such as from a meniscal tear in the knee.

Haemarthrosis can develop spontaneously and should be suspected in patients who present with a swollen, painful joint on a background of a bleeding diathesis or anticoagulant use.

Crystal arthropathy

The two most common forms are gout (uric acid) and pseudogout (calcium pyrophosphate).

Acute gout most frequently affects the metatarsophalangeal joint of the great toe, followed by the ankle, knee, small joints of the feet/hands, wrist, and elbow. Gout causes severe pain, which reaches its peak within 12 hours of onset. The affected joint is hot, red, and swollen, with shiny overlying skin. Risk factors for gout include male gender, increasing age, alcohol excess, diuretic use, and renal stones, as well as conditions that cause high cell turnover (e.g., polycythaemia, lymphoma, psoriasis).

Acute calcium pyrophosphate–deposition arthritis (pseudogout) generally occurs in patients over 60 years, with risk increasing with advancing age. Other risk factors include hyperparathyroidism, haemachromatosis, vitamin D deficiency, previous injury or surgery to the affected joint, and electrolyte disturbance. Attacks can be precipitated by acute illness, trauma or surgery. Initial presentation may be clinically indistinguishable from an attack of gout, though chondrocalcinosis on X-ray increases the likelihood of pseudogout.

Inflammatory arthropathies

Inflammatory arthropathies are autoimmune conditions that cause joint pain, swelling, and stiffness which is worse with rest, better with activity and lasts for at least 30 minutes in the morning. All inflammatory arthropathies, including rheumatoid arthritis, could present as an acute monoarthritis, but it is more common in the spondyloarthropathies. The spondyloarthropathies (Box 18.1) are a heterogenous group of autoimmune inflammatory

---

Box 18.1 The seronegative spondyloarthropathies

Axial spondyloarthropathies (which encompass ankylosing spondylitis)
Peripheral spondyloarthritis
Psoriatic arthritis
Reactive arthritis
Inflammatory bowel disease–related spondyloarthritis
Juvenile spondyloarthritis
Enthesitis-related arthritis

---

arthritides characterized by inflammatory back pain, enthesitis (i.e., inflammation at tendon insertions), and an association with HLA-B27. Reactive and psoriatic arthritis should be specifically considered in patients presenting with a single swollen joint. Reactive arthritis should be suspected in patients who present within 4 weeks of a GI or GU infection (e.g., *Chlamydia, Camplylobacter, Yersinia, Salmonella and Shigella*). The disorder most commonly affects men between 20 and 50 years old. Cutaneous manifestations, such as keratoderma blennorrhagicum and circinate balanitis, may be present. The classic triad of reactive arthritis comprises noninfectious urethritis, conjunctivitis/anterior uveitis and arthritis. However, this is found in only a minority of patients. Note that reactive arthritis can occur following other bacterial or viral infections, but these incidences are not spondyloarthropathy-associated and will not present with the clinical features described above.

Patients with psoriatic arthritis will have a personal or family history of psoriasis. Careful examination is required to establish any subtle skin lesions (e.g., behind the ears, umbilicus), psoriatic nail changes, and features of dactylitis which would support this diagnosis.

Osteoarthritis commonly affects the hands, feet, spine and the large weight-bearing joints, such as the hips and knees. Pain is worse with activity and is associated with <30 minutes of early morning stiffness. Acute single-joint exacerbations may follow minor trauma. Osteoarthritis usually evolves insidiously over months to years but may present with an acute exacerbation.

Periarticular conditions

Bursitis is commonly caused by repetitive movement, particularly if pressure is applied over the bursa during the process. Symptoms may arise after unaccustomed activity. Less often it may result from infection, rheumatoid arthritis or gout. Common sites of bursitis are pre-/infrapatellar (knee), olecranon (elbow), trochanteric (hip), retrocalcaneal (ankle) and subacromial (shoulder). Bursitis is normally a clinical diagnosis, but aspiration of the bursa may be required if there is concern about infection, for example, low-grade fever, overlying erythema, warmth.

Tendinopathies and enthesopathies are usually caused by overuse or by repetitive minor trauma. Other causes include infection and systemic conditions, such as rheumatoid arthritis, gout/pseudogout, spondyloarthropathies. Tenderness over the tendon or at the site of tendon insertion, with discomfort aggravated by movement, is usual and crepitus may be detected. Common sites for enthesopathies are the elbow (lateral and medial epicondyles), shoulder (rotator cuff), ankle (Achilles tendon), and knee (patellar).

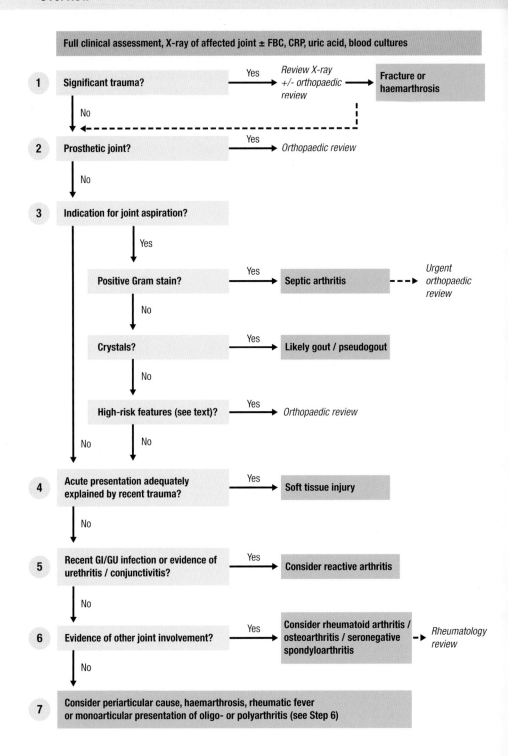

Full clinical assessment, X-ray of affected joint ± FBC, CRP, uric acid, blood cultures

1 Significant trauma? — Yes → *Review X-ray +/- orthopaedic review* → **Fracture or haemarthrosis**

No ↓

2 Prosthetic joint? — Yes → *Orthopaedic review*

No ↓

3 Indication for joint aspiration?

Yes ↓

Positive Gram stain? — Yes → **Septic arthritis** ⤍ *Urgent orthopaedic review*

No ↓

Crystals? — Yes → **Likely gout / pseudogout**

No ↓

High-risk features (see text)? — Yes → *Orthopaedic review*

No / No ↓

4 Acute presentation adequately explained by recent trauma? — Yes → **Soft tissue injury**

No ↓

5 Recent GI/GU infection or evidence of urethritis / conjunctivitis? — Yes → **Consider reactive arthritis**

No ↓

6 Evidence of other joint involvement? — Yes → **Consider rheumatoid arthritis / osteoarthritis / seronegative spondyloarthritis** ⤍ *Rheumatology review*

No ↓

7 Consider periarticular cause, haemarthrosis, rheumatic fever or monoarticular presentation of oligo- or polyarthritis (see Step 6)

1 Significant trauma?

When the patient has a history of recent trauma, examine the X-ray closely for fractures. If a fracture is identified, refer to an orthopaedic specialist.

Suspect haemarthrosis if severe joint swelling arises within 30–60 minutes of injury or occurs in a patient with impaired coagulation. Aspiration of a tense, traumatic haemarthrosis may help alleviate pain—consult an Orthopaedic specialist and correct any coagulation abnormalities prior to aspiration (under strict aseptic technique).

In the absence of a coagulation abnormality, swelling that develops 24 hours or more after joint injury is likely to represent a traumatic effusion.

2 Prosthetic joint?

In patients with a swollen/tender prosthetic joint, consult an Orthopaedic specialist. Do not aspirate a prosthetic joint without prior Orthopaedic consultation because of the risk of introducing infection. Aspiration of prosthetic joints is typically undertaken by Orthopaedic specialists in a sterile operating theatre environment.

3 Indication for joint aspiration?

Septic arthritis should be considered when trauma does not adequately explain an acutely hot, swollen, painful joint. Urgent joint aspiration is required.

Perform joint aspiration (using strict aseptic technique) with urgent Gram stain and microscopy, followed by culture and sensitivity. Aspiration of the knee is relatively simple but the other joints, especially the hip and ankle, require expert technique—seek help from Orthopaedics or Rheumatology. Never aspirate through infected overlying tissues. Once aspiration has been completed, start antibiotics as per local guidelines while awaiting results.

A joint aspirate that shows organisms on Gram stain is diagnostic of septic arthritis but is positive in only 30–50% of cases. Opaque synovial fluid, with WCC >50,000 cells/mm^3, suggests infection (Table 18.1), even if the

Table18.1 Features of inflammatory and noninflammatory joint aspirates			
Features	Noninflammatory synovial aspirate	Inflammatory synovial aspirate	Infective synovial aspirate
Macroscopic			
Appearance	Clear, straw-coloured	Translucent or opaque	Opaque due to pus
Viscosity	High (hyaluronate present)	Low (hyaluronate breakdown)	Variable
Microscopic			
Cellularity	Low	High	High
WBC (cells/mm^3)	200	2,000–50,000 >50% neutrophils	>50,000 >75% neutrophils
Crystals	Absent	Gout: negatively birefringent monosodium urate crystals Pseudogout: positively birefringent CPP crystals	Absent
Glucose	Slightly lower than serum	Slightly lower than serum	Significantly lower than serum
Protein	Normal	Elevated	Elevated
Gram stain	No organisms	No organisms	May be positive
Microbiological culture	Negative	Negative	Positive

18

Gram stain fails to demonstrate organisms—seek expert advice.

Crystal-induced arthropathy is suggested by the microscopic identification of monosodium urate crystals in gout or calcium pyrophosphate dihydrate (CPPD) crystals in pseudogout (Table 18.1). However, this does not rule out a superimposed infection, and it may be necessary to await synovial fluid cultures prior to stopping antibiotics depending on the clinical picture.

In the absence of crystals or a positive Gram stain, seek Orthopaedic review if the aspirate is bloody or there is any ongoing suspicion of septic arthritis, such as typical clinical presentation, consistent aspirate (Table 18.1) or an immunocompromised patient.

4 Acute presentation adequately explained by recent trauma?

A significant proportion of acute large joint swellings in the context of trauma with a normal X-ray are soft-tissue injuries with variable degrees of ligamentous/cartilaginous/tendinous injury. If the history is diagnostic, the X-ray is reassuring, and joint examination features are consistent with a soft-tissue injury, manage the patient conservatively. Depending on the severity of injury and the speed of the subsequent recovery, further imaging with MRI and onward referral may be necessary.

5 Recent GI/GU infection or evidence of urethritis/conjunctivitis?

In a young patient with nontraumatic acute arthritis in whom septic arthritis has been excluded, a recent history of any of the following features is highly suggestive of reactive arthritis:
- Diarrhoea
- Urinary frequency
- Dysuria or urgency

- Urethral discharge within the preceding 6 weeks (typically 1–3 weeks)
- Genital ulceration or circinate balanitis
- Symptoms/signs of conjunctivitis or iritis, for example, pain, irritation, tearing, discharge or redness.

6 Evidence of other joint involvement?

Examine all joints carefully, looking for evidence of swelling and/or tenderness; note the distribution and symmetry of additional joint involvement. Suspect rheumatoid arthritis in patients with symmetrical polyarthritis affecting the small joints of the hands. Examine for evidence of psoriasis, psoriatic nail changes, reduced range of back movements, enthesitis and dactylitis, that would suggest a spondyloarthropathy. Patients with osteoarthritis will have evidence of joint space narrowing, osteophytes, subchondral sclerosis and subchondral cysts on X-ray, and may have hard, nodular swellings on the distal and proximal interphalangeal joints.

Unless the diagnosis is clearly osteoarthritis, refer to Rheumatology for specialist assessment.

7 Consider other causes

Specifically consider and examine for periarticular causes of swelling. If there is diagnostic doubt, onward referral for further imaging and review is required. Evaluate for rheumatic fever if there is a flitting arthritis associated with other characteristic features (Box 26.2). Patients with atraumatic monoarthritis without an explanation should be referred to Rheumatology for further assessment. Less common causes to consider include connective tissue diseases, such as systemic lupus erythematosus, autoinflammatory conditions such as adult-onset Still Disease, sarcoidosis, Lyme disease, disseminated TB and intra-articular or synovial membrane tumours.

Low back pain is defined as posterior pain between the lower rib margin and the buttock creases; it is acute if the duration is <6 weeks, persistent if it lasts for 6 weeks to 3 months, and chronic if it is present for >3 months. In 90% of patients, no specific underlying cause is found—the pain is thought to originate from muscles and ligaments and is often termed 'mechanical'.

Radicular pain ('sciatica') originates in the lower back and radiates down the leg in the distribution of ≥1 lumbosacral nerve roots (typically L4–S2), with or without a corresponding neurological deficit (radiculopathy).

A thorough history and examination, supplemented where necessary by appropriate spinal imaging, is critical to identify patients with low back pain who have serious and/or treatable pathology.

Mechanical back pain

This is by far the most common cause of low back pain. The pain tends to be worse during activity, relieved by rest and is not associated with sciatica, leg weakness, sphincter disturbance, claudication or systemic upset. An acute episode is often precipitated by bending, lifting or straining. In most cases, the pain resolves after a few weeks, but recurrence or persistent low-grade symptoms are relatively common.

Lumbar disc herniation

This is the most common cause of sciatica. It predominantly affects young and middle-aged adults, often following bending or lifting. Symptoms may be exacerbated by sneezing, coughing or straining. The diagnosis is largely clinical and most cases resolve within 6 weeks. Imaging is essential for patients with persistent pain and/or neurological deficit.

Cauda equina syndrome

Associated with significant morbidity, cauda equina is considered an emergency and must be excluded in patients presenting with low back pain. It should be suspected in any patient with back pain with associated bladder dysfunction, bowel dysfunction, or bilateral neurological signs or symptoms. Presentations relate to compression of the collection of nerve roots at the base of the spine due to central disc prolapse, trauma or haematoma and warrant emergency referral to neurosurgery for decompression.

Lumbar spine stenosis

Narrowing of the lumbar spinal canal typically occurs in patients >50 years old as a result of degenerative spinal changes and may cause lumbosacral nerve root compression. Patients often have longstanding, nonspecific low back pain before developing dull or cramping discomfort in the buttocks and thighs, which is precipitated by prolonged standing or walking and eased by sitting or lying down (neurogenic claudication).

Vertebral trauma and fracture

This most commonly follows a traumatic injury (e.g., fall, road traffic accident or sporting injury) but may occur with minimal or no trauma in patients with osteoporosis or spinal conditions, such as ankylosing spondylitis. Patients with localized back pain following trauma or patients with low back pain and risk factors for vertebral fracture require imaging to evaluate instability and involvement of the spinal canal/cord.

Axial spondyloarthritis

Axial spondyloarthritis is one of the seronegative spondyloarthropathies (Box 18.1). All

Box 19.1 Features of inflammatory back pain

- Morning stiffness lasting >30 minutes
- Improvement of symptoms with exercise but not rest
- Nocturnal back pain that arises in the second half of the night
- Alternating buttock pain
- Restricted lumbar spine movements
- Sacroiliac tenderness

Box 19.2 Red flags for possible spinal cancer

- New-onset pain in a patient >55 years
- Active or previous cancer
- Constant, unremitting or night pain
- Focal bony tenderness
- Unexplained weight loss
- Fever, sweats, malaise, anorexia

the seronegative spondyloarthropathies can potentially present with inflammatory back pain (Box 19.1), but inflammatory back pain is required to make a diagnosis of axial spondyloarthritis. Axial spondyloarthritis predominantly affects the sacroiliac joints and axial skeleton and encompasses ankylosing spondylitis (AS), where there are established erosive changes to the sacroiliac joints on X-ray, and nonradiographic axial spondyloarthritis. Spondyloarthritis should be suspected in patients <40 years with insidious onset of inflammatory back pain. Associated features may include enthesitis (inflammation at tendon insertions), peripheral arthritis, uveitis, inflammatory bowel lesions, pulmonary fibrosis, and aortic valve lesions.

Box 19.3 Factors that increase the risk of spinal infection

- Diabetes mellitus
- General debility
- Indwelling vascular catheters
- IV drug misuse
- Previous TB infection
- Immunosuppression, such as HIV infection, chronic steroid therapy

Spinal tumour

Metastatic disease in the spine, particularly from breast, lung, prostate or renal cancer, are far more common than primary vertebral or other spinal tumours. The spine is frequently involved in patients with multiple myeloma. Red flag features (Box 19.2) may suggest the diagnosis, which is best confirmed with MRI.

Spinal infections

Pyogenic vertebral osteomyelitis, epidural abscess, 'discitis' or vertebral tuberculosis (TB)

may produce severe, progressive pain, often with localized tenderness and reduced range of movement. Typical associated features include fever, malaise and raised inflammatory markers. Risk factors for spinal infection are shown in Box 19.3. MRI is sensitive for detecting infection and differentiating from malignancy.

Other causes

- Spondylolisthesis (forward slippage of one vertebra on another): may cause back and radicular pain, and occasionally requires operative decompression.
- Pelvic pathology, for example, prostate cancer, pelvic inflammatory disease
- Renal tract pathology, for example, stones, cancer, pyelonephritis
- Abdominal aortic aneurysm
- Shingles
- Pregnancy

Clinical tool
Examination of the lumbar spine

- Examine for abnormal posture (scoliosis/loss of lordosis) from the back and side when the patient is standing.
- Palpate for tenderness over the bony prominences and paraspinal muscles.
- Observe extension, flexion and lateral flexion of the lumbar spine (Fig. 19.1).
- Assess spinal flexion using the Schober test: Locate the line between the posterior superior iliac crests (L3/L4 interspace); mark two points 10 cm above and 5 cm below this line. Ask the patient to bend forward as far as possible, with the knees extended. Lumbar flexion is restricted if the points separate by <5 cm.

- Test for sciatic nerve root compression (Fig. 19.2): With the patient supine, slowly flex the hip to 90° with the knee fully extended; limitation of flexion by pain radiating down the back of the leg to the foot (increased by dorsiflexing the ankle) indicates L4/L5/S1 nerve root tension (usually due to L3/4, L4/5 or L5/S1 lumbar disc herniation).
- Test for femoral nerve root compression (Fig. 19.3): With the patient prone, flex the knee to 90°; then, if pain-free, slowly extend the hip. Pain radiating from the back down the front of the leg to the knee indicates L2/L3/L4 nerve root tension.

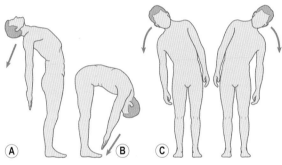

Fig. 19.1 Movements of the spine. (A) Extension. (B) Flexion. (C) Lateral flexion. From Ford MJ, Hennessey I, Japp A. Introduction to clinical examination, 8th ed. Edinburgh: Churchill Livingstone, 2005.

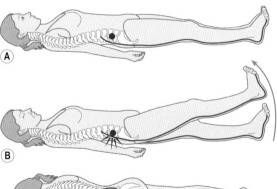

Fig. 19.2 Stretch test—sciatic nerve roots. (A) Neutral; nerve roots slack. (B) Straight leg raising limited by tension of root over prolapsed disc. From Ford MJ, Hennessey I, Japp A. Introduction to clinical examination, 8th ed. Edinburgh: Churchill Livingstone, 2005.

19

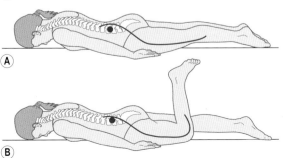

Fig. 19.3 Stretch test—femoral nerve. (A) Patient prone and free from pain because femoral roots are slack. (B) When femoral roots are tightened by flexion of the knee ± extension of the hip pain may be felt in the back. From Ford MJ, Hennessey I, Japp A. Introduction to clinical examination, 8th ed. Edinburgh: Churchill Livingstone, 2005.

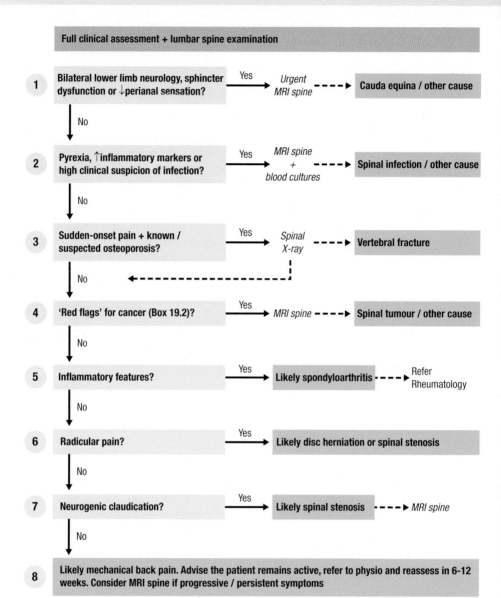

Full clinical assessment + lumbar spine examination

1 Bilateral lower limb neurology, sphincter dysfunction or ↓perianal sensation? — Yes → *Urgent MRI spine* ----▶ **Cauda equina / other cause**

No ↓

2 Pyrexia, ↑inflammatory markers or high clinical suspicion of infection? — Yes → *MRI spine + blood cultures* ----▶ **Spinal infection / other cause**

No ↓

3 Sudden-onset pain + known / suspected osteoporosis? — Yes → *Spinal X-ray* ----▶ **Vertebral fracture**

No ↓

4 'Red flags' for cancer (Box 19.2)? — Yes → *MRI spine* ----▶ **Spinal tumour / other cause**

No ↓

5 Inflammatory features? — Yes → **Likely spondyloarthritis** ----▶ Refer Rheumatology

No ↓

6 Radicular pain? — Yes → **Likely disc herniation or spinal stenosis**

No ↓

7 Neurogenic claudication? — Yes → **Likely spinal stenosis** ----▶ *MRI spine*

No ↓

8 Likely mechanical back pain. Advise the patient remains active, refer to physio and reassess in 6-12 weeks. Consider MRI spine if progressive / persistent symptoms

1   Bilateral lower limb neurology, sphincter dysfunction or ↓perianal sensation?

This is a potential medical emergency. It is critical to ask specifically about:
- Episodes of urinary/faecal incontinence
- Change in urinary frequency/urgency
- Any new difficulty in starting or stopping micturition
- A change in the sensation of toilet paper when wiping after defecation, new lower limb weakness/altered sensation

Examine the legs carefully for reduced power, diminished reflexes and sensory disturbance. If there is any suspicion of bowel/bladder dysfunction, perform a PR examination to assess anal tone and perianal sensation. It may also be helpful to measure bladder volume immediately after voiding by bedside USS or catheterization; >200 mL suggests urinary retention.

Arrange an urgent MRI spine to exclude cauda equina syndrome in any patient with low back pain (irrespective of its characteristics) associated with any of the following:
- Urinary or faecal incontinence
- Bladder dysfunction (significant postvoid residual urine, ↑bladder volume with no urge, new urgency)
- Altered perianal sensation/reduced anal tone
- Bilateral lower limb neurological signs or symptoms.

Request emergency Orthopaedic/Neurosurgical review if MRI confirms cauda equina compression.

2   Pyrexia, raised inflammatory markers or high clinical suspicion of infection

Suspect spinal infection in patients with localized spinal tenderness, a history of night sweats or fever, X-ray features suggestive of osteomyelitis, a known focus of infection (e.g., abscess), raised inflammatory markers (e.g., WBC/CRP), or other risk factors (Box 19.2). Take three sets of blood cultures and arrange an urgent MRI spine.

3   Sudden-onset pain + known/suspected osteoporosis?

Perform plain X-rays to look for lumbar compression fractures if the patient has new and abrupt onset of pain and known/suspected osteoporosis. Suspect osteoporosis if:
- >65 years of age with loss of height, kyphosis or previous radial/hip fracture
- Long-term systemic steroids have been taken

Seek an alternative cause if the X-ray reveals no fracture or one that does not correspond to the level of pain. Consider further investigation if there are any red flag features (see below).

4   'Red flags' for cancer?

Consider an underlying malignancy in any patient who presents with back pain and 'red flag' symptoms for cancer (Box 19.2), especially if they have a history of active or previous lung/prostate/breast/renal/thyroid cancer. MRI whole spine is the investigation of choice for assessment of metastatic spread in the marrow cavity, extension of tumour, and involvement of surrounding structures. A radioisotope bone scan should then be arranged to assess the function of bone and tumour cells. In cases where the origin of the primary tumour is unclear, perform a breast examination and myeloma screen, and ensure measurement of PSA (in males), Ca^{2+} and ALP in addition to routine blood tests.

5   Inflammatory features?

Perform plain X-rays of the spine and sacroiliac joints and check inflammatory markers if gradual onset of low back pain and stiffness.

Refer to Rheumatology for further evaluation of possible spondyloarthropathy if the history is consistent with inflammatory back pain (Box 19.1), there are X-ray features of spondylitis, (e.g., squaring of the vertebral bodies/sacroiliitis), there are peripheral or systemic manifestations of spondyloarthropathy (e.g., psoriasis, enthesitis, synovitis), or inflammatory markers are raised with no alternative explanation.

6   Radicular pain?

Pain is 'radicular' if it radiates to the lower limb beyond the knee with any of the following:
- Dermatomal distribution (Fig. 14.1)

19

- Evidence of radiculopathy (compression of a nerve root to cause a range of symptoms including pain, weakness, altered sensation)
- Positive sciatic or femoral stretch test (Figs 19.2 and 19.3)

Suspect lumbar disc herniation in acute-onset radicular pain, especially if the nerve stretch test is positive. In the absence of features of spinal infection, spinal tumour or cauda equina syndrome, reassess after 6–12 weeks of analgesia ± physiotherapy.

Suspect lumbar spinal stenosis if the patient is >50 years with a slow progressive onset of symptoms and/or features of neurogenic claudication (see below).

Consider referral to Orthopaedics/Neurosurgery for further investigation if:

- Persistent pain
- Evidence of >1 nerve root involvement
- Major disability
- Suspected lumbar spinal stenosis

7 Neurogenic claudication?

Consider neurogenic claudication if low back pain is accompanied by bilateral thigh or leg discomfort (e.g., burning, cramping, tingling) that arises during walking or on standing and is rapidly relieved by sitting, lying down or bending forward.

Evaluate first for vascular claudication if the patient has a history of atherosclerotic disease, vascular risk factors (e.g., diabetes mellitus, smoking, hypertension, high cholesterol) or signs of peripheral arterial disease (e.g., diminished pulses, femoral bruit, trophic skin changes). Check the ankle-brachial pressure index (ABPI) and discuss with the vascular surgery team if appropriate.

If neurogenic claudication is still suspected, arrange an MRI spine to confirm the presence of lumbar spinal stenosis and discuss with Orthopaedics/Neurosurgery.

8 Likely mechanical back pain. Consider MRI spine if progressive/persistent symptoms

In the absence of neurological, structural, infective, red flag or radicular features, provide reassurance and analgesia, recommend that the patient stay active, refer to physiotherapy, and reassess after a period of 6–12 weeks. Seek specialist input if there are persistent or progressive disabling symptoms.

Leg swelling 20

The most common cause of leg swelling is oedema—the abnormal accumulation of fluid within the interstitial space. Oedema may result from:

- ↑ Hydrostatic pressure in the venous system due to ↑ intravascular volume or obstruction
- ↓ Plasma proteins, mainly albumin, that retain fluid within the vascular compartment (↓ 'oncotic' pressure)
- ↑ Capillary permeability or
- Obstruction to lymphatic drainage: 'lymphoedema'

Unilateral oedema usually indicates localized pathology, such as venous or lymphatic obstruction. Bilateral oedema may be due to a local cause but more often represents the combination of generalized fluid overload and gravity causing oedema to pool at the lowest point. Oedema is frequently multifactorial, so search for additional causes, even if you identify a possible culprit.

Generalized oedema

Cardiogenic causes

Cardiogenic lower limb oedema is typically accompanied by other signs of volume overload ± structural heart disease (Fig. 20.1). In congestive cardiac failure (CCF), salt and water retention due to persistent neurohormonal activation leads to an ↑ in intravascular volume. High systemic venous hydrostatic pressure may also be caused by high right ventricular filling pressures if there is concomitant right heart failure. Right heart failure may arise from biventricular failure, pulmonary hypertension (e.g., chronic lung disease, thromboembolism or primary pulmonary vascular disease), pericardial disease (e.g., constriction, tamponade) or primary right heart pathology (e.g., pulmonary/tricuspid valve disease, right ventricle infarction, arrhythmogenic right ventricle cardiomyopathy).

Renal failure

In advanced renal failure, ↓ salt and water excretion results in fluid retention and ↑ systemic venous hydrostatic pressure. Chronic renal failure and heart failure commonly coexist (cardiorenal syndrome) and both may contribute to generalized oedema.

Hypoalbuminaemia

Hypoalbuminaemia produces oedema by ↓ plasma oncotic pressure. Causes include nephrotic syndrome (↑ albumin loss in urine); systemic inflammatory processes (leakage of albumin from the intravascular space due to increased capillary permeability ± persistent synthesis of acute-phase proteins, such as CRP in preference to albumin); protein-losing enteropathy (leakage of albumin into the gut due to lymphatic obstruction or mucosal disease); and advanced malnutrition.

Cirrhosis

Liver cirrhosis causes oedema through a combination of hypoalbuminaemia and ↑ hydrostatic pressure secondary to ↑ intravascular volume. Hypoalbuminaemia is caused by reduced hepatic synthesis of albumin. Intravascular volume increases due to salt and water retention as a result of neurohormonal activation in response to splanchnic and systemic vasodilation.

Iatrogenic causes

Box 20.1 lists common pharmacological causes of oedema.

Local causes of oedema

Deep vein thrombosis

DVT causes local oedema due to physical obstruction of venous drainage. Clinical features may include swelling, pain, warmth, and erythema but are unreliable; D-dimer and/or

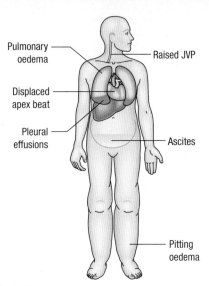

Pulmonary oedema

Displaced apex beat

Pleural effusions

Raised JVP

Ascites

Pitting oedema

Fig. 20.1 Clinical features of heart failure.

Box 20.1 Drugs causing oedema

- Calcium channel blockers
- IV fluids
- Corticosteroids
- Mineralocorticoids (fludrocortisone)
- Thiazolidinediones ('glitazones')
- Gabapentin/Pregabalin
- Withdrawal of diuretics
- NSAIDs
- Oestrogens
- Progestogens
- Testosterone
- Growth hormone

Box 20.2 Skin changes in chronic venous insufficiency

- Haemosiderin pigmentation
- Atrophy
- Hair loss
- Varicose eczema
- Induration and fibrosis of subcutaneous tissues
- Ulceration

Doppler ultrasound are integral to diagnosis. Rarely, bilateral or inferior vena caval thrombosis may cause bilateral swelling. Identification of DVT is essential as it could lead to a potentially fatal PE.

Chronic venous insufficiency

Chronic venous insufficiency is the most common cause of chronic unilateral and bilateral leg swelling. Incompetent valves in the deep and perforating veins impair venous return with a rise in hydrostatic pressure. There may be varicose veins and characteristic skin changes (Box 20.2, Figure 20.2).

Immobility

In patients with prolonged immobility, the loss of the venous pumping action of skeletal muscle causes ↑ venous hydrostatic pressure and oedema. This can be unilateral (e.g., post-stroke) or bilateral (e.g., critical care patients).

Pelvic mass

A pelvic mass may obstruct local venous drainage and increase hydrostatic pressure by directly compressing pelvic veins. With ovarian tumours, oedema is usually unilateral. Bilateral oedema is common in pregnancy because of ↑ blood volume and bilateral venous compression by the gravid uterus, but the diagnosis is usually obvious; suspect DVT if there is a sudden increase in leg swelling, particularly in the third trimester.

Lymphoedema

Lymphoedema is commonly caused by malignancy (lymphatic invasion or lymphoma), previous lymph node surgery or radiotherapy, filariasis and congenital lymphatic abnormalities. Early lymphoedema may be pitting and indistinguishable from other forms of oedema; with progression it becomes firm and nonpitting with characteristic skin changes (see below).

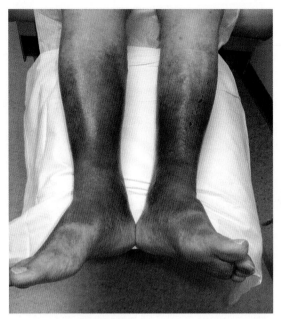

Figure 20.2 Skin changes in chronic venous insufficiency—haemosiderin pigmentation and small venous ulcers.
(From Creager MA, Beckman JA, Loscalzo J. Vascular medicine: a companion to Braunwald's heart disease, 3rd ed. Philadelphia: Elsevier; 2020.)

▌ Other causes

Compartment syndrome (↑ pressure, vascular compromise and tissue injury within a fascial compartment), rupture of a Baker cyst (a swelling of the semi-membranous bursa at the back of the knee), superficial thrombophlebitis and cellulitis may all present with an acutely painful, swollen leg.

Pretibial myxoedema is an abnormal dermal accumulation of connective tissue components in Graves disease. It causes areas of nonpitting oedema on the anterior or lateral aspects of the legs, with pink/purple plaques or nodules. Most patients will have evidence of Graves ophthalmopathy.

20

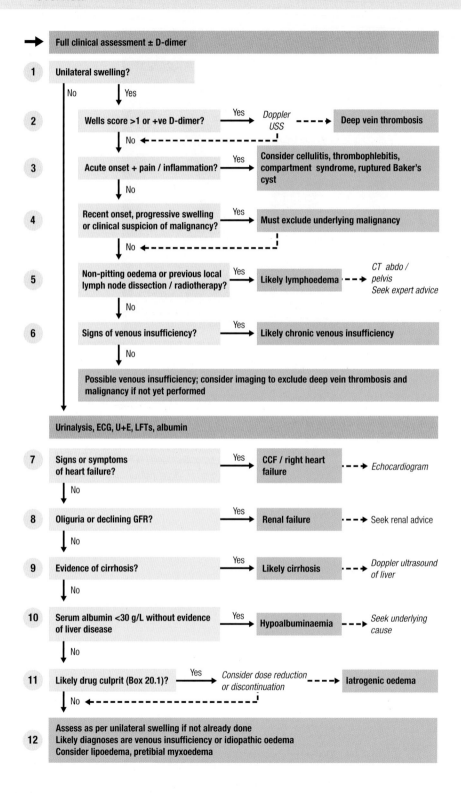

Full clinical assessment ± D-dimer

1 Unilateral swelling?

No   Yes

2 Wells score >1 or +ve D-dimer?   Yes → *Doppler USS* - - - → **Deep vein thrombosis**

No ← - - - - - - - - - - - - - -

3 Acute onset + pain / inflammation?   Yes → **Consider cellulitis, thrombophlebitis, compartment syndrome, ruptured Baker's cyst**

No

4 Recent onset, progressive swelling or clinical suspicion of malignancy?   Yes → **Must exclude underlying malignancy**

No ← - - - - - - - -

5 Non-pitting oedema or previous local lymph node dissection / radiotherapy?   Yes → **Likely lymphoedema** - - → *CT abdo / pelvis Seek expert advice*

No

6 Signs of venous insufficiency?   Yes → **Likely chronic venous insufficiency**

No

Possible venous insufficiency; consider imaging to exclude deep vein thrombosis and malignancy if not yet performed

Urinalysis, ECG, U+E, LFTs, albumin

7 Signs or symptoms of heart failure?   Yes → **CCF / right heart failure** - - → *Echocardiogram*

No

8 Oliguria or declining GFR?   Yes → **Renal failure** - - → Seek renal advice

No

9 Evidence of cirrhosis?   Yes → **Likely cirrhosis** - - → *Doppler ultrasound of liver*

No

10 Serum albumin <30 g/L without evidence of liver disease   Yes → **Hypoalbuminaemia** - - → *Seek underlying cause*

No

11 Likely drug culprit (Box 20.1)?   Yes → *Consider dose reduction or discontinuation* - - - → **Iatrogenic oedema**

No ← - - - - - - - - - - - - - - -

12 **Assess as per unilateral swelling if not already done**
Likely diagnoses are venous insufficiency or idiopathic oedema
Consider lipoedema, pretibial myxoedema

1 Unilateral swelling?

Examine both limbs for evidence of swelling and pitting. If there is bilateral lower limb swelling, even if asymmetrical, go to step 7.

2 Wells score >1 or +ve D-dimer?

Consider DVT in any patient with unilateral limb swelling, even without apparent risk factors or other signs or symptoms. Pretest clinical prediction tools, such as Wells score (Table 20.1), can guide further investigation. Evaluate for bilateral DVT in any patient with risk factors and bilateral leg swelling.

- If Wells score is ≥2, DVT is likely—arrange a Doppler USS to confirm/refute the diagnosis.
- If Wells score is <2, perform a D-dimer blood test. If negative, DVT is excluded; if positive, arrange a Doppler USS.
- Arrange Doppler USS in all pregnant patients with suspected DVT, as exclusion

by D-dimer has not been validated in this group.

3 Acute onset + pain/inflammation?

Consider cellulitis if swelling is accompanied by a discrete area of erythema, heat, swelling and pain ± fever or ↑ WBC/CRP; negative blood cultures/skin swabs do not rule out the diagnosis. Note that bilateral cellulitis is uncommon, and bilateral leg swelling and erythema is more likely to represent chronic venous insufficiency with varicose eczema. Nonetheless, skin changes in chronic venous insufficiency can serve as an entry point for unilateral cellulitis, and this should be considered in patients with an exacerbation of their symptoms.

In superficial thrombophlebitis, signs are localized, with redness and tenderness along the course of a vein, which may be firm and palpable.

A ruptured Baker cyst may be clinically indistinguishable from DVT; USS will reveal the diagnosis and exclude DVT.

Consider compartment syndrome if unilateral limb swelling is accompanied by any of the features in Box 20.3; if suspected, check CK (rhabdomyolysis) and arrange urgent orthopaedic review.

Table 20.1 Wells score (Deep Vein Thrombosis)

Clinical feature	Score
Active cancer (treatment within last 6 months or palliative)	+1 point
Paralysis, paresis or recent plaster immobilization of leg	+1 point
Recently bedridden >3 days or major surgery under general/regional anaesthesia in previous 12 weeks	+1 point
Local tenderness along distribution of deep venous system	+1 point
Entire leg swollen	+1 point
Calf swelling >3 cm compared to asymptomatic leg (measured 10 cm below tibial tuberosity)	+1 point
Pitting oedema confined to symptomatic leg	+1 point
Collateral superficial veins (nonvaricose)	+1 point
Alternative diagnosis at least as likely as DVT, such as cellulitis, thrombophlebitis	−2 points

From Wells PS, Anderson DR, Bormanis J, et al. Value of assessment of pretest probability of deep-vein thrombosis in clinical management. Lancet 350(9094):1795–1798, 1997.

Box 20.3 Features of compartment syndrome

Clinical context

Lower limb fracture, trauma, crush injury, vascular injury
    ↓GCS score

Symptoms

Pain (especially if increasing or deep/aching)
    Paraesthesia/numbness
    Paresis/paralysis

Signs

Pain on passive muscle stretching
    Tense, firm or 'woody' feel on palpation
    ↓ Capillary refill or absent distal pulses
    Muscle contracture

Investigations

↑↑CK

20

4 Recent onset, progressive swelling or clinical suspicion of malignancy?

A pelvic or lower abdominal mass may produce leg swelling by compressing the pelvic veins or lymphatics. Exclude underlying malignancy if any of the following is present:

- Weight loss
- Previous pelvic cancer
- Features suggestive of localized pelvic cancer (e.g., haematuria, intermenstrual PV bleeding)
- A palpable mass or local lymphadenopathy
- Any new-onset, progressive, unilateral leg swelling with no clear alternative explanation

Perform a rectal ± vaginal examination, check PSA level (males) and arrange imaging with USS (transabdominal or transvaginal) or CT as appropriate.

5 Nonpitting oedema or previous local lymph node dissection/radiotherapy?

Distinguish lymphoedema from other causes of swelling, as it is unlikely to respond to conventional treatments and should prompt consideration of an underlying malignancy (new or recurrent). Consider the diagnosis if any of the following is present:

- Previous pelvic malignancy, local radiotherapy or lymph node dissection
- Known or family history of congenital lymphatic anomaly
- Oedema that is firm and nonpitting
- Inability to pinch the dorsal aspect of skin at the base of the second toe (Stemmer sign)
- Thickening of overlying skin with warty or 'cobblestone' appearance

If you suspect lymphoedema, seek expert advice and consider CT of the pelvis and abdomen to look for evidence of underlying malignancy unless there is a clear antecedent cause (e.g., lymph node dissection).

6 Signs of venous insufficiency?

Suspect chronic venous insufficiency if any of the following is present:

- Characteristic skin changes (Box 20.2)
- Prominent varicosities in the affected limb

- Previous DVT or vein stripping/harvesting in the affected limb
- Longstanding pitting oedema with diurnal variation in a patient >50 years

If none of these is present, reconsider the need to exclude underlying DVT and malignancy, and assess as described for bilateral leg swelling to look for a cause of generalized oedema.

7 Signs or symptoms of heart failure?

↑ JVP signifies high central venous pressure (due to volume overload and/or ↑cardiac filling pressures) and therefore implies a cardiogenic/renal cause for bilateral pitting oedema. Assume CCF if patients also have suggestive symptoms (orthopnoea, paroxysmal nocturnal dyspnoea, recent-onset exertional dyspnoea), a background of left ventricle dysfunction, MI or left-sided valve disease or (irrespective of the JVP) clinical or CXR features of pulmonary congestion. Bear in mind the possibility of right heart failure secondary to pulmonary hypertension (or less commonly right heart disease) in patients with severe chronic lung disease or clear lung fields. Arrange an echocardiogram to assess for cardiac structure and function and consider referral to the appropriate specialty.

8 Oligouria or declining GFR?

Reduced salt and water excretion in advanced renal failure results in volume overload even in patients without heart failure. Presenting features may include ↑ JVP, bilateral oedema, hypertension, and symptoms and signs of pulmonary congestion (e.g., dyspnoea, paroxysmal nocturnal dyspnoea, orthopnoea, and bilateral lung crepitations).

Consider renal impairment as a cause or contributor to fluid retention if oliguric, GFR <30 mL/minute or GFR rapidly falling. Seek renal advice.

9 Evidence of cirrhosis?

Suspect oedema secondary to cirrhosis in patients with:

- Jaundice
- Ascites

- Peripheral stigmata of liver disease (Box 12.3)
- Hepatosplenomegaly
- LFT derangement
- Coagulopathy
- Hypoalbuminaemia

If these features are present, arrange Doppler US of the liver and consider referral to Hepatology.

| 10 | **Serum albumin <30 g/L without evidence of liver disease?** |

Hypoalbuminaemia may cause or contribute to oedema, particularly when <25 g/L. Search for an underlying cause.

Screen for nephrotic syndrome by urinalysis, looking for proteinuria. If the test is positive, perform a spot urine protein-creatinine ratio (PCR); a result >300 mg/µmol is diagnostic. Refer patients with diagnostic PCRs to Renal.

A persistent acute-phase response (resulting in ↓albumin synthesis) may occur in chronic infection, inflammatory illness or occult malignancy. Suspect this if the patient has a persistently ↑CRP/ESR, recurrent pyrexia, lymphadenopathy, constitutional upset (fever, sweats, malaise, weight loss) or local signs or symptoms, such as palpable mass, active synovitis—investigate as for fever/pyrexia of unknown origin (Chapter 26).

Consider protein-losing enteropathy, and seek GI advice if there is a history or symptoms of GI disorder. Malnutrition must be prolonged and severe to cause a significant decrease in serum albumin and is a diagnosis of exclusion.

| 11 | **Likely drug culprit (see Box 20.1)?** |

Potential drug causes are listed in Box 20.1. Where feasible, review after trial discontinuation.

| 12 | **Assess as per unilateral swelling. Likely venous insufficiency or idiopathic oedema** |

When there is bilateral swelling, first return to step 1 and assess for 'unilateral' causes, such as bilateral DVT.

Venous insufficiency is the likeliest cause in patients >50 years or in those with skin changes/predisposing factors. Dependent oedema may occur with longstanding immobility.

If pitting is absent, consider lipoedema or pretibial myxoedema.

20

Medicine of the Elderly

Confusion: delirium and dementia

Confusion is an impairment of cognitive function. In older patients presenting with confusion, it is important to distinguish between delirium and dementia as, despite its reversibility, delirium increases risk of medical complications, accelerated cognitive and functional decline, institutionalization and death.

Delirium is an acute decline in cognition that follows a fluctuating course and is accompanied by impaired attention (e.g., easily distracted, unable to maintain focus), and disturbed consciousness ('hyperalert'/agitated or drowsy/↓awareness). Common associated features include reversal of the sleep–wake cycle, hallucinations, delusions and altered emotion/psychomotor behaviour.

Dementia is an often progressive decline in an individual's function across one or more cognitive domains that impairs their ability to independently perform activities of daily living. Memory is normally impaired, but other cognitive domains that can be affected include executive function, language, attention, social cognition, and perceptual-motor skills. To diagnose dementia, cognitive changes must not be attributable to delirium.

The initial challenge with confused patients is identifying them. Agitated, restless patients rapidly attract attention, but those with 'hypoactive delirium' are quiet, withdrawn and easily missed. In patients with preexisting dementia, delirium may be overlooked unless baseline cognitive function is established.

Disorders such as depression, deafness, dysphasia, psychosis, and amnesic syndromes may also mimic confusion.

Delirium

Delirium occurs as the outcome of the interaction between predisposing patient factors (Box 21.1) and precipitating insults. Frailty is a common predisposing factor and should be considered in all patients presenting with delirium (Clinical Tool). Severe illness can cause delirium in any patient, but it is more likely to develop in response to relatively minor physiological insults in those with predisposing factors.

Potential precipitants for delirium are wide ranging and include almost any acute physical, mental or environmental insult. It is often triggered by more than one coexisting cause. Management involves identifying and treating all potential precipitants. Some causes are listed below.

Drugs

- Alcohol[a]
- Opioids[a]
- Benzodiazepines[a]
- Anticonvulsants
- Tricyclic antidepressants[a]
- Anticholinergics
- Antihistamines
- Antipsychotics[a]
- Lithium
- Corticosteroids (especially high-dose)
- Baclofen
- Levodopa/dopamine agonists
- Digoxin

Metabolic/physiological disturbance

- Hypoxia
- Hypercapnia
- Shock
- Hypo-/hyperthermia
- Hypo-/hyperglycaemia
- Hyponatraemia
- Hypo-/hypercalcaemia
- Dehydration
- Uraemia

---

[a] Indicates that confusion may arise from either drug effects or withdrawal

---

Box 21.1 Predisposing factors for delirium

- Age > 70 years
- Frailty
- Comorbid medical conditions, particularly neurological disease
- Dementia
- Visual or hearing impairment
- Depression
- History of delirium
- Alcohol misuse
- Polypharmacy

- Metabolic acidosis
- Hepatic encephalopathy
- Hypo-/hyperthyroidism

Infection

- Sepsis
- CNS infection:
  - Meningitis (bacterial, viral, fungal, tuberculosis)
  - Encephalitis
  - Cerebral abscess
- Non-CNS infection:
  - Pneumonia
  - Urinary tract
  - Biliary/intra-abdominal
  - Endocarditis

Intracranial causes

- Seizures (postictal state)
- Haemorrhage
- Ischaemic stroke
- Space-occupying lesion
- Head injury
- ↑ Intracranial pressure

Other causes

- Pain
- Postoperative
- Change in environment
- Constipation
- Urinary retention

- Acute abdominal pathology (pancreatitis, appendicitis)
- MI
- Carbon monoxide toxicity
- Acute thiamine deficiency (Wernicke encephalopathy)
- Sleep deprivation
- Unusual stimuli and sensory impairment

Dementia/chronic cognitive impairment

Most cases of dementia are caused by either neurodegenerative conditions or vascular disease. However, there are some subacute presentations of dementia which are reversible. Identification and treatment of these is essential to restore cognitive function.

Common causes

- Alzheimer's disease
- Vascular dementia
- Lewy body dementia

Reversible causes

- Vitamin B_{12}/folate deficiency
- Subdural haemorrhage
- Brain tumour
- Hypothyroidism
- Normal-pressure hydrocephalus
- HIV
- Neurosyphilis
- Wilson's disease
- Acute intermittent porphyria
- Cerebral vasculitis
- Lyme disease

Other causes

- Frontotemporal dementias
- Korsakoff psychosis
- Multiple sclerosis
- Progressive supranuclear palsy
- Heavy metal exposure
- (Variant) Creutzfeldt–Jakob disease
- Huntington's disease

Clinical tool
Diagnosing frailty and the Comprehensive Geriatric Assessment

Frailty

Frailty is a state of increased vulnerability to sudden decline in health or functional status in response to stressor events. Many elderly patients are not frail, but frailty should be specifically considered in any patients presenting with the 'frailty syndromes' of:

- Falls
- Immobility
- Delirium and dementia
- Urinary incontinence
- Susceptibility to side effects of medication

In patients in whom frailty is suspected, use the Clinical Frailty Scale (CFS, Fig. 21.1) to identify the patient's level of frailty 2 weeks prior to your assessment. Local guidelines will vary, but consider referral of patients who score ≥5 for Comprehensive Geriatric Assessment (CGA).

CGA is the gold standard for identifying and managing frailty. The CGA is a multidisciplinary assessment of a patient's physical and psychological health, mental capability, and functional ability in order to develop a detailed problem list with an associated management and follow-up plan. Frail inpatients who receive CGA have improved functional outcome, are more likely to be discharged home and are less likely to die in hospital.

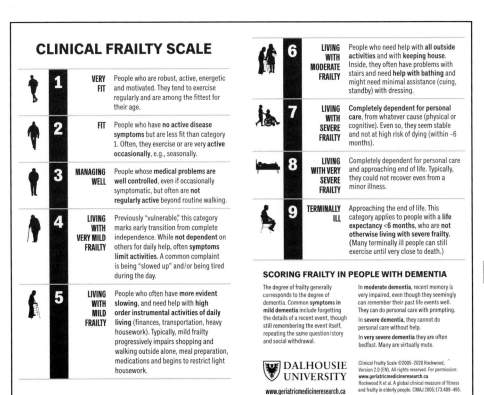

Fig. 21.1 **Clinical Frailty Scale.** (Note for Creative Commons: This figure appears as Fig. 17.1 in Rockwood K, O Theou O. Using the Clinical Frailty Scale in allocating scarce resources. Canadian Geriatrics Journal 23:211;2020.)

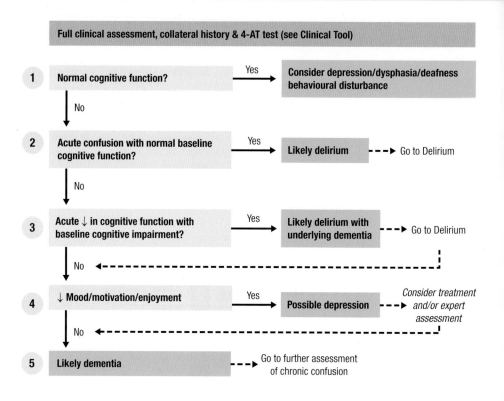

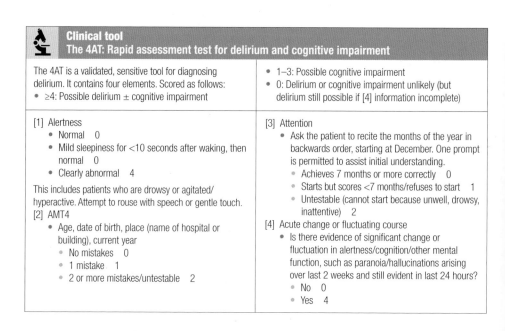

1 Normal cognitive function?

Disorientation, forgetfulness and muddled thinking may be apparent from normal conversation but confirm with an objective assessment, such as the 4AT (Clinical tool). Use this tool to screen for confusion in all patients with predisposing factors for delirium (Box 21.1). Ensure that apparent cognitive impairment is not due to communication problems (e.g., deafness, dysarthria, language barriers) or an isolated disorder of comprehension (receptive dysphasia), word-finding difficulty (expressive dysphasia), memory (amnesic syndrome), behaviour or mood. Optimize any communication difficulties prior to assessing cognition. Patients with depression often score poorly in formal testing through refusal to volunteer answers rather than making mistakes—if these patients are encouraged (or treated), performance may improve.

2 Acute confusion with normal baseline cognitive function?

In any patient with confusion, establish baseline cognitive function. Confused patients will not be able to reliably report their normal level of cognitive function, so a collateral history from relatives/friends/carers is essential. If cognitive assessments have previously been performed, they will also be helpful in establishing cognitive baseline. Thorough questioning is important as relatives may have the impression that baseline cognition was normal – as the patient was in a familiar environment, seeing familiar people, talking about familiar topics and not being pressed on recent events – even if baseline cognition was, in fact, impaired.

In patients with acute confusion, use the 4AT assessment test (Clinical tool) to diagnose delirium. A score of ≥ 4 in a patient with a normal baseline cognitive function is suggestive of delirium.

3 Acute ↓cognitive function with baseline cognitive impairment?

When impaired baseline cognitive function is established, look for any evidence of an acute change. Delirium is frequently superimposed on dementia (acute on chronic confusion)—look for important clues such as sudden decline in cognitive abilities, alteration of consciousness, fluctuating course, and difficulty concentrating. Spend time speaking with the patient and their family and observing behaviour. Seek evidence of fluctuation through discussion with nursing staff or review of overnight reports. A 4AT score of ≥4 on a background of cognitive impairment suggests delirium with underlying dementia.

4 ↓Mood/motivation/enjoyment?

Depression can mimic or exacerbate dementia. Ask patients if they feel low in mood but also enquire about things they take pleasure in (Do they still enjoy them?), as well as biological symptoms (e.g., early morning waking, ↓ appetite, ↓ weight). During conversation, note expressions of guilt, worthlessness, pessimism, and other negative thoughts (especially if exaggerated or incongruent with circumstances) and look for psychomotor slowing, lack of depth or variety in affect, and poor eye contact. Scoring systems, such as the Geriatric Depression Scale (GDS), may assist diagnosis. If uncertain, refer for specialist evaluation or reassess after a trial of treatment.

5 Likely dementia

21

There is no absolute division between acute and chronic confusion in terms of timing or causes. Even if the cause has been removed, it can take months for a delirium to resolve fully. Further, chronic confusion can fluctuate. However, if confusion has persisted for >12 weeks without an obvious acute cause or evidence of improvement, see Further assessment of chronic confusion.

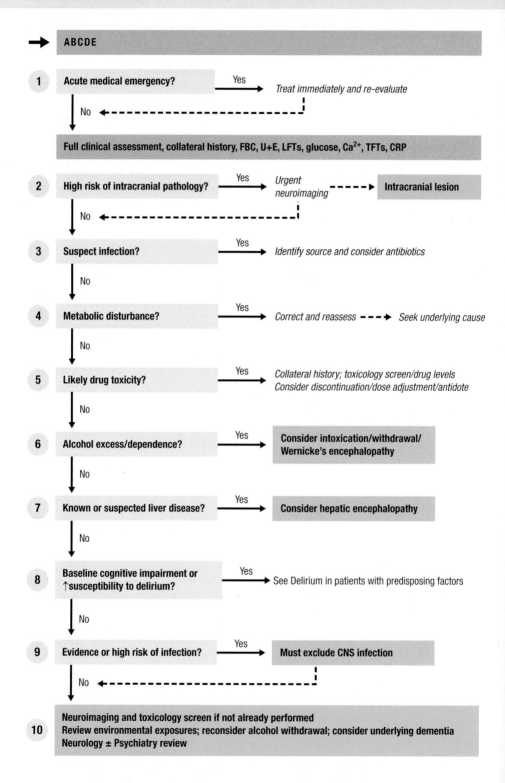

ABCDE

1 **Acute medical emergency?** — Yes → *Treat immediately and re-evaluate*

No

Full clinical assessment, collateral history, FBC, U+E, LFTs, glucose, Ca²⁺, TFTs, CRP

2 **High risk of intracranial pathology?** — Yes → *Urgent neuroimaging* - - - → **Intracranial lesion**

No

3 **Suspect infection?** — Yes → *Identify source and consider antibiotics*

No

4 **Metabolic disturbance?** — Yes → *Correct and reassess* - - → *Seek underlying cause*

No

5 **Likely drug toxicity?** — Yes → *Collateral history; toxicology screen/drug levels Consider discontinuation/dose adjustment/antidote*

No

6 **Alcohol excess/dependence?** — Yes → **Consider intoxication/withdrawal/ Wernicke's encephalopathy**

No

7 **Known or suspected liver disease?** — Yes → **Consider hepatic encephalopathy**

No

8 **Baseline cognitive impairment or ↑susceptibility to delirium?** — Yes → See Delirium in patients with predisposing factors

No

9 **Evidence or high risk of infection?** — Yes → **Must exclude CNS infection**

No

10 **Neuroimaging and toxicology screen if not already performed Review environmental exposures; reconsider alcohol withdrawal; consider underlying dementia Neurology ± Psychiatry review**

1 Acute medical emergency?

Evaluate and treat respiratory failure (Chapter 4), shock (Chapter 2), depressed consciousness (Chapter 15), hypothermia and seizure (Chapter 24) before considering other causes of delirium. Exclude new or worsening hypercapnia in any patient with chronic type 2 respiratory failure or significant chronic lung disease. If the capillary blood glucose is <4.0 mmol/L, send blood for laboratory glucose measurement but treat immediately, without waiting for the result. Reassess if confusion persists despite effective correction.

2 High risk of intracranial pathology?

Consider urgent CT brain to exclude a structural CNS cause if any of the following are present:
- New focal neurological signs or ataxia
- First seizure
- Drowsiness (if you suspect opioid toxicity, give a trial of naloxone before CT)
- Recent head injury
- Sudden severe headache
- Any fall/trauma in a patient on anticoagulation

In patients with active malignancy, immunosuppression or recent falls, look for other causes of delirium, but have a low threshold for early neuroimaging to exclude intracranial metastases/abscess/haemorrhage.

3 Suspect infection?

Infection is a common cause of delirium, and delirium may be the only presenting feature of infections in patients with predisposing factors (Box 21.1). Evaluate for infection as described in Chapter 26, but note that frail patients may not present with typical symptoms or signs and may not have fever. In this group, consider empirical antibiotic treatment if there is a convincing focus of infection even in the absence of ↑ temperature/WBC/CRP, but weigh the likelihood of bacterial infection against complications such as GI upset or *Clostridium difficile* diarrhoea. Be careful when attributing delirium to UTI in the elderly as asymptomatic bacteriuria is common. Ensure that there are no

other precipitants for delirium, and treat only if there is sufficient evidence of infection (e.g., fever, dysuria, new incontinence).

Meningitis/encephalitis is a less common cause of delirium in vulnerable patients but should be higher up the differential list in young, fit people presenting with delirium. Assume meningitis/encephalitis if the patient has meningism (Box 13.2), a purpuric rash or a febrile illness with headache, seizures, focal neurological signs or no obvious alternative source. Initiate management as described in Chapter 13.

4 Metabolic disturbance?

Review blood chemistry for metabolic disturbance; check laboratory glucose, even if capillary BG is within the normal range. The healthy brain is relatively resistant to metabolic insult so do not attribute confusion solely to modest biochemical derangement. However, delirium is likely to be explained by hypoglycaemia, hypothyroidism or, if severe, dehydration, acidosis, ↓Na^+ (especially <120 mmol/L), ↑Ca^{2+} (>3.0 mmol/L) or hyperglycaemia (e.g., hyperosmolar hyperglycaemic state; Table 25.2). In patients with severe AKI, confusion due to toxic accumulation of medication or uraemic encephalopathy should be considered.

Patients predisposed to delirium are more sensitive to metabolic derangement; even mild dehydration, renal impairment or glycaemic/electrolyte/thyroid disturbance may impair cognition. Correct any disturbances but continue to search for additional contributing factors.

See Further assessment of hyponatraemia in any patient with unexplained ↓Na^+.

5 Likely drug toxicity?

Illicit drug use or poisoning

Substance misuse is a common cause of acute confusion/psychosis in younger patients. Assess as described in the chapter on Poisoning (Chapter 28).

Prescribed medication

Anticonvulsants, opioids, sedatives and lithium can cause confusion, even in normally healthy

21

patients. Many other drugs may precipitate delirium in vulnerable patients (Box 21.1), especially tricyclic antidepressants, anticholinergics, opiates, benzodiazepines, and antihistamines. Even if they are normally well tolerated, these agents may contribute to delirium in the context of other acute insults. Benzodiazepines can have a paradoxical effect, worsening confusion and agitation. Abrupt withdrawal of benzodiazepines and opioids can also precipitate delirium, often several days after stopping.

Verify all drugs and dosages with the patient/relatives/carers. Check how frequently PRN medications, especially benzodiazepines and opioids, are used at home and ensure they have not been inadvertently omitted, reduced, or reinstated in hospital. Consider a trial cessation or ↓ dose of any drug with potential CNS side effects, especially when recently introduced or increased. Weigh the likelihood of toxicity against ongoing treatment benefit and predictable problems on discontinuation. Where necessary, taper the dose gradually to avoid withdrawal symptoms.

6 Alcohol excess/dependence?

Acute alcohol intoxication

Acute alcohol intoxication is the most common cause of altered mental status presenting in the emergency department but may coexist with other pathology, such as head injury, liver injury, nutritional deficiency. Confirm the presence of alcohol with breath or blood tests but always search for additional causes of confusion.

Alcohol withdrawal

This may present early (e.g., 6–12 hours after cessation of drinking) or late (e.g., 2–3 days after hospital admission). Typical symptoms include confusion, agitation, hallucinations and adrenergic overstimulation (tremor, sweating, tachycardia). The diagnosis is obvious in patients with a florid presentation and clear history of alcohol excess/dependence but consider it in all cases of unexplained delirium. Screen all patients for alcohol problems (Box 21.2). If in doubt, obtain a collateral history. Seizures may complicate

---

> **Box 21.2 Features of alcohol dependence in the history**
>
> - A strong, often overpowering, desire to take alcohol
> - Inability to control starting or stopping drinking and the amount that is drunk
> - Drinking alcohol in the morning
> - Tolerance, where increased doses are needed to achieve the effects originally produced by lower doses
> - Withdrawal state when drinking is stopped or reduced, including tremor, sweating, rapid heart rate, anxiety, insomnia and occasionally seizures, disorientation or hallucinations (delirium tremens). It is relieved by more alcohol.
> - Neglect of other pleasures and interests
> - Continuing to drink in spite of being aware of the harmful consequences

severe withdrawal but consider neuroimaging if first fit, focal neurological signs or evidence of head injury.

Wernicke encephalopathy

Consider thiamine deficiency and give supplementation in all patients with acute confusion on a background of chronic alcohol excess. Consider a diagnosis of Wernicke encephalopathy if there is short-term memory loss, diplopia, gaze palsy, nystagmus, ataxia, or severe malnutrition.

7 Known or suspected liver disease?

Suspect hepatic encephalopathy in any patient with an existing diagnosis or clinical features of cirrhosis. Constructional apraxia (inability to draw a star) and/or asterixis, together with the absence of florid hallucinations/adrenergic features, may differentiate hepatic encephalopathy from alcohol withdrawal in patients with alcoholic liver disease. If you suspect encephalopathy, seek and treat potential precipitants as described in Chapter 12.

8 Baseline cognitive impairment or ↑susceptibility to delirium?

The diagnostic approach now depends on the patient's threshold for developing delirium. If any feature in Box 21.1 is present, proceed to Delirium in patients with predisposing factors.

9   Evidence or high risk of infection?

If not already carried out, perform neuroimaging and LP to exclude CNS infection and structural djsease. If CT is nondiagnostic, consider MRI brain.

10   Neuroimaging and toxicology screen. Consider other causes. Consider underlying demetia. Neurology ± Psychiatry review.

Consider causes of subacute presentations of confusion such as B_{12}/folate deficiency, HIV, neurosyphilis, Lyme disease, Wilson disease, porphyria and heavy metal poisoning, and investigate with blood and urine tests if appropriate.

Check carboxyhaemoglobin levels for CO toxicity if there is associated headache or if the patient has been exposed to smoke/exhaust fumes (though levels may correlate poorly with symptoms).

If the cause is still not apparent, seek expert Neurological ± Psychiatric input. EEG may assist in the diagnosis of atypical seizures, toxic encephalopathies or unusual neurodegenerative diseases.

In frail, elderly patients, it is possible for delirium to persist for months despite optimal management. Delirium increases the risk of subsequent cognitive impairment, and it may unmask an underlying dementia. Expert input from Old-age Psychiatry may be required to differentiate between persistent delirium and a new permanent cognitive impairment. In patients who have dementia, a new delirium may result in a permanent decline in mental and physical functioning.

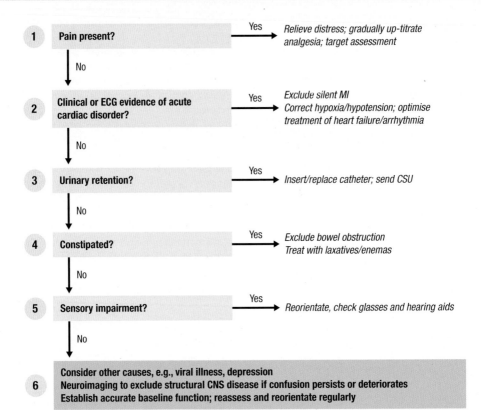

1 Pain present? — Yes → *Relieve distress; gradually up-titrate analgesia; target assessment*

No ↓

2 Clinical or ECG evidence of acute cardiac disorder? — Yes → *Exclude silent MI*
Correct hypoxia/hypotension; optimise treatment of heart failure/arrhythmia

No ↓

3 Urinary retention? — Yes → *Insert/replace catheter; send CSU*

No ↓

4 Constipated? — Yes → *Exclude bowel obstruction*
Treat with laxatives/enemas

No ↓

5 Sensory impairment? — Yes → *Reorientate, check glasses and hearing aids*

No ↓

6 **Consider other causes, e.g., viral illness, depression**
Neuroimaging to exclude structural CNS disease if confusion persists or deteriorates
Establish accurate baseline function; reassess and reorientate regularly

1 Pain present?

Pain can cause or contribute to delirium in vulnerable patients and may be difficult to assess if the patient is agitated or muddled. Have a high index of suspicion for bony injury (e.g., hip fracture) in patients who have a history of recent falls. Wherever possible, identify and treat the underlying cause using simple analgesia/nonpharmacological measures as first-line treatment but do not leave patients in distress. Where opioids are required, carefully up-titrate and monitor.

2 Clinical or ECG evidence of acute cardiac disorder?

Occasionally, MI presents as delirium. Seek urgent cardiology input if the ECG meets the criteria for ST-elevation MI. Check troponin and assess further for acute coronary syndrome if there are other indicative ECG changes (Box 3.2). Cardiac failure may contribute to delirium through hypoxia or cerebral hypoperfusion. Avoid hypotension where possible (review medication) and correct hypoxia and anaemia. Treat any brady- or tachyarrhythmias and consider diuretic if there is fluid overload.

3 Urinary retention?

Delirium may be the only sign of urinary retention in older adults. Retention may be suggested by a palpable bladder on abdominal examination. Arrange a postvoid bladder scan. If there is a postvoid residual volume of >300 mL, insert a urinary catheter and send a CSU. Assess for potential causes of urinary retention as per Chapter 23.

4 Constipated?

Establish how regularly the patient moves their bowels. If there is concern about constipation, perform a PR to assess for faecal impaction. Start laxatives and consider suppositories/enemas if the rectum is full.

5 Sensory impairment?

Patients with moderate to severe dementia are at high risk of becoming acutely confused when presented with unusual surroundings, people and stimuli. Provide frequent reassurance and reorientation, encourage visits from family members, check that patients have their normal glasses and hearing aids, and ensure adequate lighting.

6 Reassess, consider rarer causes

Once all potential precipitants for delirium have been identified and treated, it can take weeks for delirium to improve. However, worsening or prolonged delirium should prompt a full reassessment, paying particular attention to medications, pain, untreated infection, constipation, and metabolic disturbance. Consider rarer causes as described in Delirium: overview if no precipitant is identified or the patient's condition is deteriorating.

21

Further assessment of hyponatraemia

Step 1 Confirm true hyponatraemia

Apparent hyponatraemia may result from drip-arm contamination, laboratory/labeling error, or 'pseudohyponatraemia' due to hyperlipidaemia, hyperproteinaemia, hyperglycaemia or high plasma ethanol. Check plasma osmolality (usually normal in pseudohyponatraemia) and recheck Na^+ if the result appears spurious.

Step 2 Estimate the rate of Na^+ decline

A rapid ↓ in plasma Na^+ may lead to life-threatening cerebral oedema and requires prompt correction. In contrast, a gradual ↓ in Na^+ allows osmotic adaptation by cerebral neurons, and rapid correction may lead to irreversible brainstem damage (central pontine myelinolysis).

It is therefore critical to distinguish acute (<72 hours) from chronic (>72 hours) hyponatraemia. Suspect chronic if any of the following features are present:

- Recent U+E results demonstrating a progressive decline in plasma Na^+
- Lowly progressive onset of symptoms, such as anorexia, lethargy, confusion
- Asymptomatic or only mild symptoms with a plasma Na^+ ≤125 mmol/L
- No clear cause for a sudden decrease in plasma Na^+ (see below)

In these patients, correct Na^+ with extreme care. Recheck U+E every 2–4 hours and aim for a rise in plasma Na^+ of ≤10 mmol/L in the first 24 hours, and ≤8 mmol/L every 24 hours after that until a serum Na of 130 mmol/L is achieved.

Suspect acute hyponatraemia if:

- Abrupt onset of symptoms within the last 48 hours OR
- Major symptoms (severe confusion, ↓GCS, seizures) with Na^+ ≥120 mmol/L, especially with a history of sudden increase in free water intake, such as excessive IV dextrose administration (especially postoperatively) or polydipsia

Review for medications that can precipitate acute hyponatraemia, such as thiazides, cyclophosphamide, oxytoxin, desmopressin and terlipressin.

If you suspect acute hyponatraemia, or a patient has major symptoms of hyponatraemia, seek urgent expert advice but, in an emergency, aim to increase plasma Na^+ by 5 mmol/L in the first hour with hypertonic saline.

Step 3 Assess volume status

Clear evidence of either ↑ or ↓ extracellular fluid (ECF) volume is very helpful in determining the underlying cause. Categorize the patient as:

- Hypervolaemic if there is evidence of fluid overload, such as oedema, ↑JVP, ascites.
- Hypovolaemic if there is evidence of fluid depletion, such as dry mucous membranes, ↓skin turgor, thirst, ↓JVP.
- Euvolaemic if neither of the above is present.

The most common causes of hypervolaemic hyponatraemia are cardiac failure, cirrhosis, oliguric renal failure and nephrotic syndrome. If the cause is not obvious, check for proteinuria, perform an echocardiogram and assess for evidence of cirrhosis (Chapter 12).

In hypovolaemic hyponatraemia, there is Na^+ and water depletion, with relatively greater Na^+ loss. The most common causes are excessive diuretic therapy and acute diarrhoea/vomiting.

If the source of Na^+ and water loss is not obvious, measure urine sodium. The normal response of the kidneys to salt and water depletion is to minimize Na^+ excretion. If urine Na^+ is appropriately low (<20 mmol/L) suspect GI tract losses, e.g., diarrhoea, vomiting or 'third space' losses (e.g., pancreatitis, burns). If urine Na^+ is >20 mmol/L, then there is a contribution to salt and water depletion from renal losses, such as adrenal insufficiency, renal tubular acidosis or 'salt-wasting' renal disease.

Step 4 If euvolaemic, or if cause unclear, measure urine sodium and osmolality

If feasible, discontinue any diuretics for 10 days and recheck U+E alongside plasma and urine osmolality and urine Na^+.

Low urine Na^+ (<20 mmol/L) implies that ↓ plasma Na^+ is not due to excessive renal Na^+ losses. The cause may be hypovolaemic hyponatraemia due to extrarenal losses (see above), but without obvious clinical manifestations of hypovolaemia. In this case, urine osmolality will be ↑ (>150 mmol/kg) due to the presence of other solutes. If urine osmolality is <150 mmol/kg, the likely cause is excessive water intake. In hospitalized patients, check for recent administration of hypotonic IV fluids, e.g., 5% dextrose. In non-hospitalized patients consider psychogenic polydipsia.

If hyponatraemia is accompanied by ↑urine Na^+ (>20 mmol/L) and osmolality (>150 mmol/kg), consider diuretic use, adrenal insufficiency, hypothyroidism, salt-wasting renal disease and the syndrome of inappropriate antidiuretic hormone secretion (SIADH).

Check TFTs and a 9 a.m. cortisol. High or high–normal plasma urea/uric acid may indicate subtle ↓ ECF volume; if present, consider salt-wasting diseases or occult diuretic use. Otherwise, the likely diagnosis is SIADH.

If you suspect SIADH, look for an underlying cause (Box 21.3). Consider trial cessation of any suspected causative agent. If the cause remains unclear, request a CXR and CT brain and assess the response to fluid restriction (<1 L/day).

Box 21.3 Causes of SIADH

- Tumours, especially small-cell lung cancer
- CNS disorders: stroke, trauma, infection
- Pulmonary disorders e.g., pneumonia, tuberculosis
- Drugs
  - Anticonvulsants, e.g., carbamazepine
  - Psychotropics, e.g., haloperidol
  - Antidepressants, e.g., fluoxetine
  - Cytotoxics, e.g., cyclophosphamide
  - Hypoglycaemics, e.g., chlorpropamide
  - Opioids, e.g., morphine
  - Proton-pump inhibitors, e.g., omeprazole
- Sustained pain, stress, nausea, e.g., postoperative state
- Acute porphyria
- Idiopathic

Further assessment of chronic confusion

The approach to progressive cognitive decline over a period of months to years differs from the approach to acute confusion. Exclude the reversible causes (as described in Delirium) with a CT brain and blood tests; if no reversible cause is identified, refer for specialist evaluation and care.

Consider psychiatric illness

Perform an objective measure of cognition (e.g., Mini-Mental State Examination, Montreal Cognitive Assessment) to ensure the presentation fits with a chronic decline in cognition. Depression can mimic or exacerbate dementia and may be difficult to diagnose. Consider using tools such as the Cornell Scale for Depression in Dementia to assist diagnosis and, if you suspect depression, reassess cognitive function after a trial of antidepressant therapy.

Assess for reversible causes

Perform a CT brain in every patient with chronic confusion. This may identify reversible causes, for example, subdural haemorrhage or normal pressure hydrocephalus (ataxia and incontinence should raise the index of suspicion), or suggest possible aetiological factors, such as vascular disease. Measure TFTs in all patients, as hypothyroidism can present as dementia and responds to treatment. Take a careful alcohol history and consider Wernicke–Korsakoff syndrome in any patient with chronic alcohol misuse (Box 21.2). Look for and correct nutritional deficiencies, e.g., B_{12}, folate.

Consider rare causes

Perform a more intensive work-up if the patient has an unusual pattern of cognitive impairment, (e.g., preserved recent memory or personality/speech change), unexplained neurological findings on examination, a rapid course of cognitive decline or onset at a young age. This should usually include an HIV test, copper studies, Lyme/syphilis serology, MRI brain and LP ± further specialist assessment.

21

Patients may present with falls, difficulty mobilizing or complete immobility. Younger patients can usually be rapidly categorized into an underlying aetiology, but evaluation of elderly patients is more complex. Falls in the elderly are common and associated with increased mortality, morbidity and higher risk of hospitalization and institutionalization. Normal physiological changes of ageing (e.g., increased body sway, reduced muscle bulk [sarcopenia] and impaired reaction time) increase the likelihood of mobility problems. Moreover, mobility problems may be self-reinforcing as reduced activity leads to loss of muscle function and confidence. A thorough, systematic approach is essential to identify adverse consequences of immobility, serious underlying pathology, and potentially reversible contributing factors.

Accidental trip

Some falls are the unavoidable consequence of a trip. In the absence of significant injury, recurrent mobility problems or other concerns, these patients do not require detailed assessment. However, many elderly patients exhibit post hoc rationalization of their fall ('I must have tripped on the carpet'), so falls should be classified as accidental only when there is unequivocal evidence for this.

Reduced mobility secondary to chronic disorder

Immobility and instability may occur as a consequence of chronic illness or sensory impairment. Cardiovascular, neurological, psychiatric and musculoskeletal disease can all impact on a patient's mobility. Specific conditions within each system that can contribute to immobility and falls can be found in Box 22.1. Assessment should focus on identifying the cause of the fall so that contributory conditions can be optimized and risk of falls reduced.

Reduced mobility secondary to acute illness

In frail patients (Clinical tool, Diagnosing Frailty and the Comprehensive Geriatric Assessment, Chapter 21) a sudden decline in mobility (e.g., acute fall, inability to mobilize) may be the principal manifestation of any acute medical, surgical or psychiatric illness. Acute delirium (Chapter 21) is a common cause of falls and immobility in the elderly; delirium and its precipitants should be considered in patients presenting with mobility problems. In those with chronic underlying mobility problems, a relatively minor insult may lead to a major deterioration in mobility.

Reduced mobility secondary to medications

Certain medications (Box 22.2) increase the risk of falls and immobility, with antipsychotics, antidepressants and benzodiazepines all being strongly linked with increased falls. Polypharmacy also contributes to immobility, with use of five or more regular medications being linked with a 30% increased risk of falls for older adults in the community.

Multifactorial mobility problems

In patients with recurrent falls or other chronic mobility problems, there is often no single identifiable cause but rather multiple contributing factors. As well as the factors already described, consider muscle weakness, balance disorders, nutritional status, risks from the patient's environment, and fear of falling. A comprehensive and multidimensional approach to assessment is essential.

Box 22.1 Chronic conditions associated with reduced mobility and falls

Neurological

- Stroke
- Vestibular disorders
- Peripheral neuropathy
- Neurodegenerative disorders (e.g., Parkinson's disease [PD], MS)
- Radiculopathy

Cardiovascular

- Orthostatic hypotension
- Syncope (Chapter 24)

Psychiatric

- Dementia
- Depression

Musculoskeletal

- Osteoarthritis
- Inflammatory arthritis
- Previous joint injury/fracture
- Footwear and foot problems

Genitourinary

- Urinary incontinence

Box 22.2 Drugs associated with increased risk of falls

- Alcohol
- Anticonvulsants
- Antidepressants
- Antihypertensives
- Antipsychotics
- Anticholinergics
- Benzodiazepines
- Hypnotics
- Diuretics
- Digoxin
- Opioids
- Diabetes medications (oral hypoglycaemics, insulin)

Clinical tool
How to perform Gait Speed and Timed Up and Go assessments

Gait speed	Timed Up and Go
• Clinician marks out 9 metres on a flat surface, with the first 2.5 and last 2.5 metres highlighted. • Patient walks the 9-metre distance at their normal speed with their walking aid if they use one. • Clinician uses a stopwatch to measure the time taken for the patient to travel across the middle 4 metres, allowing the patient to accelerate for the first 2.5 and decelerate for the final 2.5 metres. • Faster of two trials is recorded. • Gait speed in m/s is calculated as 4 divided by time in seconds. • Gait speed of <0.8 m/s suggests impairment.	• Patient begins sitting in a standard chair. • Distance 3 metres from the patient is marked by the clinician. • Patient asked to stand up from chair, walk to mark, turn around, walk back, and sit down in chair, using their walking aid if they have one. • Clinician measures the time taken to perform this using a stopwatch. • Older adults who take ≥12 seconds to complete task are at increased risk of falling.

22

FALLS AND IMMOBILITY

Mobility problems: overview

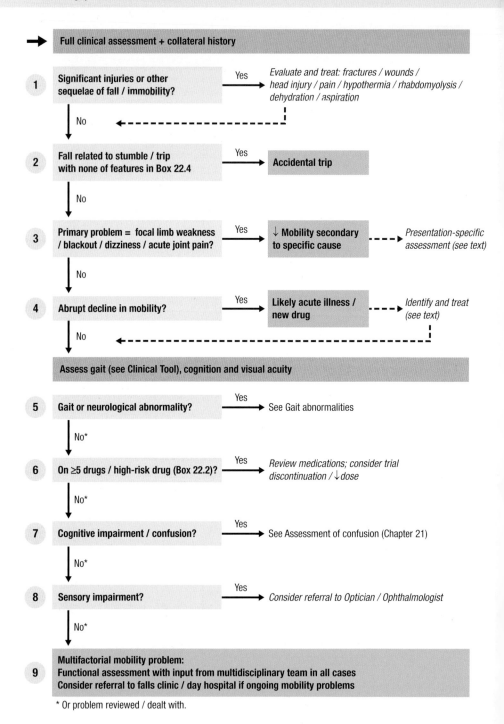

Full clinical assessment + collateral history

1 Significant injuries or other sequelae of fall / immobility? — Yes → *Evaluate and treat: fractures / wounds / head injury / pain / hypothermia / rhabdomyolysis / dehydration / aspiration*

No ↓

2 Fall related to stumble / trip with none of features in Box 22.4 — Yes → **Accidental trip**

No ↓

3 Primary problem = focal limb weakness / blackout / dizziness / acute joint pain? — Yes → **↓ Mobility secondary to specific cause** --→ *Presentation-specific assessment (see text)*

No ↓

4 Abrupt decline in mobility? — Yes → **Likely acute illness / new drug** --→ *Identify and treat (see text)*

No ↓

Assess gait (see Clinical Tool), cognition and visual acuity

5 Gait or neurological abnormality? — Yes → See Gait abnormalities

No* ↓

6 On ≥5 drugs / high-risk drug (Box 22.2)? — Yes → *Review medications; consider trial discontinuation / ↓ dose*

No* ↓

7 Cognitive impairment / confusion? — Yes → See Assessment of confusion (Chapter 21)

No* ↓

8 Sensory impairment? — Yes → *Consider referral to Optician / Ophthalmologist*

No* ↓

9 Multifactorial mobility problem:
Functional assessment with input from multidisciplinary team in all cases
Consider referral to falls clinic / day hospital if ongoing mobility problems

* Or problem reviewed / dealt with.

1 Significant injuries or other sequelae of fall/immobility?

In all patients who have fallen (or who have been found on the floor), perform a rapid but thorough survey of the entire body for injuries. Fractures, lacerations or bruising may be not immediately apparent, and the cognitively impaired patient may not bring them to your attention. Assess the perfusion and function of any limb with bruising, deformity, pain or swelling and consider the need for X-rays. Pain will compound any existing mobility problems, and so it is imperative to ensure it is adequately treated. If there is a history of head injury, arrange neuroimaging if any of the features in Box 22.3 are present.

In patients with a prolonged period of immobility, such as, lying on the floor or confined to bed, check temperature to exclude hypothermia, look for clinical and biochemical evidence of dehydration and examine the heels/sacrum for pressure sores. Consider aspiration/hypostatic pneumonia in patients with hypoxia, lung crepitations or radiological changes on CXR. If there has been significant soft-tissue pressure damage or any prolonged time on the floor, check CK and urinary myoglobin (suggested by haematuria on urinalysis with no red cells on microscopy) to exclude rhabdomyolysis, and be vigilant for compartment syndrome (Box 20.3).

In patients in whom a fragility fracture is identified, or those who have risk factors for fragility fracture, a fracture risk assessment should be carried out using the QFracture tool (https://qfracture.org/). It is important to arrange a dual-energy X-ray absorptiometry (DEXA) scan in all patients who have had a fragility fracture and in those with a 10% risk of fracture in the next 10 years.

2 Fall related to stumble/trip with none of the features in Box 22.4?

Take care in making this diagnosis—a simple trip on a loose carpet tile at walking pace is usually not 'normal', and the visual impairment that led to the trip or the poor balance that turned it into an injurious fall might be reversible. On the other hand, exhaustive assessment is inappropriate in patients with a genuinely accidental fall and no underlying mobility problems. Have a low threshold for further evaluation if any of the features in Box 22.4 are present or events leading up to the fall are unclear. In elderly patients presenting with a fall without the features present in Box 22.4, take the opportunity to assess for impairment of gait and balance, using either the Gait Speed or Timed Up and Go test (Clinical Tool: How to perform Gait Speed and Timed Up and Go assessments). If an impairment is identified, patients are likely to benefit from Physiotherapy referral and education on falls prevention.

3 Primary problem = focal limb weakness/blackout/dizziness/acute joint pain?

If you identify new limb weakness on examination, assess as described in Chapter 14.

If mobility problems are related to dizziness, evaluate first for symptomatic postural

---

Box 22.3 Criteria for performing a CT head scan for patients presenting with head injury

CT head within 1 hour

- GCS score ≤12 on initial assessment
- GCS score <15 at 2 hours after the injury
- Suspected open or depressed skull fracture
- Signs of basal skull fracture
- Post-traumatic seizure
- Focal neurological deficit
- >1 Episode of vomiting

If loss of consciousness or amnesia since the injury, perform a CT head within 8 hours of injury if:

- Age ≥65
- Any current bleeding or clotting disorders (including anticoagulation)
- Dangerous mechanism of injury
- 30 minutes of retrograde amnesia

Box 22.4 Features not consistent with a diagnosis of simple accidental trip

- Recurrent or multiple falls
- Recent decline in mobility or functional status
- Inability to get up from the ground
- Implausible mechanism for fall
- Witnessed period of unresponsiveness
- Inability to recall landing on ground
- Facial injuries

22

hypotension: a fall of ≥20 mmHg in systolic BP or ≥10 mmHg in diastolic BP within 3 minutes of changing from a lying to standing position, accompanied by a feeling of light-headedness/presyncope. If this is detected, search for underlying causes, e.g., antihypertensives, dehydration, autonomic neuropathy. Otherwise, assess as in Chapter 17.

Consider whether an apparent fall could have been a blackout. Beware of accepting rationalizations for the event ('I must have tripped') and make every attempt to obtain an eyewitness account of the current episode or previous ones. If patients cannot recall how they came to be lying on the ground, assess, in the first instance, as per transient loss of consciousness (Chapter 24). Also suspect transient loss of consciousness if the patient was witnessed as having a period of unresponsiveness, sustained facial injuries during the fall (most conscious patients can protect the face) or experienced palpitation, chest pain, breathlessness or a presyncopal prodrome prior to 'falling'. Have a lower threshold for further evaluation of possible syncope in patients with ECG abnormalities or a history of major cardiac disease.

If mobility problems are secondary to an acutely painful joint, assess as in Chapter 18.

4   Abrupt decline in mobility?

An abrupt decline in mobility (e.g., acute fall, new onset of recurrent falls or being 'off legs') is one of the classic atypical presentations of acute illness in frail patients (Clinical tool, Chapter 21). Characteristic signs/symptoms of the specific precipitant may be absent and 'screening' investigations (Box 22.5) are often required to uncover the problem or identify a focus for further assessment. Have a high index of suspicion for an acute infection causing a deterioration in mobility.

Review all drugs (including over-the-counter products), particularly those started within the previous weeks, and consider trial discontinuation of any high-risk agents (Box 22.2).

If significant loss of mobility was preceded by a fall, consider the possibility of fracture or head injury—ensure that pain is adequately treated, and organize appropriate imaging.

> **Box 22.5 Screening investigations to identify acute illness in elderly patients**
>
> - Capillary BG
> - Urine dipstick and MSU/CSU (avoid diagnosing a urinary tract infection purely on the basis of abnormal dipstick results)
> - Blood tests: FBC, U+Es, LFTs, glucose, CRP, TFTs, Ca^{2+}
> - CXR
> - ECG

An abrupt decline in mobility on a background of weight loss, muscle wasting, hypoalbuminaemia or chronic anaemia may suggest a progressive disorder 'coming to a head'. Aim to diagnose and reverse any acute precipitants for the deterioration, before investigating for any progressive disease that has not already been identified. Once this has been addressed, complete a full assessment to identify underlying mobility problems and reversible risk factors for falling.

In patients with a background of progressive mobility decline/increasing frailty, the acute precipitant may be minor. Do not overemphasize it in comparison with the underlying contributory factors.

5   Gait or neurological abnormality?

Assessment of walking pattern is key to understanding mobility problems. It is a fundamental element of the neurological examination and can reveal abnormalities not elicited on gross testing of individual modalities. It may also unmask impaired-effort tolerance due to cardiorespiratory or lower limb disease. Finally, the gait assessment is an opportunity to assess falls risk, even in the absence of specific findings. Check that patients are safe to mobilize, equip them with their normal walking aid and follow the steps in Clinical tool: How to perform a gait assessment.

6   On ≥5 drugs/high-risk drug (Box 22.2)?

Medications are one of the most readily modifiable of all factors influencing mobility problems, but indiscriminate changes may do more harm than good. Individual medications that may increase the risk of falling are

Clinical tool
How to perform a gait assessment

- Ask patient to stand from sitting position.

  Look for: need for assistance; necessary use of upper limbs.

- Ask patient to continue standing.

  Ask about: light-headedness/sensation of spinning or movement.
  Look for: ability to continue standing safely/unsteadiness/stooped posture.

- Ask patient to move feet together; ensure he/she is standing close by.

  Look for: increasing unsteadiness.

- Ask patient to close eyes (Romberg test).

  Look for: increasing unsteadiness (Be ready to catch patient).

- Ask patient to open eyes, walk 3 metres, then turn around and walk back, using an aid if required.

  Look for: overall safety and stability; unilateral gait abnormality (stroke, peripheral nerve lesion, joint disease, pain); short, shuffling steps (PD[1], diffuse cerebrovascular disease); high-stepping gait (foot-drop, sensory ataxia); broad-based/unsteady gait (cerebellar lesion, normal pressure hydrocephalus).

- Ask the patient to walk for a longer distance.

  Ask about: chest pain, calf pain, breathlessness, fatigue.
  Look for: ↑RR, laboured breathing, need to stop.

- Repeat, if necessary, after correction of any reversible factors—for example, treatment of acute illness, effective pain control, rehydration, removal of offending drug

[1]Other features of Parkinsonian gait include reduced arm-swing, stooped posture and, sometimes, difficulty in starting and stopping ('festinating' gait).

---

listed in Box 22.2. Polypharmacy (≥5 regular medications) is also a risk factor for falls. Review the indications for all drugs and consider whether they are still required. Look for opportunities to rationalize treatment, consider alternatives and consider decreasing the dose.

A gradual approach will allow the impact of individual changes to be assessed and is essential with psychotropic medication, from which abrupt withdrawal may be worse than the toxic syndrome. Explore a possible contribution from alcohol in all cases. In patients with underlying mobility/balance problems, it may critically impair stability even when consumed within recommended limits.

7 Cognitive impairment/confusion?

Acute delirium should be specifically considered as it may not be readily apparent if it is hypoactive or superimposed on chronic impairment. Vigilance and collateral history are essential counterparts to objective measures of cognitive function. Chronic cognitive impairment is also a risk factor for falls but difficult to ameliorate. Consider silent precipitants of wandering/getting out of bed, such as urinary urgency or nicotine withdrawal. Further assessment of confusion is detailed in Chapter 21.

8 Sensory impairment?

Visual impairment increases the risk of falls and may be reversible, such as with refractory errors, cataracts. Screen for reduced visual acuity. If detected, refer to an optician or ophthalmologist, as appropriate. Hearing loss may also contribute to instability and increased risk of falling, particularly in combination with some of the other risk factors. If suspected, refer to an Audiologist.

9 Multifactorial mobility problem: arrange multidisciplinary team assessment

All patients with serious falls, recurrent falls or reduced mobility should undergo a multifactorial falls-risk assessment so that targeted interventions based on individual risk can be implemented. This requires contribution from the multidisciplinary team, with physiotherapy and occupational therapy input to assist with assessment of functional ability, environmental contributors to the presentation, and scope for benefit from measures such as walking aids/strength and balance training/home alarms. In patients with ongoing problems, especially when there is evidence of frailty, refer to the day hospital or a specialist falls clinic for comprehensive geriatric assessment (Clinical tool).

22

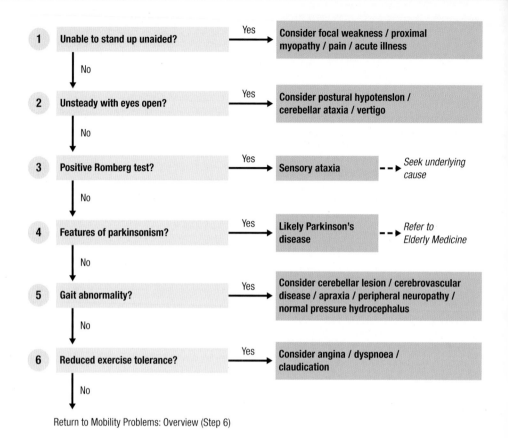

Return to Mobility Problems: Overview (Step 6)

1 Unable to stand up unaided?

Lower limb weakness may limit the ability to rise from a chair or necessitate use of the chair arms or pulling on nearby furniture. Systemic illness, toxic insults or metabolic derangement may cause mild generalized weakness. If weakness is persistent, asymmetrical, or associated with wasting/neurological abnormalities, see Chapter 14.

2 Unsteady with eyes open?

Check lying/standing BP if the patient feels faint or light-headed. Consider vertigo if the patient has a sensation of spinning or movement. Observe standing posture, identify reduction in joint function, and evaluate pain. If patients can remain standing without assistance, ask them to move their feet close together—inability to do so indicates ataxia. Look for associated features of cerebellar disease, such as intention tremor, dysdiadochokinesis, dysmetria (past-pointing), dysarthria, nystagmus.

3 Positive Romberg test?

A marked increase in unsteadiness after eye closing is a positive test, suggesting a sensory (proprioceptive or vestibular) rather than cerebellar cause of ataxia. Reduction in sensation may be a normal part of ageing, such as reduced vibration sense in the feet is common and of limited significance in the older patient. Examine the patient during walking for an unsteady, ataxic or 'stomping' gait. The list of possible causes of peripheral neuropathy is vast but screen routinely for diabetes mellitus, alcohol excess, liver disease, malnutrition (vitamin B$_{12}$ deficiency) or iatrogenic causes, e.g., anticonvulsants, chemotherapy.

4 Features of parkinsonism?

Look for the typical features of PD:
- Tremor: coarse, slow (5 Hz) and usually asymmetrical; present at rest, absent during sleep; decreased by voluntary movement; increased by emotion; adduction–abduction of the thumb with flexion–extension of the fingers ('pill-rolling')
- Increased tone: 'lead-pipe' rigidity or, in the presence of tremor, 'cog-wheel' with a jerky feel
- Bradykinesia: slow initiation of movement, ↓speed of fine movements, expressionless face
- Gait: delayed initiation, ↓arm swing, stooped posture, short, shuffling steps, difficulty turning

The presence of these features makes idiopathic PD more likely, but parkinsonism has other causes, most commonly, diffuse cerebrovascular disease. The classic description of vascular parkinsonism is of signs of PD below the waist, with relative sparing of the arms.

New presentations or progression of PD are usually assessed in an outpatient setting by a movement disorders specialist. Mobility-related admissions in patients with PD are more likely to be connected with a superimposed acute illness or a medication problem. Make certain that hospitalized patients with PD receive their medication at the correct dose and time to ensure that their mobility does not deteriorate further.

5 Gait abnormality?

Gait screening is sensitive for neuromotor, sensory and musculoskeletal abnormalities in the lower limbs because walking is a complex task in comparison with the tests of neurological function used in the standard screening examination.

The gaits associated with parkinsonism and sensory ataxia are described above. Suspect cerebellar ataxia if the gait is unsteady and broad-based with an inability to heel–toe walk (as if inebriated with alcohol). A hemiplegic gait is usually obvious and will be associated with focal neurological signs. Bilateral lower limb proximal muscle weakness may produce a 'waddling' gait.

Pain can limit exertion or alter gait, leading to a decrease in function or an increased risk of falling. The patient will typically place the foot of the affected side delicately on the floor for as little time as possible to avoid the pain of weight-bearing ('antalgic' gait). Osteoarthritis is frequently responsible but is usually chronic and slowly progressive, and thus unlikely to lead to hospital admission without additional factors. Acutely painful joints require careful assessment (Chapter 18).

Consider gait apraxia if no specific neurological abnormality or gait pattern is noted but the gait is nonetheless abnormal. Apraxia, the inability to conduct learned, purposeful movements properly (in the absence of a focal insult), is a result of general or frontal cerebral insults, such as dementia, cerebrovascular disease, normal-pressure hydrocephalus, sedation or metabolic derangement.

Psychological causes of reduced mobility (especially the fear of falling) can also reduce mobility and increase the risk of falls and may be elicited only by asking the patient to mobilize greater distances.

6 Reduced exercise tolerance?

22

Observe for/ask about exertional dyspnoea, chest discomfort and claudication. The latter may be due to peripheral vascular disease (e.g., diminished pulses, skin changes, vascular disease elsewhere), but consider neurogenic claudication secondary to spinal stenosis, especially if the discomfort responds to postural change, for example, bending over, sitting down, more quickly than standing still.

Urinary incontinence (UI) is the involuntary leakage of urine. Estimates of prevalence vary, but it affects 25–45% of women and is three times more common in women than men. Prevalence increases with older age. UI can have a serious impact on patients' quality of life due to reduced levels of activity, social withdrawal and depression. In frail patients (Clinical tool, Chapter 21), it increases the risk of falls, UTIs, pressure sores, and institutionalization. Despite the prevalence and impact of the condition, it tends to be underreported and underrecognized in clinical practice. UI is frequently multifactorial, particularly in frail patients, so seek to identify all potentially modifiable contributing factors (Box 23.1). Take care also to evaluate the impact of symptoms on daily activities and quality of life.

Stress incontinence

Urine leakage is provoked by an increase in intra-abdominal pressure, such as during coughing, sneezing, effort or exertion. It is usually due to insufficient urethral support from the pelvic floor muscles but can also be caused by intrinsic weakness of the urethral sphincter, such as post-pelvic surgery. Stress incontinence is far more common in females than males and most often relates to obstetric trauma. It frequently accompanies pelvic organ prolapse and may also occur with atrophic vaginitis. Stress incontinence in males is usually a complication of prostatectomy.

Urge incontinence

Urine leakage occurs due to intense bladder contraction and is preceded by the sensation of urgency. This can result from neurological disease (e.g., multiple sclerosis, stroke, spina bifida) but is more often due to intrinsic bladder activity ('detrusor overactivity').

Mixed incontinence

A combination of stress and urge incontinence; treatment should be aimed at the more dominant aspect.

Overflow incontinence

This describes the involuntary passage of urine from an overfull bladder, which may or may not be accompanied by a sensation of urgency. Incomplete bladder emptying may result from:

- Bladder outflow obstruction, for example, benign prostatic hyperplasia (BPH), prostate cancer, bladder tumour, urethral stenosis, cystocele or postsurgery to correct incontinence
- Bladder atonia in neurological disease, e.g., cauda equina compression, conus medullaris compression or autonomic neuropathy
- Drugs with anticholinergic effects, such as antipsychotics or antidepressants

Treatment of overflow incontinence is with relief of obstruction (e.g., resection of prostate cancer, medical treatment of BPH) or intermittent catheterization. An indwelling catheter may be required depending on patient preference, their ability to self-catheterize or, in frail patients, due to concerns about skin integrity.

Continuous incontinence

Constant leakage of urine throughout the day (and night) suggests the presence of a fistula between the bladder and the urethra or vagina. Underlying causes include urogynaecological cancer, previous pelvic surgery/radiotherapy or obstetric trauma.

Box 23.1 **Aggravating factors**

- Polydipsia/polyuria, including poorly controlled diabetes mellitus, diabetes insipidus, hypercalcaemia, and psychogenic polydipsia
- Caffeine
- Alcohol overuse/misuse
- Constipation
- Medications (Box 23.2)
- Mobility problems (Chapter 22)
- Visual impairment
- Obesity
- Respiratory disease
- Smoking
- Cognitive impairment, such as delirium or dementia (Chapter 21)

Box 23.2 **Medications potentially aggravating incontinence**

- Diuretics
- Drugs with cholinergic effects[a]
- Drugs with anticholinergic effects[b]
- Alpha-blockers[a]
- Alpha-agonists[b]
- Calcium channel blockers
- Beta agonists
- Sedatives
- Lithium

[a]*May cause or aggravate urge incontinence*
[b]*May cause or aggravate overflow incontinence*

Functional incontinence

As well as effective urinary storage and voiding mechanisms, continence requires adequate cognition, motivation, mobility, dexterity and access to the bathroom. Functional incontinence occurs when the person is unable to get to the toilet due to one or more physical, cognitive or environmental reasons.

Transient incontinence

Several conditions can cause transient UI, which can be corrected by treating the underlying disorder. Urinary tract infections may present with new incontinence accompanied by fever and dysuria. Constipation and faecal impaction may precipitate bladder outflow obstruction, resulting in overflow incontinence. Neuropsychiatric conditions such as delirium, psychosis and depression may result in functional incontinence. Systemic conditions such as poorly controlled diabetes mellitus, diabetes insipidus and hypercalcaemia cause polyuria, which increases risk of incontinence. Medication changes that could contribute to incontinence should also be considered (Box 23.2)

23

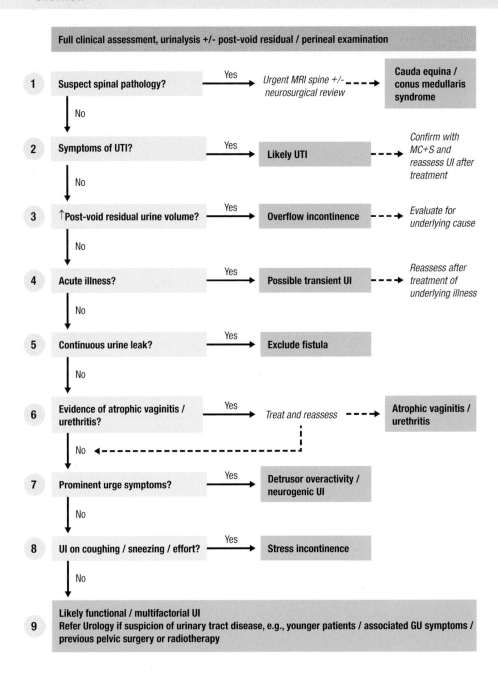

Full clinical assessment, urinalysis +/- post-void residual / perineal examination

1 Suspect spinal pathology? — Yes → *Urgent MRI spine +/- neurosurgical review* - - - → **Cauda equina / conus medullaris syndrome**

No ↓

2 Symptoms of UTI? — Yes → **Likely UTI** - - - → *Confirm with MC+S and reassess UI after treatment*

No ↓

3 ↑Post-void residual urine volume? — Yes → **Overflow incontinence** - - - → *Evaluate for underlying cause*

No ↓

4 Acute illness? — Yes → **Possible transient UI** - - - → *Reassess after treatment of underlying illness*

No ↓

5 Continuous urine leak? — Yes → **Exclude fistula**

No ↓

6 Evidence of atrophic vaginitis / urethritis? — Yes → *Treat and reassess* - - - → **Atrophic vaginitis / urethritis**

No ← - - - - - - - - - - - - - - - - - - ↓

7 Prominent urge symptoms? — Yes → **Detrusor overactivity / neurogenic UI**

No ↓

8 UI on coughing / sneezing / effort? — Yes → **Stress incontinence**

No ↓

9 Likely functional / multifactorial UI
Refer Urology if suspicion of urinary tract disease, e.g., younger patients / associated GU symptoms / previous pelvic surgery or radiotherapy

1 Suspect spinal pathology?

Arrange an urgent spinal MRI to exclude cauda equina/conus medullaris syndrome in any patient with recent onset of UI associated with lower limb weakness, altered perianal/perineal sensation, faecal incontinence or new low back or leg pain (Chapter 14). Seek immediate Neurosurgical/Neurology input if concerning imaging features or unexplained neurological findings.

2 Symptoms of UTI?

Suspect a UTI if there is a short history of UI accompanied by fever, dysuria, frequency, or malodourous urine.

In women <65 years: The absence of leukocytes and nitrites on dipstick makes UTI unlikely. If dipstick testing is positive or there is strong clinical suspicion, send an MSU for culture. It may be appropriate to wait for culture results prior to initiating treatment, but consider empirical treatment when symptoms are severe or there is a high risk of complication. Following treatment, reevaluate to ensure that UI resolves.

In men and patients >65 years: Urine dipstick is unreliable and MSU should be sent if there is suspicion of UTI. Antibiotics should be started empirically in men with suspected UTI and in women >65 years with severe symptoms or at high risk of complications. Empirical antibiotics should be based, if possible, on previous urine culture results. Evaluate for prostatic disease in men with a UTI (Step 3) and arrange renal tract imaging (USS initially) in any patient with recurrent UTI. Be aware of red flags which could suggest genitourinary cancer (Box 23.3).

3 ↑ Postvoid residual (PVR) urine volume?

Using a bedside bladder USS, measure PVR in all patients with UI. Suspect overflow incontinence due to incomplete bladder emptying if the PVR is >100 mL (or >50 mL in younger patients). In men, ask about other symptoms of bladder outlet obstruction such as hesitancy and poor stream, examine the prostate and check a PSA (prior to rectal exam). Exclude constipation/faecal impaction as an underlying cause, particularly in frail elderly patients. Seek a neurological opinion when there is a history of neurological disorder or associated symptoms/signs of neurological

---

Box 23.3 Red flags for genitourinary cancer

- Haematuria either without UTI or persists following treatment of UTI in patients aged >45 years
- Dysuria with unexplained nonvisible haematuria in patients aged >65 years
- Unexplained nonvisible haematuria with raised WCC in patients aged >65 years
- Unexplained recurrent or persistent UTI in patients aged >65 years
- Asymmetrical, firm or nodular prostate on digital rectal examination
- Raised age-adjusted PSA

Adapted from NICE 2015 (Suspected cancer: recognition and referral). Available from www.nice.org.uk/guidance/ng12. All rights reserved. Subject to Notice of rights. NICE guidance is prepared for the National Health Service in England. It is subject to regular review and updating and may be withdrawn. NICE accepts no responsibility for the use of its content in this product/publication.

---

disease, such as lower limb weakness. Otherwise, refer to Urology for further assessment and investigation, such as cystoscopy.

4 Acute illness?

Suspect transient UI as a nonspecific manifestation of illness in frail patients (Clinical tool, Chapter 21) who are acutely unwell, have experienced an abrupt decline in function, mobility or cognition or who have evidence of newly deranged physiology. Seek and treat the underlying illness, then reevaluate continence once the patient has returned to baseline status.

5 Continuous urine leak?

Suspect a fistula between the bladder (or ureter) and the vagina/urethra if UI is continuous rather than intermittent, especially if there is a history of previous pelvic surgery/radiotherapy or a complex obstetric history. Refer to Urology for specialist assessment.

6 Evidence of atrophic vaginitis/urethritis?

Suspect this as a cause of UI (usually stress-type) in postmenopausal women with symptoms of urethral irritation (e.g., burning, frequency, painful intercourse) but negative urine dipstick and culture or with mucosal pallor or erythema on perineal examination. Reassess symptoms after treatment with topical oestrogen for at least 14 days. Continue to seek other causes of UI unless symptoms fully resolve.

23

7 Prominent urge symptoms?

Evaluate as urge incontinence if the patient reports a clear and consistent history of urgency to void prior to leakage of urine. Consider using the 3 IQ questionnaire (Box 23.4) or a voiding diary if the history is unclear or the pattern of UI is variable.

Ensure you have excluded urinary retention: repeat a post-void bladder scan if initial results are equivocal and perform post-void catheterization if there is a strong clinical suspicion. Consider neurogenic aetiology and obtain specialist input in patients with a history of neurological disorder (e.g., multiple sclerosis, spina bifida) or associated neurological signs or symptoms.

In the absence of urinary retention or neurological features, assume detrusor overactivity as the likely diagnosis. Refer for specialist urological assessment (e.g., urodynamic studies) if the diagnosis is uncertain or symptoms fail to respond to standard treatments.

8 UI on coughing/sneezing/effort?

Evaluate as stress incontinence if urine leakage consistently coincides with manoeuvres that increase intra-abdominal pressure (e.g., coughing, sneezing, laughing, sitting/standing-up) especially if there is no associated sensation of urgency. Where the history is unclear, inspect for leakage of urine while asking the patient to cough or, again, consider using the 3 IQ questionnaire (Box 23.4) or a voiding diary.

Refer to Gynaecology if there is uterine/vaginal prolapse. Consider potentially aggravating factors such as chronic lung disease (cough) or medications (Box 23.2). In women with uncomplicated stress UI, reassess after simple measures such as pelvic muscle retraining, but consider referral to Urogynaecology if symptoms remain severe. Refer male patients with stress UI for Urology assessment.

9 Likely functional/multifactorial UI. Specialist urological assessment in selected cases

In frail or elderly patients, UI is often due to a constellation of factors that prevent timely

---

Box 23.4 IQ questionnaire

1. During the past 3 months, have you leaked urine (even a small amount)?
   - Yes – move to question 2
   - No – stop questionnaire.
2. During the past 3 months, did you leak urine:
   - When performing physical activity (coughing, sneezing, lifting, exercising)?
   - When you felt an urge to empty your bladder, but were not able to get to the toilet in time?
   - Neither of the above circumstances.
3. During the past 3 months, did you leak urine MOST often:
   - When performing physical activity (coughing, sneezing, lifting, exercising)? **Stress incontinence predominant**
   - When you felt an urge to empty your bladder, but were not able to get to the toilet in time? **Urge incontinence predominant**
   - Neither of the above circumstances. **Other cause** (neither urge incontinence nor stress incontinence)
   - Both of the above circumstances equally as often. **Mixed UI.**

---

toileting (functional incontinence) rather than a single specific urinary tract pathology. Consider specialist urological assessment/investigation if there are associated GU symptoms such as haematuria or pelvic pain, a complex obstetric history, previous pelvic surgery or radiotherapy, or where functional incontinence seems unlikely, such as in younger patients or those without significant comorbidity.

Otherwise, systematically address all factors that may be contributing to UI (Box 23.1). Review medications (Box 23.2) and amend where necessary. Establish whether the patient has awareness of the need to void. If not, try prompted toileting (particularly after diuretics). If the patient has awareness of the need to void but cannot reach the toilet in time, assess mobility (Chapter 22) and consider the need for walking aids, a downstairs toilet or commode. Evaluate the effectiveness of continence aids such as pads, urisheaths or a commode. Finally, determine the level of distress caused by symptoms and the overall impact on quality of life. Consider referral for comprehensive geriatric assessment.

Miscellaneous

Transient loss of consciousness (TLOC) presents a particular diagnostic challenge. The event has usually resolved by the time of assessment, and since critical elements of the history are unknown to the patient, witness accounts are crucial. It is often helpful if witnesses have used their mobile phone to video the event, and this should be encouraged if there are recurrent events of unclear cause. Risk stratification of patients should be used to identify those with potentially life-threatening causes of TLOC who require hospital admission for further investigation, while differentiating from those at lower risk who can be managed as outpatients.

Syncope

Syncope denotes TLOC resulting from global cerebral hypoperfusion, typically associated with a BP <60 mmHg for ≥6 seconds. It is characterized by rapid onset, short duration and spontaneous complete recovery.

Syncope can be divided into four aetiological subtypes:
- Arrhythmia-related—due to transient compromise of cardiac output by a tachy- or bradyarrhythmia, e.g., ventricular tachycardia, complete heart block
- Cardiac—due to structural heart disease, especially left ventricular outflow obstruction, e.g., severe aortic stenosis, hypertrophic obstructive cardiomyopathy.

Acute pulmonary embolism or aortic dissection may also cause syncope.
- Orthostatic—due to failure of homeostatic maintenance of BP on standing, e.g., caused by antihypertensive medications or autonomic neuropathy
- Reflex (neurally mediated)—reflex vasodilatation and/or bradycardia occurs in response to a particular trigger, e.g., vasovagal or carotid sinus syncope.

Seizure

A seizure is a sudden burst of abnormal excessive neuronal activity in the brain. The clinical features experienced by the patient can be varied and include abnormalities in tone and movement, loss of awareness or altered behaviour, occurring with or without loss of consciousness. Common types of seizure include:
- Focal seizure—abnormal electrical activity is localized to one area of the brain. The clinical presentation of a focal seizure will depend on the area of the brain affected. Awareness may be impaired (focal impaired-awareness seizures) or retained (focal aware seizures). Focal seizures can progress to bilateral tonic-clonic seizures. Possible clinical features can be found in Table 24.1.
- Generalized seizure—abnormal electrical activity occurs on both sides of the brain, usually resulting in loss of consciousness.

Table 24.1 Typical features of common types of seizure

Factor	Focal seizures	Bilateral tonic-clonic seizures	Psychogenic non-epileptic seizures
Seizure appearance	Variable. Can include: – Tonic and/or clonic movements – Disturbances of vision, smell, speech, or taste – Abnormal sensations In focal impaired awareness seizures: – Staring – Reduced awareness of surroundings – Automatisms (e.g., lip smacking)	Typical sequence: 1. Tonic posturing 2. Bilateral rhythmic jerking—initially fast and low amplitude, becoming slower and higher amplitude as the seizure progresses 3. Stertorous breathing as seizure resolves	May display: – Asynchronous twitching/jerking movements – Pelvic thrusting – Back arching – Head shaking from side to side – Variable amplitude of convulsions – Intelligible verbal communication – Weeping – Stuttering – Rapid breathing as seizure resolves
Awareness	Present in focal aware seizures Reduced in focal impaired awareness seizures	No	May display: – Preserved awareness – Purposeful movement – Interaction with examiner – Convulsions modified by presence of examiner – Recollection of event
Onset	Rapid	Rapid	Commonly gradual
Observations	↓ SpO_2 ↑Heart rate	↓ SpO_2 May be cyanotic ↑Heart rate	Normal
Duration	<2 minutes	<2 minutes	>5 minutes
Frequency	Variable	Variable	High frequency Can have multiple attacks in a single day
Eyes closed	No	No	Yes May resist eye opening
Tongue biting	No	Lateral tongue biting	Anterior tongue biting possible
Postictal period	5 minutes to several hours	5 minutes to several hours	Absent
Aura	Yes	No	No

24

Bilateral tonic-clonic seizures are the most common. Possible clinical features can be found in Table 24.1.

- Convulsive status epilepticus—defined as a single tonic-clonic seizure lasting >5 minutes or a succession of tonic-clonic seizures, without recovery in between, for >5 minutes. This is a medical emergency and requires urgent treatment to terminate seizure activity.

Seizures may arise as a single event which is often provoked by an external factor, or they may be recurrent, at which point a diagnosis of epilepsy would be considered.

Provoked seizures are those that occur because of electrolyte disturbances (e.g., hypoglycaemia, hyponatraemia), toxins (e.g., antidepressant overdose), withdrawal syndromes (e.g., drugs or alcohol), traumatic head injury, stroke, neoplasms or inflammatory processes. Unprovoked seizures occur in the absence of any underlying precipitating cause, or as a result of a preexisting brain lesion or neurological condition (distinguishing it from an acute provoked seizure). Recurrent unprovoked seizures define epilepsy.

Hypoglycaemia

Hypoglycaemia may cause impairment of consciousness that resolves with prompt correction of capillary blood glucose. Many cases are iatrogenic, from treatment of diabetes with insulin or glucose-lowering drugs. Other causes of hypoglycaemia include alcohol, liver failure, insulinoma and adrenal insufficiency.

Functional neurological disorders (FNDs)

Functional neurological disorders can present with a wider variety of symptoms that may be physical, sensory or cognitive. Psychogenic nonepileptic seizures may be associated with collapse and loss of consciousness with or without shaking activity. Many different terms have been used to define these events (e.g., pseudoseizures, pseudosyncope), which can be confusing. However, they all describe episodes that resemble seizure or syncope but do not have an underlying somatic mechanism, that is, no epileptiform activity or cerebral hypoperfusion. They can present major diagnostic difficulty, with the diagnosis often being a gradual process rather than a single event where all the relevant information is unlikely to be available. Many patients with these conditions are misdiagnosed, with the associated risk of being started on unnecessary medications. Hence, specialist input from a neurologist with an interest in functional disorders is usually necessary. Features that suggest a nonepileptic seizure, and how they can be differentiated from epileptic seizures, can be found in Table 24.1. However, note that these are not hard-and-fast rules, and distinguishing epileptic from nonepileptic seizures can be extremely challenging.

Other causes

Other causes which may present with TLOC include falls, drug/alcohol intoxication, cataplexy, narcolepsy, or concussion following head trauma. Transient ischaemic attacks (TIAs) present with focal neurological signs and symptoms and very rarely cause TLOC.

24

Transient loss of consciousness: overview

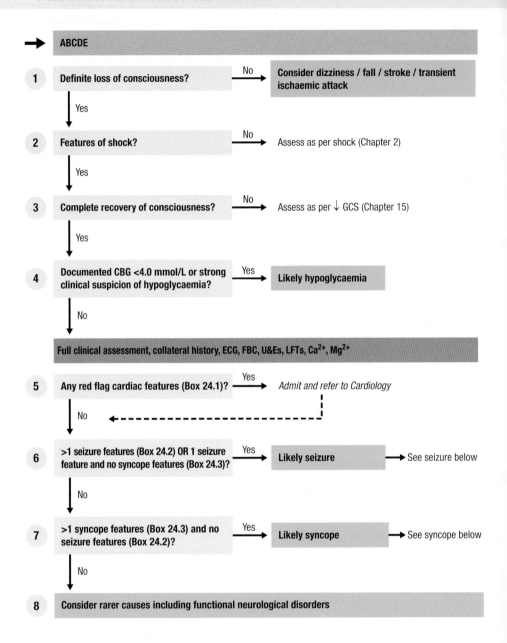

1 Definite loss of consciousness?

In the absence of a clear witness account, this may be difficult to establish. Ask the patient to recount the events in as much detail as possible.

Assume TLOC if:
- A witness confirms a period of unresponsiveness
- The patient describes 'waking up' or 'coming to' on the ground, especially if there is no recollection of falling
- There are facial injuries (most conscious patients can protect their face as they fall).

TLOC is unlikely if:
- There was no loss of postural tone
- The patient recalls landing on the ground
- A witness account suggests interaction with or awareness of the environment throughout the episode.

2 Features of shock?

Syncope may be a manifestation of major haemodynamic compromise, e.g., massive PE, severe GI bleed. If you find evidence of shock (Box 2.1) during the ABCDE assessment, evaluate further as per Chapter 2.

3 Complete recovery of consciousness?

The diagnostic pathway below is appropriate only for a transient episode of loss of consciousness. If there is evidence of persistently ↓GCS score during the ABCDE assessment, evaluate in the first instance as described in Chapter 15.

4 Documented CBG <4.0 mmol/L or strong clinical suspicion of hypoglycaemia?

Attributing an episode of reduced consciousness to hypoglycaemia requires:
- Demonstration of low blood glucose in association with TLOC
- Recovery with restoration of normoglycaemia

Corroborate a low CBG with a formal lab glucose measurement whenever feasible but do not wait for the result to initiate treatment. Patients may have had corrective treatment prior to assessment without a CBG, e.g.,

from ambulance crew. In these circumstances, suspect hypoglycaemia if the episode resolved with administration of carbohydrate/glucagon and was preceded by symptoms of autonomic activation (e.g., sweating, trembling, hunger)/neuroglycopenia (e.g., poor concentration, confusion, incoordination) or occurred in a patient taking insulin or a glucose-lowering drug. If treatment has not already been initiated, give a fast-acting carbohydrate, intramuscular glucagon, or IV dextrose as appropriate. It is critical to continue to monitor blood sugar regularly following an episode of hypoglycaemia. A long-acting carbohydrate should be given as soon as possible after the patient recovers and their blood sugar is >4 mmol/L.

5 Any red flag cardiac features (Box 24.1)?

Always exclude a serious underlying cardiac cause for TLOC if any of the features in Box 24.1 are present. Continue through the diagnostic pathway but admit the patient to hospital for continuous cardiac monitoring and discuss with a cardiologist.

Box 24.1 Red flag cardiac features

- TLOC during exertion
- Severe valvular heart disease, coronary artery disease or cardiomyopathy
- Family history of unexplained premature sudden death
- Previous ventricular arrhythmia or high risk for ventricular arrhythmia, such as prior MI or ventricular surgery
- Sustained or nonsustained ventricular tachycardia on telemetry
- High-risk ECG abnormality:
  - Bifascicular or trifascicular block (Fig. 24.1)
  - New T-wave or ST-segment changes (Box 3.2)
  - Sinus bradycardia <50 bpm or sinus pause >3 seconds
  - Second-degree atrioventricular (AV) block or complete heart block (Figs. 24.2 and 24.3)
  - Evidence of preexcitation (Fig. 5.3)
  - Marked QT interval prolongation, such as QTc >500 msec
  - Brugada pattern: RBBB with ST elevation in leads V_1–V_3 (Fig. 24.4)

24

Transient loss of consciousness: step-by-step assessment

Box 24.2 **Clinical features strongly suggestive of seizure**

- TLOC preceded by typical aura, e.g., unusual smell, 'rising' sensation in abdomen, déjà vu
- A witness account of abnormal tonic-clonic limb movements that are:
  - Coarse and rhythmic
  - Maintained for >30 seconds (ask witness to demonstrate movements)
- A witness account of head-turning to one side, unusual posturing, cyanosis or automatisms such as chewing or lip-smacking during the episode
- Bitten lateral border of tongue
- A prolonged period (>5 minutes) of confusion or drowsiness after the episode

---

6 | **>1 seizure feature (Box 24.2 *OR* 1 seizure feature and no syncope features (Box 24.3)?**

Differentiating between seizure and syncope is a key step in the assessment process. Features that suggest seizure are listed in Table 24.1. Descriptions of 'jerking', 'twitching' or 'fitting' are unhelpful since 'seizure-like' movements may occur in up to 90% of syncopal episodes. In contrast to seizure, the abnormal movements in syncope are usually nonrhythmic and brief (<15 seconds).

The episode of TLOC is highly likely to have been a seizure if >1 of the features in Box 24.2 are present. Seizure is also likely if any of these features are present and there are no specific pointers to syncope (Box 24.3). In both cases, proceed to Seizure assessment (below).

7 | **≥1 syncope features (Box 24.3) and no seizure features (Box 24.2)**

Suspect syncope if any of the features in Box 24.3 and none of those in Box 24.2 are present. Proceed to Syncope assessment (below).

Where differentiation between seizure and syncope is not straightforward, other clinical features may be helpful: amnesia for events before and after the episode, and headache or aching muscles after the episode suggest a seizure diagnosis; previous episodes of presyncope, witnessed pallor during TLOC, known cardiovascular disease and an abnormal ECG favour syncope. Urinary incontinence is not a useful discriminating feature.

8 Consider rarer causes including functional neurological disorders

If all other causes have been ruled out, then consider rarer causes of TLOC, including FNDs, particularly if atypical features are present (Table 24.1). Note that distinguishing between functional and organic causes of seizure/syncope can be very challenging, and sometimes there are few clinical features to suggest the underlying cause of TLOC. Have a low threshold for specialist input if the cause remains unclear.

Box 24.3 Clinical features strongly suggestive of syncope

- TLOC preceded by chest pain, palpitations, dyspnoea, light-headedness or typical 'presyncopal' prodrome, e.g., light-headedness, warmth, nausea, vomiting
- TLOC after standing up, after prolonged standing, during exertion or following a typical precipitant, e.g., unpleasant sight, sound, smell or pain, venipuncture, micturition, cough, large meal
- Brief duration of TLOC (<1 minute)
- Rapid return of clear-headedness after TLOC

24

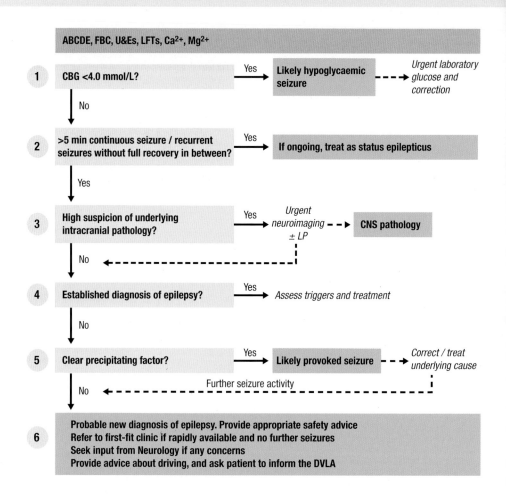

1   CBG <4.0 mmol/L?

Consider hypoglycaemia at the outset and correct urgently if <4.0 mmol/L because it:

- Is easily identified and corrected
- Will cause permanent neurological damage if not corrected
- Needs to be excluded prior to assessment for other causes.

2   >5 min continuous seizure/recurrent seizures without full recovery in between?

Status epilepticus is a medical emergency requiring urgent intervention. Provide appropriate anticonvulsant therapy. First-line therapy is with a benzodiazepine administered via either the buccal or rectal route if IV access is not immediately available. Once established, ongoing benzodiazepine treatment should be administered via the IV route. For a seizure that persists despite this treatment, second-line therapies include IV levetiracetam or phenytoin under the guidance of senior clinicians. Rapidly exclude or correct reversible factors (below) and seek urgent input from ICU ± the Neurology team. In some scenarios (e.g., seizures in the context of an overdose of a cardiotoxic agent), phenytoin is contraindicated (Chapter 28). Where seizures are persistent or recurrent following an overdose, is important to seek specialist toxicological advice on management.

3 High suspicion of underlying intracranial pathology?

Seizure may be a manifestation of important underlying intracranial pathology, such as haemorrhage, infarction, infection or space-occupying lesion.

Arrange urgent neuroimaging with a CT in the first instance if the patient is at risk of these pathologies (Box 24.4). Consider neuroimaging to exclude new intracranial pathology in any patient with known epilepsy with a change in seizure type/pattern without an apparent precipitating factor.

If any features suggest CNS infection (e.g., fever, meningism, rash), perform a lumbar puncture following CT, provided there are no contraindications (Clinical tool, Chapter 13).

4 Established diagnosis of epilepsy?

In patients with known epilepsy, address all factors that may have lowered seizure threshold (Box 24.5) or triggered the event. Measurement of anticonvulsant drug levels is not routinely indicated but consider it if there has been a recent change in medication or you suspect noncompliance.

5 Clear precipitating factor?

Important causes of seizure in adults without epilepsy include alcohol (excess or withdrawal), metabolic disturbance (e.g., $\downarrow Na^+$, $\downarrow Mg^{2+}$, $\downarrow Ca^{2+}$), recreational drug misuse or drug overdose, and CNS infection. Look for these factors and refer for specialist neurological evaluation (see below) if none is evident.

6 Probable new diagnosis of epilepsy. Refer to a neurologist as inpatient or outpatient

Admit any patient with repeated seizures or a significant causative factor that requires inpatient treatment. Consider early discharge only when patients have fully recovered, exhibit no neurological abnormalities and have a responsible adult to accompany and stay with them. Seek advice from Neurology if you have any concerns.

Arrange neuroimaging for all first-seizure episodes. Depending on local resources, imaging may be performed as an outpatient provided

---

Box 24.4 Indications for urgent neuroimaging in seizure

- Status epilepticus
- Focal or partial onset seizure
- Confusion, $\downarrow$GCS or focal neurological signs >30 minutes post-fit
- Recent head injury
- Acute severe headache preceding seizure
- Known malignancy with potential for brain metastases
- Immunosuppression (especially HIV)
- Meningism, fever or persistent headache and suspicion of CNS infection
- Anticoagulated or bleeding disorder

Box 24.5 Trigger factors for seizures

- Alcohol excess or withdrawal
- Recreational drug misuse
- Sleep deprivation
- Physical/mental exhaustion
- Intercurrent infection
- Metabolic disturbance ($\downarrow Na^+$, $\downarrow Mg^{2+}$, $\downarrow Ca^{2+}$, uraemia, liver failure)
- Noncompliance with medication or drug interaction
- Flickering lights

---

there are no indications for urgent imaging (Box 24.4) and a first seizure follow-up service is available. Further investigation may not be required in patients with a preexisting diagnosis of epilepsy who have fully recovered following a typical, uncomplicated fit.

A new diagnosis of an isolated seizure and/or epilepsy has significant lifestyle implications for patients. Patients should be warned about common seizure triggers or precipitating factors, such as alcohol or stress or lack of sleep (Box 24.5). They should avoid unsupervised activities that may pose a risk with sudden loss of consciousness (e.g., swimming or working at heights). Finally, there are strict criteria for driving. In the UK, the Driving and Vehicle Licensing Agency (DVLA) provides detailed guidance on the rules and regulations about driving with certain medical conditions, including seizures (https://www.gov.uk/government/publications/assessing-fitness-to-drive-a-guide-for-medical-professionals). Patients should be instructed to inform the DVLA.

24

Syncope: overview

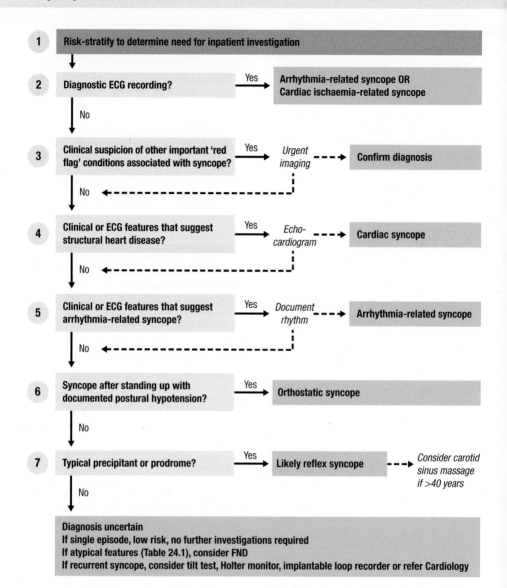

1 **Risk-stratify to determine need for inpatient investigation**

2 **Diagnostic ECG recording?** — Yes → **Arrhythmia-related syncope OR Cardiac ischaemia-related syncope**
No ↓

3 **Clinical suspicion of other important 'red flag' conditions associated with syncope?** — Yes → *Urgent imaging* - - - → **Confirm diagnosis**
No ↓

4 **Clinical or ECG features that suggest structural heart disease?** — Yes → *Echo-cardiogram* - - - → **Cardiac syncope**
No ↓

5 **Clinical or ECG features that suggest arrhythmia-related syncope?** — Yes → *Document rhythm* - - - → **Arrhythmia-related syncope**
No ↓

6 **Syncope after standing up with documented postural hypotension?** — Yes → **Orthostatic syncope**
No ↓

7 **Typical precipitant or prodrome?** — Yes → **Likely reflex syncope** - - - → *Consider carotid sinus massage if >40 years*
No ↓

Diagnosis uncertain
If single episode, low risk, no further investigations required
If atypical features (Table 24.1), consider FND
If recurrent syncope, consider tilt test, Holter monitor, implantable loop recorder or refer Cardiology

1 Risk-stratify to determine need for inpatient investigation

Admit all syncopal patients with red flag cardiac features (Box 24.1) and discuss promptly with the Cardiology team. Consider discharge with outpatient investigation (preferably in a syncope clinic if available) if the patient has recovered fully and has no other medical problems or no red flag features; otherwise, admit for a period of observation and investigation (monitoring ± ambulatory monitoring and ECG).

2 Diagnostic ECG recording?

Mobitz type II 2nd degree AV block (Fig. 24.2), complete heart block (Fig. 24.3), prolonged pauses, ventricular tachycardia or very rapid supraventricular tachycardia (>180/min) on the presenting ECG or telemetry establish an arrhythmic cause of syncope. Arrhythmia-related syncope is also highly likely with persistent sinus bradycardia <40 bpm, alternating left and right bundle branch block (LBBB and RBBB) or pacemaker malfunction with pauses.

ECG evidence of acute ischaemia suggests an arrhythmia secondary to ischaemia, for example, ventricular tachycardia, or cardiac ischaemia-related syncope. Acute coronary syndrome (ACS) is unlikely in the absence of chest pain or ECG evidence of ACS.

Discuss urgently with Cardiology if any of the above features is present.

3 Clinical suspicion of other important 'red flag' conditions associated with syncope?

These conditions may present with syncope, but this is rarely the predominant symptom. Exclude PE and aortic dissection if syncope occurs in the context of sudden-onset chest pain with no obvious alternative explanation. Also consider PE in syncopal patients with dyspnoea, hypoxia, evidence of DVT or major thromboembolic risk factors. Suspect aortic dissection if there is a new early diastolic murmur, pulse deficit or widened mediastinum on CXR (Chapter 3). Consider subarachnoid haemorrhage if there is associated headache (Chapter 13) and ruptured ectopic pregnancy or abdominal aortic aneurysm if there is abdominal pain (Chapter 7).

4 Clinical or ECG features that suggest structural heart disease?

Assess for clinical and ECG features that may suggest a 'structural' causes of cardiac syncope (e.g., severe aortic stenosis, hypertrophic cardiomyopathy, prolapsing atrial myxoma) or conditions that predispose to arrhythmia (e.g., severe left ventricular (LV) systolic impairment.) Clinical features may include:
- Exertional syncope
- A family history of sudden unexplained death (especially <40 years)
- A new murmur
- Dyspnoea, ankle swelling, raised JVP and bilateral chest crepitations suggestive of cardiac failure
- A history of MI, cardiomyopathy, valvular heart disease or congenital heart disease

ECG features may include LV hypertrophy, left axis deviation and left bundle branch block (LBBB). If clinical or ECG findings are consistent with structural heart disease, arrange an echocardiogram. Discuss with Cardiology if any relevant abnormalities are detected.

5 Clinical or ECG features that suggest arrhythmia-related syncope?

If the echocardiogram has not been diagnostic (see above), then suspect an arrhythmic aetiology for syncope in the following circumstances:
- Sudden-onset palpitation rapidly followed by syncope
- Syncope during exertion or while supine
- Previous MI or any of the following ECG abnormalities:
  - LBBB (Fig. 3.5), bi- or trifascicular block (Fig. 24.1)
  - Sinus bradycardia <50 bpm
  - Mobitz type I 2nd degree AV block (Fig. 24.5)
  - Sinus pause >3 seconds
  - Evidence of preexcitation (Fig. 5.3)
  - Prolonged QT interval (QTc >440 msec in men or >460 msec in women)
  - Brugada pattern: RBBB with ST elevation in leads V_1–V_3 (Fig. 24.4)

24

Syncope: step-by-step assessment

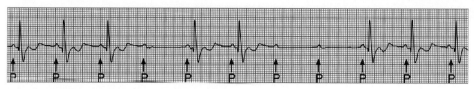

Fig. 24.1 Trifascicular block indicated by left axis deviation, 1st degree atrioventricular block and RBBB. (From Hampton JR. The ECG in practice, 5th ed. Edinburgh: Churchill Livingstone; 2008.)

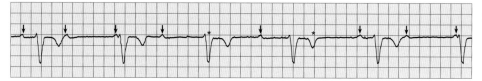

Fig. 24.2 Mobitz type II 2nd degree atrioventricular block. (From Boon NA, Colledge NR, Walker BR. Davidson's principles and practice of medicine, 20th ed. Edinburgh: Churchill Livingstone; 2006.)

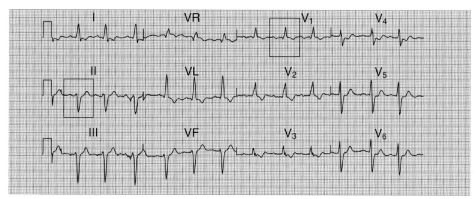

Fig. 24.3 Complete heart block. Arrows indicate P waves. (From Douglas G, Nicol F, Robertson C. Macleod's clinical examination, 12th ed. Edinburgh: Churchill Livingstone; 2009.)

- Features of arrhythmogenic right ventricular cardiomyopathy: negative T waves in leads V_1–V_3 and epsilon waves (a small deflection at the end of the QRS complex—see Fig. 24.6)
- Pathological Q wave
- Any ECG abnormality or history of cardiovascular disorder in the absence of a typical prodrome or precipitant for reflex or orthostatic syncope.

The correlation of a syncopal episode with a documented rhythm disturbance is the gold standard for diagnosis of arrhythmia-mediated syncope. This is frequently challenging, particularly when syncopal episodes are infrequent. The choice of investigation and degree of persistence depend on the risk of life-threatening arrhythmia and frequency of syncope.

Admit patients with red-flag cardiac features (Box 24.1) immediately for continuous inpatient ECG monitoring. Arrange Holter (1- to 7-day tape) or ambulatory patch monitoring (14 days) if symptoms occur relatively frequently. Consider an event recorder (external or implanted) if there is a high suspicion of arrhythmia but episodes are infrequent or prove difficult to capture by other methods.

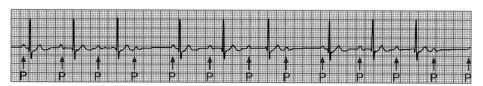

Fig. 24.4 Brugada syndrome. (From Hampton JR. The ECG in practice, 5th ed. Edinburgh: Churchill Livingstone; 2008.)

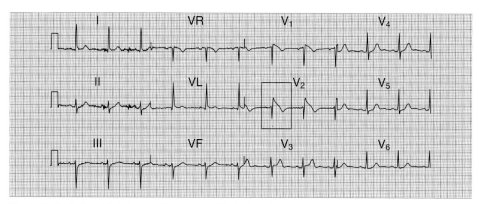

Fig. 24.5 Mobitz type I 2nd degree atrioventricular block. (From Boon NA, Colledge NR, Walker BR. Davidson's principles and practice of medicine, 20th ed. Edinburgh: Churchill Livingstone; 2006.)

6 Syncope after standing up with documented postural hypotension?

Diagnose orthostatic syncope if there is:
- A history of light-headedness shortly after standing, followed by brief TLOC
- A documented postural BP drop (of ≥20 mmHg in systolic BP or ≥10 mmHg in diastolic BP within 3 minutes of moving from lying to standing)

In other circumstances, it may be difficult to distinguish orthostatic from reflex syncope, for example, when symptoms occur with prolonged standing.

Look for an underlying cause of postural hypotension. Common causes, particularly in the elderly, include drugs (e.g., antihypertensives, vasodilators [especially sublingual nitroglycerine] and diuretics), autonomic neuropathy, and Parkinsonian syndromes. In severe form it may reflect fluid loss, such as major haemorrhage or severe dehydration.

7 Typical precipitant or prodrome?

A clear precipitating trigger, such as intense emotion, venepuncture or prolonged standing (vasovagal syncope) or coughing, sneezing or micturition (situational syncope), together with typical prodromal symptoms, strongly suggests reflex syncope, especially in patients with no ECG or clinical evidence to suggest structural heart disease or arrhythmia. Consider tilt-table testing in cases of diagnostic doubt. Tilt-table testing enables the reproduction of reflex syncope in a safe laboratory setting. Carotid sinus hypersensitivity is a form of reflex syncope and is usually diagnosed with carotid sinus massage (CSM). CSM should be avoided in patients with a carotid bruit or history of stroke/TIA and requires continuous ECG monitoring; it is diagnostic when syncope is reproduced in the presence of asystole lasting >3 seconds.

24

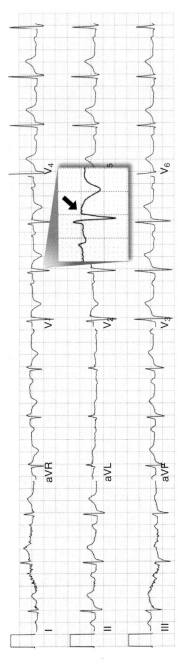

Fig. 24.6 An epsilon wave in a patient with arrhythmogenic right ventricular cardiomyopathy. (From Issa Z, Miller JM, Zipes DP. Clinical arrhythmology and electrophysiology: a companion to Braunwald's heart disease, 4th ed. Philadelphia: Elsevier; 2024. Note for Creative Commons: this figure appears as eFIG. 33.5 in Adler AM, Carlton RR, Stewart KL. Introduction to radiologic & imaging sciences & patient care, 8th ed. New York: Saunders; 2022.)

Unintentional weight loss of >5% body weight within the preceding 12 months requires investigation. Lesser degrees of weight loss may also signify underlying pathology, particularly in the frail elderly. Establish how much weight has been lost and over what time frame; whether there has been a change in clothes size; and whether there has been a corresponding change in appetite. If present, use 'system-specific' symptoms or signs (e.g., haemoptysis, altered bowel habit) to narrow the differential diagnosis and guide appropriate investigation.

Malignancy

In patients with unintentional weight loss, an underlying malignancy is the first diagnosis to consider. Approximately 50% of patients presenting with unintentional weight loss secondary to malignancy have GI cancers. Weight loss in non-GI cancers tends to be associated with more advanced disease.

Nonmalignant GI disease

Weight loss is frequently observed in disorders that lead to swallowing difficulty (Chapter 10), malabsorption (e.g., coeliac disease, pancreatic insufficiency) or persistent inflammation (e.g., inflammatory bowel disease). In peptic ulcer disease, chronic mesenteric ischaemia and chronic pancreatitis, the pain associated with eating may lead to weight loss through avoidance of food. However, weight loss is not an expected feature of functional GI disorders, such as irritable bowel syndrome.

Endocrine disorders

Persistent hyperglycaemia due to uncontrolled or undiagnosed diabetes causes weight loss, alongside polydipsia and polyuria. In thyrotoxicosis, weight loss occurs despite normal or increased appetite. Patients with hypercalcaemia may experience weight loss due to underlying malignant disease or the direct effects of $\uparrow Ca^{2+}$, such as osmotic diuresis, anorexia, nausea and vomiting. Weight loss is also one of several nonspecific presenting symptoms in chronic adrenal insufficiency (Box 11.2).

Chronic disease

In severe nonmalignant disease, such as advanced COPD, heart failure or chronic kidney disease, several mechanisms may contribute to weight loss, including poor appetite, persistent catabolic state and polypharmacy. Weight loss is frequently a presenting feature of chronic inflammatory states (e.g., inflammatory arthritis, connective tissue disease, vasculitis). Prominent weight loss is also a feature of chronic infection, such as tuberculosis, infective endocarditis and HIV.

Neurological disorder

Motor neuron disease, Parkinson's disease, multiple sclerosis and stroke may lead to weight loss through dysphagia (Chapter 10). Limb weakness and impaired functional abilities can present a significant barrier to food preparation and consumption. Multifactorial weight loss is also common in dementia, particularly in advanced stages.

Medication

Drug side effects such as anorexia, dry mouth, altered taste sensation, nausea, vomiting or sedation may result in reduced calorie intake (Box 25.1). Certain drugs may be misused to facilitate weight loss, such as laxatives or thyroxine.

Psychiatric

Low mood can lead to low appetite or a lack of motivation to prepare meals, resulting in weight loss. This is a more common phenomenon in elderly people with mood disorders. Depression is an underrecognized phenomenon in older adults and is particularly

---

Box 25.1 Drug causes of weight loss

Direct weight loss effect

- Diuretics ('pseudo' weight loss)
- Levothyroxine (if excessive dosage)
- Topiramate (mechanism uncertain)
- Appetite suppressants, such as lorcaserin
- Glucagon-like peptide-1 (GLP-1) analogues, such as semaglutide
- Sympathomimetic agents, such as methylphenidate
- Sodium-glucose co-transporter-2 (SGLT-2) inhibitors, such as empagliflozin

Other drug-induced mechanisms of weight loss

- Nausea and vomiting: Box 11.1
- Altered sense of taste, such as allopurinol, zopiclone, metronidazole
- Dry mouth, such as anticholinergics, clonidine, diuretics
- Sedation, such as opiates, benzodiazepines, antipsychotics

---

common in those living in institutional settings. Addressing the underlying depressive illness can lead to improved oral intake and weight gain. Primary eating disorders (anorexia and bulimia) are most common in younger females but are increasingly recognized in young men; the patient may deny that a problem exists, and concerns are often raised by relatives and friends who have noticed a change in eating behaviour or physical appearance. Substance misuse disorders, including alcohol dependence, may result in weight loss due to multifactorial malnutrition.

Other

Explore possible social causes for weight loss, such as lack of money to buy food, lack of access to food and social isolation. Poor dentition or ill-fitting dentures may also contribute.

Unintentional weight loss is a concerning but nonspecific symptom. Refer, initially, to the relevant chapter if one of the following symptoms is present: Dysphagia (Chapter 10), GI haemorrhage (Chapter 8), Haemoptysis (Chapter 6), Jaundice (Chapter 12). Return to this pathway if no cause for weight loss is identified.

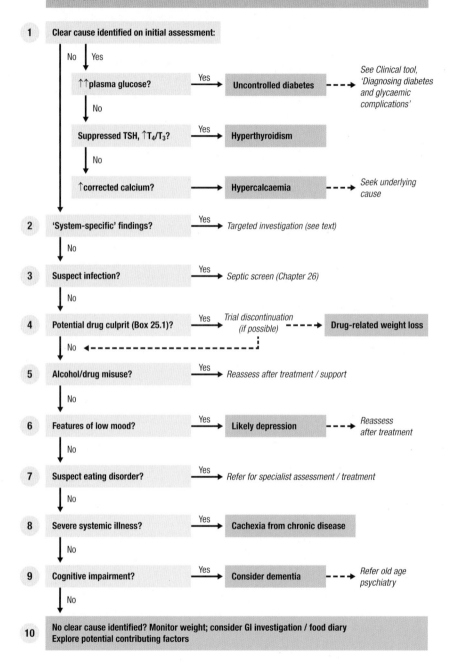

Full clinical assessment, breast, genital & rectal examination, FBC, U&E, LFT, calcium, glucose, TFT +/- CXR

1 Clear cause identified on initial assessment:

No / Yes

↑↑plasma glucose? — Yes → **Uncontrolled diabetes** - - - → *See Clinical tool, 'Diagnosing diabetes and glycaemic complications'*

No

Suppressed TSH, ↑T₄/T₃? — Yes → **Hyperthyroidism**

No

↑corrected calcium? → **Hypercalcaemia** - - - → *Seek underlying cause*

2 'System-specific' findings? — Yes → *Targeted investigation (see text)*

No

3 Suspect infection? — Yes → *Septic screen (Chapter 26)*

No

4 Potential drug culprit (Box 25.1)? — Yes → *Trial discontinuation (if possible)* - - - → **Drug-related weight loss**

No ◄- - - - - - - - - - - - - - - - - - - ┘

5 Alcohol/drug misuse? — Yes → *Reassess after treatment / support*

No

6 Features of low mood? — Yes → **Likely depression** - - - → *Reassess after treatment*

No

7 Suspect eating disorder? — Yes → *Refer for specialist assessment / treatment*

No

8 Severe systemic illness? — Yes → **Cachexia from chronic disease**

No

9 Cognitive impairment? — Yes → **Consider dementia** - - - → *Refer old age psychiatry*

No

10 No clear cause identified? Monitor weight; consider GI investigation / food diary
Explore potential contributing factors

1   Clear cause identified on initial screening?

Hyperglycaemia

Consider new-onset diabetes in patients without a preexisting diagnosis (Clinical tool): check for diabetes-related ketoacidosis (DKA) and hyperosmolar hyperglycaemic state (HHS) and, if present, admit for urgent treatment.

In the absence of hyperglycaemic emergencies, refer to your local diabetes service for treatment initiation. Remember that a mild, transient increase in blood glucose level may occur in any acute illness and is typically a marker of disease severity (stress hyperglycaemia). In older patients with new-onset diabetes and weight loss, consider underlying pancreatic malignancy, especially when there is associated abdominal pain.

In patients with known diabetes, use plasma HbA1c to gauge recent glycaemic control;

consider hyperglycaemia as a contributor to weight loss if control is suboptimal (especially in type 1 diabetes) but continue to search for alternative causes.

Thyrotoxicosis (TSH)

Suppressed TSH with $\uparrow T_4/T_3$ level is diagnostic of hyperthyroidism. Look for associated clinical features, including tachycardia, tremor, poor sleep, heat intolerance and increased bowel activity ± eye and skin changes in Graves disease. Check thyroid receptor antibody (TRAB) levels to help identify the underlying aetiology and refer to Endocrinology.

Hypercalcaemia

Check plasma parathyroid hormone (PTH) levels to identify the likely cause. PTH should be suppressed by hypercalcaemia, so $\uparrow$PTH or 'inappropriately normal' PTH suggests primary

---

Clinical tool
Diagnosing diabetes and glycaemic complications

Diagnosis of diabetes

Typical presenting symptoms of diabetes include thirst, polyuria, blurred vision, and unexplained weight loss. These will be more prominent and have a shorter history in type 1 diabetes due to absolute insulin deficiency. In type 2 diabetes, there may be little in the way of symptoms, or they may go unnoticed due to their insidious onset. Biochemical cut-offs to clinch the diagnosis are described in Table 25.1. In symptomatic patients, one laboratory measure is required to confirm diabetes. In asymptomatic people, repeat testing, preferably with the same test, is recommended as soon as possible to confirm the diagnosis.

Assessment of long-term glycaemic control

Guidelines for targeting HbA1c in the ongoing management of diabetes vary between <48 mmol/mol (6.5%) and <58 mmol/mol (7.5%), depending on local authority. Nonetheless, the aim is to achieve the lowest HbA1c possible for the individual patient, with consideration of their risk of hypoglycaemia and comorbidities.

Acute complications of diabetes

Hyperglycaemic crises

DKA is a medical emergency and involves a triad of hyperglycaemia, ketosis and acidosis. It is the result of insulin deficiency (absolute—type 1 diabetes/pancreatic disease; or relative—poorly controlled type 2 diabetes). It develops rapidly over hours, and associated mortality is <1% (with higher rates in developing countries). Diagnostic

criteria can be found in Table 25.2. Seek a precipitating cause (e.g., poor compliance with treatment, intercurrent illness, new diagnosis of type 1 diabetes mellitus), and initiate urgent treatment.

HHS is usually a complication of poorly controlled type 2 diabetes, often with insidious onset over days to weeks. Blood glucose is very high, with high osmolality and hypercoagulability. It is life threatening, with a 5–15% mortality rate. Frail elderly patients are most at risk. It can be complicated by myocardial infarction, stroke or peripheral arterial thrombosis. In addition, overly rapid correction of metabolic abnormalities can lead to complications such as seizures, cerebral oedema and central pontine myelinolysis. It is therefore vital to correct abnormalities gradually and to carefully monitor the plasma osmolality during treatment.

Hypoglycaemia

Whilst there is no clear consensus on the biochemical definition of hypoglycaemia, it is largely accepted that a blood glucose level <4 mmol/L (72 mg/dL) would be an appropriate level to trigger treatment in a person with diabetes. Severe hypoglycaemia is defined by the requirement for external assistance to restore normal blood glucose (whether relatives or emergency services). Symptoms (Table 25.3) will usually alert a person with diabetes to the development of hypoglycaemia, but some people lose their hypoglycaemia warning symptoms, known as impaired hypoglycaemia awareness, and they are at high risk of severe hypoglycaemia as a result.

25

Table 25.1 Biochemical criteria for diagnosis of diabetes mellitus

Diabetes	Measurement
Fasting plasma glucose	≥7.0 mmol/L (126 mg/dL)
Random plasma glucose	≥11.1 mmol/L (200 mg/dL)
2-hour plasma glucose on OGTT[a]	≥11.1 mmol/L (200 mg/dL)
HbA1c[b]	≥48 mmol/mol (6.5%)
Impaired fasting glycaemia	
Fasting plasma glucose	6.1–6.9 mmol/L (110–125 mg/dL)
Impaired glucose tolerance	
2-hour plasma glucose on OGTT	7.8–11.0 mmol/L (140–200 mg/dL)

[a]OGTT—Oral glucose tolerance test: venous plasma glucose in fasting state, administer 75g oral glucose load, repeat venous plasma glucose at 2 hours.
[b]Not suitable as a diagnostic test in children and young people or in the context of suspected type 1 diabetes, symptoms for <2 months, acute illness, pregnancy, treatment with medications that cause rapid glucose rise (e.g., steroids, antipsychotics) or acute pancreatic damage/surgery.

Table 25.3 Symptoms of hypoglycaemia

Autonomic	Neuroglycopenic	Non-specific
Palpitation	Confusion	Tiredness
Sweating	Weakness	Nausea
Tremor	Dizziness	Headache
Hunger	Reduced concentration	—
Anxiety	Incoordination	—
—	Drowsiness	—
—	Speech difficulty	—

Table 25.2 Criteria for diagnosis of DKA and HHS

	DKA	HHS
Plasma glucose[a]	>11 mmol/L	>30 mmol/L
Osmolality	—	>320 mOsm/kg
Arterial pH	<7.3	>7.3
Serum bicarbonate	≤15 mmol/L	>15 mmol/L[b]
Blood ketones (capillary sample)	≥ 3 mmol/L	< 3 mmol/L
Urine ketones	++ Positive	Negative/small
Mental status	Alert or drowsy	Altered cognition

[a]If a patient with DKA has started treatment with supplementary insulin, they may present with a normal blood glucose but still have ketosis and acidosis and be at risk of clinical deterioration.
[b]In some patients, metabolic acidosis may be present due either to relative insulin deficiency (check ketones) or to intercurrent acute illness (lactic acidosis or AKI).
Adapted from Joint British Diabetes Societies for Inpatient Care guidelines: Management of Diabetic Ketoacidosis in Adults (2023) and The Management of Hyperosmolar Hyperglycaemic State (HHS) in Adults (2022).

hyperparathyroidism. If ↓PTH, consider malignancy (e.g., skeletal metastases, multiple myeloma or tumour secretion of PTH-related peptide). Other causes, particularly if hypercalcaemia is mild, include sarcoidosis, thiazide diuretics and vitamin D analogues.

2   'System-specific' findings?

Consider underlying malignancy in any patient with unexplained weight loss. Look for clues in the history, physical examination and routine tests that may help to target further investigation.

Request an urgent CXR in patients with persistent respiratory symptoms (>3 weeks) or in those >40 years with a history of smoking or asbestos exposure. Refer for respiratory investigation (usually CT chest ± bronchoscopy) in patients with an abnormal CXR, respiratory symptoms for >6 weeks despite a normal CXR, or clinical features and risk factors suggestive of lung cancer.

Refer patients with concerning GI symptoms or unexplained iron deficiency anaemia (see Clinical Tool: Further Assessment of Anaemia) for urgent endoscopic evaluation. Upper GI endoscopy is indicated if dysphagia, vomiting or upper abdominal pain/discomfort are present; colonoscopy if there is altered bowel habit, tenesmus or lower abdominal pain/discomfort; and upper and lower GI endoscopy in the presence of iron-deficiency anaemia. CT colonogram provides a less-invasive alternative to colonoscopy and may be more appropriate in selected patients, such as the frail or multimorbid.

In patients with diarrhoea and weight loss, consider non-malignant GI causes. Inflammatory bowel disease (IBD) may present with abdominal pain with associated persistent bloody diarrhoea. Malabsorption presents with abdominal bloating, diarrhoea, steatorrhoea and nutritional deficiencies. Send coeliac serology and faecal elastase as baseline investigations. Patients with suspected IBD or unexplained malabsorption symptoms should be referred to Gastroenterology.

Arrange appropriate imaging if you palpate an abdominal or pelvic mass. USS is often a helpful initial investigation, particularly for pelvic masses, but CT is frequently required for further characterization ± staging of malignant tumours.

Check a PSA level in males with prostatic symptoms. Measure PSA prior to the rectal exam to avoid false-positive tests. Refer patients with a hard irregular prostate or a raised age-adjusted PSA for urgent urological assessment. Bear in mind that localized prostate cancer is unlikely to account for significant weight loss, so continue to seek alternative causes unless there are features of advanced disease, such as bone pain, biochemical evidence of skeletal metastases (e.g., ↑ALP) or a markedly ↑PSA (>20 ng/mL).

Lymphadenopathy, either local or generalized, may signify infection, inflammation, haematological malignancy or solid organ cancer with lymphatic involvement. Check LDH (often ↑ in haematological malignancy), blood film, and screen for infection and autoimmune disease. Consider specific clinical examinations depending on the scenario (e.g., breast examination, testicular examination). In persistent lymphadenopathy, consider CT chest/abdomen/pelvis and arrange lymph node biopsy to establish a tissue diagnosis.

3   Suspect infection?

Perform a septic screen in patients with fever or elevated WCC/inflammatory markers (Clinical tool, A Septic Screen, Chapter 26). Ask about foreign travel, infectious contacts, and risk factors for HIV and TB. Examine carefully and repeatedly for murmurs and peripheral stigmata of endocarditis.

4   Severe systemic illness?

Assess the severity and trajectory of chronic disease (e.g., heart failure, COPD, degenerative neurological disease or renal failure) using symptom status, functional performance, frequency of hospitalization and objective markers (e.g., GFR, FEV1). Weight loss and anorexia may occur in advanced disease. Seek specialist input to optimize management but consider the need for dietetic and/or palliative care input. Consider autoimmune causes for

25

Clinical tool
Further assessment of anaemia

Step 1 Use the mean cell volume (MCV) to narrow the differential diagnosis

Microcytic anaemia (MCV <80 fL) is most commonly due to iron deficiency.

First, confirm iron deficiency. Serum ferritin is more indicative of total body iron than serum iron but may be increased by liver disease or systemic inflammation.
- ↓ferritin (<15 ng/mL) confirms iron deficiency.
- If ferritin is between 15 and 150 ng/mL but there is suspicion of systemic inflammation, transferrin saturation <16% suggests iron deficiency.
- Iron deficiency is unlikely if ferritin >150 ng/mL.

If iron deficiency is confirmed, identify the underlying cause.
- Review the patient's diet and consider inadequate iron intake, especially in vegetarians.
- Ask about blood loss: menorrhagia, haematemesis, melaena, haemoptysis, epistaxis, haematuria, trauma.
- Arrange UGIE and colonoscopy unless there is a clear non-GI source of bleeding, such as menorrhagia, haematuria.
- Exclude coeliac disease: serology ± duodenal biopsy at the time of UGIE.
- If the cause remains unclear, refer to GI for further investigation, such as capsule endoscopy.

Reassess symptoms and FBC after iron supplementation and treatment of the underlying cause.

Refer patients with a ↓MCV and normal iron stores to Haematology for investigation of alternative diagnoses, such as thalassaemia, sideroblastic anaemia.

In patients with a *macrocytic anaemia* (MCV >100 fL), measure vitamin B_{12} and fasting serum folate. Folate deficiency is likely to be due to poor dietary intake (fruit, leafy vegetables), but always check coeliac serology. B_{12} deficiency is unlikely to be due to dietary deficiency unless the patient is a strict vegetarian/vegan. Consider causes of malabsorption, such as coeliac disease, IBD and previous gastrectomy or small bowel resection. Investigate for pernicious anaemia; intrinsic factor antibodies are diagnostic but present in only 50% of cases; antiparietal cell antibodies are nonspecific but their absence makes pernicious anaemia less likely (present in 85% of cases). Seek Haematology advice in difficult cases.

If B_{12} and folate are normal, exclude hypothyroidism, pregnancy, alcohol excess and chronic liver disease, and then evaluate for haemolysis (Step 2) and myelodysplasia (Step 3), as described below.

In patients with a *normocytic anaemia*, measure iron studies and vitamin B_{12}/folate as combined iron and B_{12} or folate deficiencies (e.g., nutritional deficiency, small bowel disease) may result in a normocytic picture. Normocytic anaemia, however, is most commonly a result of anaemia of chronic disease and typically occurs in older patients.

Step 2 Investigate for haemolysis

Consider haemolysis in patients with normal or ↑MCV. Haemolytic anaemia should be suspected in any patient with anaemia and:
- Raised bilirubin/LDH—suggests increased red cell destruction
- Reticulocytosis—suggests a compensatory increase in red cell production
- Reduced haptoglobin—haptoglobin binds free haemoglobin released by haemolysis

Causes of haemolytic anaemia can be classified as intravascular or extravascular. Distinguishing intravascular from extravascular haemolysis helps to narrow the differential diagnosis. Intravascular haemolysis occurs when red cells are destroyed within the vasculature, releasing free haemoglobin into the plasma. Clinical features that suggest intravascular haemolysis include positive urinalysis for blood (due to haemoglobinuria) and red cell fragments (schistocytes) on a blood film. With extravascular haemolysis, there is increased destruction of red blood cells by the reticuloendothelial system (e.g., the spleen). Clinical features that suggest extravascular haemolysis include splenomegaly and spherocytosis on a blood film. Causes of both types of haemolysis can be found in Box 25.2.

The cause of haemolysis may be suggested by the initial blood film (e.g., sickle cells), but it is likely that further investigation will be required. Screen for autoimmune haemolytic anaemia with a direct antiglobulin test (DAT) if extravascular haemolysis is identified. Refer all patients with haemolytic anaemia to Haematology to guide further investigation and management. Emergency referral is required if you suspect haemolytic uraemic syndrome (diarrhoeal illness with AKI), thrombotic thrombocytopenic purpura (neurological symptoms, AKI, fever) or disseminated intravascular coagulation (deranged clotting, low fibrinogen, concomitant severe illness).

Step 3 Seek evidence of bone marrow failure or haematological malignancy

Review the FBC and blood film for:
1. Deficiencies in other cell lines (↓WBC, ↓platelets)
2. Increased WBC, such as chronic myeloid leukaemia, chronic lymphocytic leukaemia
3. Atypical cells, such as blasts

Ask about symptoms of bleeding, fever, weight loss or night sweats. Examine for lymphadenopathy, splenomegaly, petechiae and ecchymosis. Refer all patients with a suspicion of haematological malignancy or bone marrow failure to Haematology for further investigation, such as bone marrow evaluation.

Look for evidence of multiple myeloma: send serum for protein electrophoresis and urine for measurement of Bence Jones protein. Discuss with Haematology if these

Clinical tool—cont'd
Further assessment of anaemia

are positive or if there is clinical suspicion, for example, bone pain, pathological fracture, lytic bone lesions, unexplained ↑Ca^{2+} or ESR.

Step 4 Consider chronic nonhaematological disease

The most common cause of normocytic anaemia is chronic inflammatory disease, e.g., rheumatoid arthritis, polymyalgia rheumatica, chronic infection or malignancy. Consider the diagnosis if:
- Other causes of ↓Hb have been excluded (including iron, B_{12}, folate deficiency)
- There is no evidence of active bleeding
- Anaemia is mild, such as Hb>80 g/L, and
- ↑ESR/CRP or ↓albumin

Search for an underlying cause and maintain a high suspicion for malignancy, particularly when there is underlying weight loss.

Consider chronic kidney disease as a potential cause for normocytic anaemia (↓erythropoietin production) if GFR <60 mL/min/1.73 m^2, and especially if <30 mL/min/1.73 m^2. Measure ferritin and transferrin saturation to ensure that the patient is iron-replete and discuss with a nephrologist.

Step 5 Refer to a haematologist

Seek input from Haematology if the cause of anaemia is still unclear, you suspect a serious or unusual haematological disorder, or the patient fails to respond to therapy.

---

weight loss in patients with fever and weight loss in the absence of infection. Enquire about symptoms of inflammatory arthritis, connective tissue disease and vasculitis and send the relevant immunology.

5   Potential drug culprit?

Review all medications, prescribed and non-prescribed, including any over-the-counter medications and supplements. In patients with reduced dietary intake, ask about symptoms such as dry mouth, drowsiness, altered taste sensation or nausea and look for potential drug culprits (Box 25.1). If you suspect a drug cause, reassess weight and symptoms after discontinuation.

6   Alcohol/drug misuse?

Enquire about alcohol intake and recreational drug use. Where possible seek collateral history from friends or family (who may have raised the concerns regarding weight loss). Explore associated factors that may be contributing to weight loss, such as appetite suppression, replacement of meals with alcohol/drug intake, lack of money to buy food or coexistent mood disorders.

7   Features of low mood?

Look for evidence of low mood, such as anhedonia (loss of pleasure in life), undue pessimism or feelings of guilt/worthlessness, as well as biological features of depression, such as lack

---

Box 25.2 Causes of haemolytic anaemia

Intravascular causes

Mechanical stress
- Prosthetic heart valves
- March haemoglobinaemia
- Microangiopathic haemolysis such as thrombotic thyrombocytopenic purpura, disseminated intravascular coagulation, haemolytic uraemic syndrome

Infections
- Bacterial toxins such as *Clostridium perfringens*
- Intracellular pathogens such as malaria

Drug-induced

Acquired membrane disorder such as paroxysmal nocturnal haemoglobinuria

Oxidative stress such as glucose-6-phosphate dehydrogenase deficiency

Extravascular causes

Warm antibody autoimmune haemolytic anaemia
- Primary (idiopathic)
- Secondary—drug-induced, associated with malignancy or autoimmune disease

Cold antibody autoimmune haemolytic anaemia
- Primary (idiopathic)
- Secondary – infection (e.g., mycoplasma), lymphoma

Hypersplenism

Hereditary spherocytosis

Sickle cell anaemia

---

of energy, poor sleep (early morning waking), and reduced libido. Consider undertaking a depression score, such as the Geriatric Depression Scale in the elderly or the Patient Health Questionnaire-9 (PHQ-9) in younger adults. If you suspect depression as the cause of weight

25

loss, reassess weight and other symptoms after a period of treatment.

8 Suspect eating disorder?

Consider the possibility of an eating disorder, particularly in younger women with amenorrhoea or a background of psychiatric or psychological problems. Be alert to important clues such as distorted attitudes to weight or body image (e.g., underplaying the seriousness of weight loss, fear of gaining weight, preoccupation with weight issues) or concerns raised by friends/family members (e.g., skipping meals, concealing food). Be sensitive and tactful but persistent in questioning and refer to specialist services if significant concern.

9 Cognitive impairment?

Assess cognition formally with a Mini-Mental State Examination or Addenbrooke's Cognitive Examination-III in patients with either established or suspected or cognitive impairment. Wherever possible, obtain a collateral history from friends, relatives or carers to evaluate the contribution from cognitive impairment to weight loss e.g., forgetting meals, inability to prepare food, paranoid ideas about food. In patients with more advanced dementia, enquire about the patient's ability to transfer food from plate to mouth and any swallowing problems. Refer patient for specialist evaluation, such as psychiatry of old age.

10 Consider further investigation and/or food diary. Explore factors contributing to reduced food intake

If weight loss persists with no clear cause, consider GI investigation/referral ± CT if not already performed. Use a food diary to record calorie intake. Reconsider the possibility of a primary eating disorder or depression. Explore possible contributing factors to inadequate food intake, including inadequate dentition, swallowing problems, lack of motivation (or money), impaired mobility (unable to get to shop), or subtle cognitive impairment. Refer frail, elderly patients for comprehensive geriatric assessment. In those with unexplained weight loss, ensure follow-up over time in case new symptoms suggesting an underlying cause become apparent.

In clinical practice, fever (or pyrexia) is a body temperature of ≥38°C. Extreme fever (>41°C) is life threatening and tends to occur with gram-negative bacteraemia, severe toxidromes, intra-cranial pathology (leading to central tempera-ture dysregulation) or extreme environmental conditions. Pyrexia of unknown origin is an intermittent fever of ≥38.3°C that persists without explanation for 3 weeks despite appropriate investigation.

Fever occurs most commonly as part of the acute phase response to infection. Sepsis is defined as 'life-threatening organ dysfunction due to a dysregulated host response to infection'.[1] It carries a significant mortality and must be recognized and managed quickly. Other groups of conditions which cause fever are malignancies, inflammatory diseases, drug reactions and miscellaneous causes. A nonexhaustive list of conditions from each group that should be considered in a patient with fever follows.

Infection

Respiratory system

- Acute bronchitis
- Bronchiolitis
- Pneumonia
- Influenza
- Empyema
- Infective exacerbation of bronchiectasis/COPD
- Tuberculosis (TB)

GI causes

- Gastroenteritis
- Appendicitis
- Biliary sepsis
- Viral hepatitis
- Diverticulitis
- Intra-abdominal abscess

Skin/soft tissue

- Cellulitis
- Necrotizing fasciitis
- Pyomyositis
- Infected pressure sore
- Wound infection

Musculoskeletal causes

- Septic arthritis (native and prosthetic joint)
- Osteomyelitis
- Discitis
- Epidural abscess

Genitourinary tract

- Lower urinary tract infection (UTI), such as cystitis, prostatitis
- Upper UTI (pyelonephritis)
- Perinephric collection
- Pelvic inflammatory disease
- Epididymo-orchitis
- Sexually transmitted infections (STIs)

1. Singer M, Deutschman CS, Seymour CW, et al. The third international consensus definitions for sepsis and septic shock (sepsis-3). JAMA. 2016:23;315(8):801-10.

CNS

- Meningitis (bacterial, viral, fungal, TB)
- Encephalitis
- Cerebral abscess

ENT

- Upper respiratory tract infection (RTI), such as tonsillitis
- Otitis media
- Quinsy
- Dental abscess
- Mumps/parotitis
- Glandular fever (Epstein–Barr virus; EBV)
- Sinusitis

Immunocompromised patients

- *Pneumocystis jiroveci (carinii)* pneumonia
- Aspergillosis
- TB
- Atypical mycobacterial infection, such as *Mycobacterium avium intracellulare*
- Cytomegalovirus (CMV) infection
- Toxoplasmosis
- Cryptococcal meningitis
- *Crytosporidium* infection
- Disseminated herpes/fungal infection

Returning travelers

- Malaria
- Typhoid

- Infective diarrhoea, for example, cholera, amoebiasis, *Shigella*
- Amoebic liver abscess
- *Rickettsiae*
- Schistosomiasis
- Dengue
- Chikungunya
- Leptospirosis

Other infectious causes

- Infective endocarditis
- Brucellosis
- Lyme disease
- Q fever
- HIV
- Fungal infection
- Measles, rubella
- Herpes zoster infection (chickenpox or shingles)

Malignancy

- Haematological malignancy, including lymphoma, leukaemia, and myeloma
- Solid tumours, especially renal, liver, colon, pancreas

Inflammatory diseases

- Large vessel vasculitis (e.g., giant cell arteritis, Takayasu arteritis)

- Medium vessel vasculitis (e.g., polyarteritis nodosa)
- ANCA-associated vasculitis (e.g., granulomatosis with polyangiitis, microscopic polyangiitis)
- Polymyalgia rheumatica
- Inflammatory arthritis
- Systemic lupus erythematosus
- Inflammatory myopathy
- Adult-onset Still's disease
- Familial Mediterranean fever
- Pancreatitis
- Inflammatory bowel disease
- Sarcoidosis
- Rheumatic fever
- Pericarditis

Drugs

- Drug fever (almost any drug)
- Neuroleptic malignant syndrome
- Serotonin toxicity
- Stimulant and anticholinergic toxidromes

Other causes

- Transfusion-associated
- Thyrotoxicosis, thyroiditis
- Phaeochromocytoma
- Deep vein thrombosis (DVT)/pulmonary embolism (PE)
- Delirium tremens
- Erythroderma/Stevens–Johnson syndrome

26

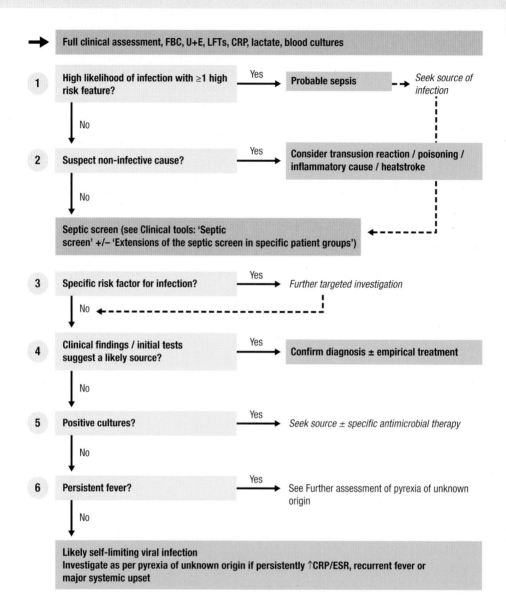

Full clinical assessment, FBC, U+E, LFTs, CRP, lactate, blood cultures

1 High likelihood of infection with ≥1 high risk feature? — Yes → Probable sepsis ⇢ *Seek source of infection*

No ↓

2 Suspect non-infective cause? — Yes → Consider transusion reaction / poisoning / inflammatory cause / heatstroke

No ↓

Septic screen (see Clinical tools: 'Septic screen' +/– 'Extensions of the septic screen in specific patient groups')

3 Specific risk factor for infection? — Yes → *Further targeted investigation*

No ↓

4 Clinical findings / initial tests suggest a likely source? — Yes → Confirm diagnosis ± empirical treatment

No ↓

5 Positive cultures? — Yes → *Seek source ± specific antimicrobial therapy*

No ↓

6 Persistent fever? — Yes → See Further assessment of pyrexia of unknown origin

No ↓

Likely self-limiting viral infection
Investigate as per pyrexia of unknown origin if persistently ↑CRP/ESR, recurrent fever or major systemic upset

1 High likelihood of infection with >1 high risk feature?

It is essential to consider sepsis due to its high associated mortality. Scores such as qSOFA, SIRS and NEWS are all used as tools to screen for sepsis, but each has its limitations, and the Surviving Sepsis Campaign recommends no single screening tool. The National Institute for Health and Care Excellence (NICE) recommends diagnosing sepsis and initiating immediate management with fluids and antibiotics if there is a high likelihood of infection and one of the following high-risk features:

- Altered consciousness
- Heart rate >130 bpm
- Respiratory rate $\geq$ 25/min OR $\geq$ 40% inspired O_2 to maintain $SpO_2 > 92\%$
- Systolic blood pressure $\leq$ 90 mmHg OR > 40 mmHg below normal
- Not passed urine in previous 18 hours OR if catheterized, passed <0.5 mL/kg/hr
- Mottled or ashen appearance
- Cyanosis of skin, lips or tongue
- Lactate >2 mmol/L
- Nonblanching rash of skin

Adapted from National Institute for Health and Care Excellence. Suspected sepsis: recognition, diagnosis and early management. 2016.

It is important to note that not all patients with sepsis will have fever, and symptoms can sometimes be nonspecific.

Manage all patients with suspected sepsis in accordance with the Surviving Sepsis guidelines (https://www.sccm.org/Surviving SepsisCampaign/Guidelines/Adult-Patients) while searching for a focus of infection; see Clinical tool: A septic screen.

Assess haemodynamic status frequently and manage as septic shock (Chapter 2) if there is persistent hypotension (mean arterial pressure [MAP] <65 mmHg) and ↑serum lactate (>2 mmol/L) despite adequate volume resuscitation. In this instance, refer to Critical Care for consideration of central venous access and vasopressor support.

2 Suspect noninfective cause for fever?

Most acute febrile illnesses are caused by infection, but the following noninfective conditions are potentially life-threatening and must be specifically considered at the outset.

Transfusion reaction: If the patient is receiving blood products, stop the transfusion, ensure the patient's ID matches that on the unit, inspect the unit of blood, and check that the ABO and RhD groups in the transfused blood are compatible with the patient. Contact the blood bank and seek immediate Haematology input if there is any suspicion of ABO incompatibility or other major transfusion reaction. If the patient is otherwise systemically well, consider restarting the transfusion with ongoing close observation of the patient and appropriate symptomatic relief.

Toxidromes: Serotonin toxicity (syndrome) and neuroleptic malignant syndrome can cause fever as a presenting feature. Further information on the assessment of these conditions can be found in the chapter on Poisoning (Chapter 28).

Inflammation: Venous thromboembolism, pancreatitis, vasculitis, inflammatory bowel disease (IBD) and Steven-Johnson syndrome are all potentially life-threatening conditions which can present with fever. They will typically present with other clinical features that will suggest the diagnosis.

Heatstroke: Suspect if the patient has had sustained exposure to very hot weather (e.g., during a heatwave) or has been undertaking prolonged severe exertion in high temperatures.

In all of the above cases, continue to evaluate for infection and other causes if there is any diagnostic doubt.

3 Specific risk factor for infection?

Infections other than those discussed above may need to be considered in patients returning to or entering the UK from abroad (especially from the tropics), those who are immunocompromised, and patients who use IV drugs.

26

Clinical tool
A septic screen

The septic screen combines clinical assessment with laboratory analysis and imaging studies to identify a source of infection. It may also reveal noninfectious causes of pyrexia, such as malignancy. The full screen may not be required in all patients, especially if there is an obvious focus of infection.

General

- ≥2 sets of blood cultures, urinalysis, FBC, U+E, LFTs, CRP, CXR

Respiratory

- Assess suspected RTI (e.g., new/worsening cough with purulent sputum or CXR consolidation) as per Chapter 4.
- Perform a pleural tap and send fluid for biochemical, microbiological and cytological analysis if unilateral pleural effusion (Chapter 4).
- Perform a viral throat swab. If other respiratory features (e.g., haemoptysis, CXR changes, hypoxia), consider further investigation (e.g., CT, bronchoscopy) to exclude atypical infection, lung cancer and PE.

Abdominal

- Send stool samples for microscopy, culture and sensitivity testing ± *Clostridium difficile* toxin if acute diarrhoea (Chapter 9).
- If persistent bloody diarrhoea, consider IBD, and refer to Gastroenterology for further investigation (Chapter 9).
- Perform an urgent ascitic tap in any febrile patient with ascites; treat empirically as spontaneous bacterial peritonitis (SBP), pending culture, if >250 neutrophils/μL ascitic fluid. Consider TB and malignancy if fluid is exudative and initial cultures negative.
- If new-onset jaundice, arrange an abdominal USS and serology for viral hepatitis (Chapter 12).
  - Treat empirically for biliary sepsis and arrange surgical review if there is a cholestatic pattern of jaundice or USS shows dilated bile ducts or cholecystitis.
- In patients with an acute abdomen (Chapter 7), check amylase, arrange erect CXR and refer to Surgery for consideration of further imaging (e.g., CT abdomen and pelvis) and operative intervention.

Urinary tract

- Send an MSU if new-onset urinary tract symptoms or an indwelling urinary catheter. Bacterial UTI is highly likely if urinalysis is positive for leukocytes/nitrites in patients <65, but urinalysis should not be used to diagnose UTI if catheterized or >65.

- Arrange an USS to exclude renal obstruction in patients with symptoms of pyelonephritis and a history of renal calculi, an acute kidney injury (AKI) or a high urinary pH. CTKUB (CT of kidneys, urinary, and bladder) may be required if a high index of suspicion remains for calculi despite normal ultrasound, or if there is a deterioration in the patient's clinical condition. Consider PR and testicular examination to assess for prostatitis and epididymo-orchitis, respectively.
- Send swabs for *Neisseria gonorrhoeae* and *Chlamydia* if urethral or PV discharge.

Skin and soft tissue

- Send swabs from any wounds or sites discharging pus.
- Suspect cellulitis if there is an area of acutely hot, erythematous and painful skin; look for potential entry sites, such as peripheral cannulae, skin breaks.
- Seek immediate surgical assessment and give IV antibiotics if any features of severe necrotizing infection, such as rapid spread, crepitus, anaesthesia over lesion, major haemodynamic compromise or pain out of proportion with clinical findings.
- Consider investigation for osteomyelitis (e.g., MRI) if persistent nonhealing ulcer.
- Examine the whole body for rashes—seek urgent Dermatology advice if blistering, mucosal involvement or pustules (Chapter 27).

CNS

- Assume CNS infection if severe headache, neck stiffness, purpuric rash, focal neurological signs, new-onset seizures or unexplained ↓GCS. Arrange urgent CT head to exclude raised ICP if the patient has focal neurological signs, papilloedema, seizures, or a GCS score ≤12. Otherwise, if safe, perform LP in the first hour of presentation before initiating treatment with antibiotics (Clinical tool: LP and CSF interpretation, Chapter 13). Do not delay antibiotics if LP cannot be performed within 1 hour, the patient has evidence of shock or severe sepsis, or there is a rapidly progressing purpuric rash.
- If meningitis is suspected, send blood for *Neisseria meningitidis* and *Streptococcus pneumoniae* PCR.

Cardiovascular

- Investigate for endocarditis (Box 26.1) with a transthoracic echocardiogram and ≥3 sets of blood cultures if new murmur, vasculitic/embolic phenomena or a predisposing cardiac lesion with no obvious alternative source of infection.

Clinical tool—cont'd
A septic screen

- Consider a transoesophageal echocardiogram if transthoracic images equivocal or persistent high clinical suspicion.

ENT

- Send a bacterial throat swab if pustular tonsillar or pharyngeal exudates.
- If parotitis or tender lymphadenopathy, consider a throat swab for mumps PCR and, if age-appropriate, check EBV serology (>95% of patients >35 years will have evidence of previous exposure).

- If tenderness over the sinus with nasal congestion, discharge, loss of smell and headache, consider sinusitis and arrange a CT of the sinuses.

Musculoskeletal

- If acutely swollen, painful joint, seek urgent specialist assessment and perform diagnostic aspiration to exclude septic arthritis (Chapter 18).
- If there is unexplained back pain with no other obvious source for fever, take ≥3 blood cultures and arrange spinal MRI to exclude discitis.

Box 26.1 Modified Duke criteria for the diagnosis of infective endocarditis

Major criteria

Positive blood culture
- Typical organism from two cultures
- Persistent positive blood cultures taken >12 hours apart
- ≥3 positive cultures taken over >1 hour

Endocardial involvement
- Positive echocardiographic findings of vegetations
- New valvular regurgitation

Minor criteria

- Predisposing valvular or cardiac abnormality
- IV drug misuse
- Pyrexia ≥38°C
- Embolic phenomenon
- Vasculitic phenomenon
- Blood cultures suggestive—organism grown but not achieving major criteria
- Suggestive echocardiographic findings
  Definite endocarditis: two major, or one major and three minor, or five minor
  Possible endocarditis: one major and one minor, or three minor

Modified from Penman ID, Ralston SH, Strachan MWJ, Hobson RP. Davidson's principles and practice of medicine, 24th ed. Edinburgh: Elsevier Limited, 2023;464.

If the patient has come from an at-risk region for viral haemorrhagic fever and has unexplained bleeding, discuss urgently with the health protection team (before admission if possible). Otherwise, complete a septic screen as per Clinical tool: Extensions to the septic screen in specific patient groups. The prevailing strains and resistance patterns of common infections such as pneumonia may differ in other parts of the world, so seek input from an ID specialist at an early stage.

Immunocompromised patients may present atypically, experience more severe sequelae from infection with common pathogens, and are at greater risk of opportunistic infections (especially with mycobacteria, viruses and fungi). Follow the additional steps for immunocompromised (Clinical tool: Extensions to the septic screen in specific patient groups) if the patient has an acquired or congenital immunodeficiency (including HIV); is receiving treatment with high-dose steroids, chemotherapy or immunosuppressants; or is neutropenic for any reason. More specific forms of immunocompromise include asplenia (↑susceptibility to encapsulated organisms and malaria) and the presence of indwelling vascular-access devices or other prosthetic material. Test for HIV in patients who are at high risk or who present with an atypical infection or other indicators of HIV; see https://www.bhiva.org/HIV-testing-guidelines.

Ask about all forms of drug use in any patient presenting with unexplained fever. If there has been IV drug use, establish frequency, duration and sites of injection. Maintain awareness of any local/national outbreaks, as unusual organisms may be implicated, such as anthrax

26

skin infections. Always consider the possibility of underlying blood-borne infection, e.g., hepatitis B or C, HIV. Discuss with the ID team if the patient is haemodynamically compromised or fails to improve on standard therapy.

4 Clinical findings/initial tests suggest a likely source?

Following appropriate investigations, treat immediately with antibiotics according to the likely source and local guidelines in patients with sepsis. If no clear source is identified or the patient has neutropenia (especially if the neutrophil count is $<1.0 \times 10^9$/L) or other significant immunocompromise, provide empirical broad-spectrum antibiotic ± antifungal therapy. The choice of antimicrobials will depend on patient factors and local resistance patterns. Check local guidelines and discuss with relevant specialties, such as Oncology, Haematology, Microbiology.

In patients with suspected sepsis without high-risk features, a rapid assessment to determine whether the acute presentation is due to an infectious or noninfectious cause and to identify the potential source should be performed within a 3-hour period. If there is still concern about sepsis at the end of this period, antibiotics to target the likely source should be initiated. When the likelihood of infection is low, or when the patient is systemically well, antibiotics can often be deferred pending the results of cultures. However, the patient will require regular reassessment to ensure that sepsis is not developing, particularly if there is a clinical deterioration.

5 Positive cultures?

Reevaluate your initial diagnosis and treatment in the light of culture results.

Positive cultures may confirm a suspected source of infection and guide the most appropriate antibiotic therapy. Blood cultures that yield an unexpected organism may challenge your working diagnosis and prompt reevaluation for an alternative source; for example, *Staphylococcus aureus* would not be consistent with suspected UTI.

In the patient with no obvious source of fever, positive blood cultures, especially in multiple bottles, confirm an infective aetiology and help to guide further investigation; blood culture results are central to the diagnosis of infective endocarditis (Box 26.1).

Persistently positive blood cultures despite appropriate antibiotic therapy suggest a deep-seated infection; the source must be identified and removed, e.g., débridement, drainage.

6 Persistent fever?

Acute fever is frequently a manifestation of self-limiting viral illnesses. In the absence of continuing pyrexia, ongoing symptoms or signs, or worrying investigation results, no further action is required.

Recurrent fever, especially with persistent elevation of inflammatory markers or significant constitutional upset, mandates further evaluation; if present, proceed to Further assessment of pyrexia of unknown origin.

Clinical tool
Extensions to the septic screen in specific patient groups

Recent travel or residence abroad

- Document exactly where the patient has been, specific dates of travel, activities undertaken (including a sexual history), unwell contacts, and onset and duration of symptoms. Ask about vaccinations/malaria prophylaxis prior to and during travel.
- Assess the patient for diarrhoea, constitutional symptoms, rash, ulceration, jaundice, lymphadenopathy and hepatosplenomegaly to help narrow the differential diagnosis.
- Investigation of any returning traveler with unexplained fever requires consultation with an ID specialist at an early stage to guide investigations and management.

Immunocompromised

- In patients living with HIV, early involvement of an ID specialist is required. Check the most recent CD4 count and repeat if >3 months ago. Fungal and viral infections are more likely if CD4 count <200 but can occur at higher counts. Check compliance with antiretroviral therapy/antimicrobial prophylaxis.
- Seek early advice from a respiratory specialist if there are respiratory symptoms or an abnormal CXR (especially cavitation) or a high suspicion of *Pneumocystis* pneumonia due to any of the following features:
  - Subacute (e.g., over 2–3 weeks) or progressive shortness of breath
  - Nonproductive cough
  - Diffuse bilateral perihilar infiltrates on CXR or non-specific changes
  - Unexplained hypoxaemia (including desaturation on exercise).
- Send three sputum samples for microscopy (acid-fast bacilli, fungal), histopathological analysis (*Pneumocystis*) and mycobacterial culture; induced sputum or other diagnostic procedures (e.g., bronchoalveolar lavage) may be necessary.

- If prominent GI symptoms, send stool for microscopy or antigen detection for *Cryptosporidium*, and investigate for CMV colitis with CMV serology, PCR and flexible sigmoidoscopy ± biopsy. Consider intra-abdominal TB.
- If CNS features, investigate as per the general septic screen but send blood for *Toxoplasma* serology; request CSF staining for *Cryptococcus, Toxoplasma,* and TB; and biopsy any space-occupying lesion.
- Request a dermatology review and biopsy of any suspicious or unusual rashes, such as cutaneous T-cell lymphomas, Kaposi sarcoma.
- Prolonged indwelling vascular access catheters (e.g., Hickman lines, tunneled lines) carry a substantial risk of bacterial/fungal infection; suspect line infection in all cases where there is no clear alternative source, even if the entry point looks clean.
  - Take blood cultures from the line and, if feasible, remove and send the tip for culture.
  - Consider echocardiography to look for endocarditis in patients with confirmed bacteraemia—especially *Staphylococcus aureus*—or persistent fever.
- Discuss early with the relevant specialty if you suspect infection of prosthetic material, such as valve prosthesis, pacemaker and prosthetic joint.

IV drug use

- Take ≥3 sets of blood cultures prior to starting antibiotic therapy.
- Look at all new and old injection sites; if inflamed or tender, consider USS to exclude an underlying abscess.
- Arrange a Doppler USS to exclude DVT if there is any groin or leg swelling.
- Exclude iliopsoas abscess by CT if there is groin or lower back pain with difficulty extending along the leg.
- Arrange an echocardiogram ± transoesophageal echocardiography if there is evidence of septic emboli on CXR or no alternative source of fever.

26

Further assessment of pyrexia of unknown origin

Due to the variety of conditions which can cause pyrexia of unknown origin, input from multiple specialties is often required to reach a final diagnosis. Begin by repeating a full clinical assessment, including travel, sexual, occupational and recreational history. Perform lymph node, skin, joint, breast, testicular, rectal and eye examination and ensure urinalysis has been done. The outcome of this assessment will determine which specialties to involve and direct further investigation.

- Send TFTs to exclude hyperthyroidism.
- If not done already, perform a CT chest/abdomen/pelvis to assess for solid organ tumours, lymphadenopathy, or abscesses. In men, send a PSA.
- Biopsy any suspicious masses, skin lesions, or lymphadenopathy detected clinically or radiologically.
- Arrange a peripheral blood film, LDH, and assess for myeloma with serum immunoglobulins, protein electrophoresis and urinary Bence-Jones protein. If a haematological malignancy is suspected, arrange Haematology review ± bone marrow biopsy.
- Use the Duke (Box 26.1) and Jones (Box 26.2) criteria to confirm or refute a suspected diagnosis of endocarditis or rheumatic fever, respectively.
- Arrange ID review. Seek advice on previous results and further investigation required based on patient risk factors. Ensure HIV serology has been performed.
- Consider a rheumatological cause for fever. Arrange Rheumatology review if indicated by symptoms and signs.
- If joint pain and stiffness, consider inflammatory arthritis and send CRP, ESR and anti-CCP.

Box 26.2 Jones criteria for the diagnosis of rheumatic fever

All patients

Supporting evidence of preceding streptococcal infection: recent scarlet fever, raised antistreptolysin O or other streptococcal antibody titre, positive throat culture, PLUS:
- Two major criteria
- One major criterion and two minor criteria

Major manifestations
- Carditis
- Polyarthritis
- Chorea
- Erythema marginatum
- Subcutaneous nodules

Minor manifestations
- Fever
- Arthralgia
- Previous rheumatic fever
- ↑ESR or CRP
- Leukocytosis
- First-degree AV block

N.B. Evidence of recent streptococcal infection is particularly important if there is only one major manifestation.

From Penman ID, Ralston SH, Strachan MWJ, Hobson RP. Davidson's principles and practice of medicine, 24th ed. Edinburgh: Elsevier Limited, 2023: 452.

- If hair loss, dry eyes and dry mouth, skin or genital ulceration, Raynaud phenomenon or photosensitive rash, consider SLE and send ANA, dsDNA and ENA.
- In patients >50 with headache and raised CRP and ESR, exclude giant cell arteritis (Chapter 16). Vasculitis should be considered in patients with a subacute history of fever, lethargy, arthralgia and myalgia, especially if they have a new purpuric rash, AKI or respiratory features such as haemoptysis. Note that the multisystem nature of vasculitis means

that its clinical presentations are hugely variable. Perform urinalysis assessing for blood and protein and send ANCA. Consider angiography of affected organs. Biopsy of an affected site may be required. If evidence of renal impairment, or urinalysis is positive for blood or protein, refer to Nephrology for further evaluation,

- Suspect adult-onset Still's disease if microbiological and autoimmune investigations are consistently negative and there are recurrent joint pains or a transient, nonpruritic, salmon-pink maculopapular rash that coincides with fever, especially if ↑↑↑ferritin.
- If abdominal pain or diarrhoea, consider IBD, and refer to Gastroenterology for

consideration of colonoscopy and biopsy (Chapter 9).

- If LFTs are persistently deranged or there is hepatomegaly without an obvious cause, discuss with Hepatology.
- Review all drugs: discontinue one at a time for 72 hours and then reinstate if fever persists.
- If the cause remains unclear, consider a whole-body PET scan to look for evidence of occult malignancy (e.g., lymphoma) or vasculitis. Think about bone marrow biopsy and liver biopsy, and consider diagnoses of exclusion, e.g., Familial Mediterranean fever, fictitious fever.

26

The accurate diagnosis of skin disease is usually based on pattern recognition developed through experience rather than a rule-based approach. This chapter is a step-by-step approach for the nonspecialist to assist identification of dermatological emergencies that require urgent advice and treatment. A glossary of key dermatology terms can be found in Box 27.1.

Acute generalized skin eruptions are common and frequently present as a symmetrical, widespread rash composed of macules, papules, and patches which start on the torso before spreading to the proximal limbs. Such eruptions are often described as maculopapular rashes, exanthematous eruptions/exanthems, and morbilliform eruptions (Fig. 27.1). Often these eruptions are secondary to drugs (Table 27.1), with the rash appearing 6 to 10 days after the introduction of the causative agent. Other causes include eruptions secondary to viruses (e.g., enteroviruses, EBV, rubella), bacterial infections (e.g., staphylococcal infection), or systemic disease. These rashes are usually self-limiting and resolve on withdrawal of the causative medication or resolution of the acute illness. However, during the evaluation of acute eruptions, it is essential to identify the features of conditions that are associated with significant morbidity or mortality and require urgent intervention.

Erythroderma

Erythroderma (red skin) describes inflammatory skin disease manifesting predominantly as erythema and involving >90% of the body surface area (BSA; Fig. 27.2). It causes loss of skin integrity resulting in dysfunctional temperature regulation; fluid, electrolyte and protein loss; and increased susceptibility to infection. All these factors contribute to a high associated mortality. The majority of cases are caused by an underlying skin condition (e.g.,

eczema, psoriasis). Other causes include drug eruptions (Table 27.1) and cutaneous lymphoma.

Severe Cutaneous Adverse Reactions (SCARs)

Toxic epidermal necrolysis and Stevens–Johnson syndrome

Toxic epidermal necrolysis (TEN) and Stevens-Johnson syndrome (SJS) are acute eruptions caused by a cell-mediated cytotoxic reaction against epidermal cells, resulting in epidermal necrosis and sloughing. TEN/SJS are characterized by detachment of epidermis from the dermis, with exposure of the inflamed dermis (Fig. 27.3). Prior to the development of epidermal sloughing, there is a prodrome of fever and constitutional upset, followed by the development of widespread tender erythematous

---

Box 27.1 Dermatology Glossary

Macule	flat area of altered color <1 cm in diameter
Patch	flat area of altered color >1 cm in diameter
Papule	raised, palpable lesion <1 cm in diameter
Pustule	a papule containing pus
Nodule	raised, palpable lesion >1 cm in diameter which involves the deeper layers of the skin/subcutaneous tissue
Plaque	palpable, thickened area of skin >1 cm in diameter. Most plaques are elevated from the skin surface.
Vesicle	clear fluid filled blister <1 cm in diameter
Bulla	vesicle >1 cm in diameter
Petechiae	pinpoint, nonblanching foci of haemorrhage into the skin
Purpura	larger, nonblanching, red or purple lesions caused by haemorrhage into the skin. Can be palpable or nonpalpable
Ecchymosis	bruise
Wheal	transient area of localized skin swelling. Often pale centrally with surrounding erythema
Erosion	sore caused by loss of superficial surface of a mucous membrane

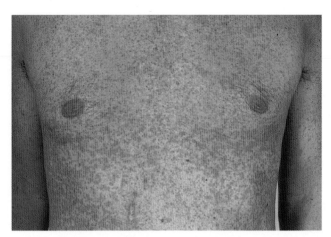

Fig. 27.1 Morbilliform drug rash due to penicillin allergy. Also known as an exanthematous eruption/
maculopapular rash. (Note for Creative Commons: This figure appears as Fig. 22.60 in Feather A, Randall D, Waterhouse
M. *Kumar and Clark's clinical medicine*, 10th ed. Philadelphia: Elsevier, 2021.)

Table 27.1 Table of drug-induced generalized eruptions and example causative agents						
	Toxic epidermal necrolysis/ Stevens-Johnson syndrome (TEN/SJS)	Acute generalized exanthematous pustulosis (AGEP)	Drug reaction with eosinophilia and systemic symptoms (DRESS)	Cutaneous vasculitis	Urticaria	Other drug eruptions
Antibiotics – Beta-lactams – Tetracyclines – Macrolides – Sulfonamides – Fluoroquinolones	✓	✓	✓	✓	✓	✓
Anticonvulsants	✓	✓	✓	✓	—	✓
Antifungals	✓	✓	—	—	—	✓
Antiretrovirals	✓	—	✓	—	—	✓
NSAIDS	✓	✓	—	✓	✓	✓
Paracetamol	✓	✓	—	—	—	—
Allopurinol	✓	—	✓	✓	—	✓
Antipsychotics	✓	—	✓	✓	—	—
Chemotherapeutic Agents	✓	—	—	—	—	✓
Diltiazem	—	✓	—	—	—	—
Hydroxychloroquine	—	✓	—	—	—	—
Anticoagulants	—	—	—	✓	—	—
Thiazide diuretics	—	—	—	✓	—	—
Biologics	—	—	—	✓	—	—
Opioid analgesics	—	—	—	—	✓	—

27

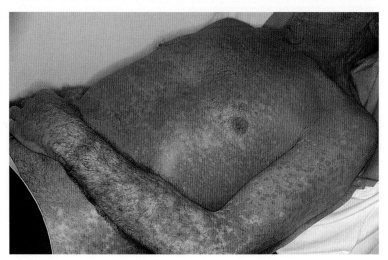

Fig. 27.2 **Erythroderma.** (From Gawkrodger DJ. *Dermatology: an illustrated colour text*, 4th ed. Edinburgh: Churchill Livingstone, 2008.)

macules and patches. In severe cases the lesions merge, resulting in more confluent erythema. The lesions subsequently develop into flaccid bullae, with the epidermis then completely detaching. Mucous membranes are involved, with erosive mucositis of the eyes, mouth, and genitals all being common (Fig. 27.3).

TEN and SJS exist on a spectrum of disease and are defined by the total body surface area (TBSA) of epidermal detachment. SJS is characterized by <10% TBSA of epidermal detachment, with TEN diagnosed when there is >30% TBSA of epidermal detachment. If 10–30% TBSA is involved, the condition is described as TEN/SJS overlap. Drugs (Table 27.1) cause >80% of cases and have usually been commenced 1–3 weeks prior to presentation. Like erythroderma, loss of skin integrity in TEN and SJS leads to a high associated mortality.

Erythema multiforme represents a similar but milder type of cytotoxic reaction. Classically, it presents with 'target' lesions, consisting of three zones: a dark or blistered centre (bull's-eye) surrounded by a pale zone and an outer rim of erythema (Fig. 27.4). The lesions predominantly occur on the hands/feet and affect <10% of the BSA. Erythema multiforme major involves mucous membranes, while erythema multiforme minor does not.

The underlying cause is more often infectious (especially herpes simplex and mycoplasma) than drug induced.

DRESS syndrome

DRESS *(drug reaction with eosinophilia and systemic symptoms)* syndrome typically presents as a morbilliform rash (Fig. 27.1) with multiple other systemic features. Systemic manifestations include fever, lymphadenopathy, hepatitis, leukocytosis, and eosinophilia. Hepatitis can progress to fulminant liver failure. Renal, respiratory, endocrine, and cardiac complications are also possible. Facial oedema is a common feature. There can be up to 8 weeks between introduction of the causative drug (Table 27.1) and development of cutaneous manifestations. Therefore, diagnosis requires a high index of suspicion and a careful medication history.

Acute generalized exanthematous pustulosis

Acute generalized exanthematous pustulosis (AGEP) is characterized by large patches of pruritic, oedematous erythema covered by small, nonfollicular, sterile pustules (Fig. 27.5). The rash often develops in skin folds or on the face. Skin manifestations are accompanied by fever and leukocytosis. Organ involvement occurs in about 20% of cases

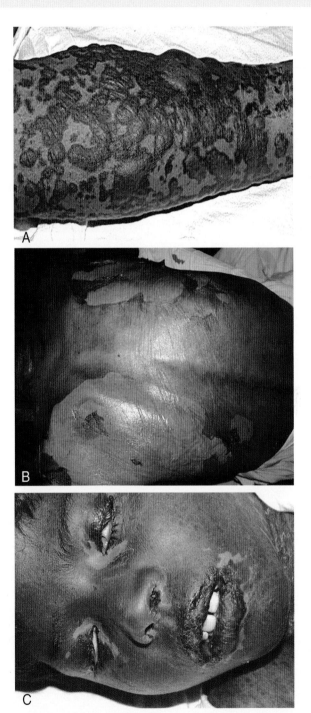

Fig. 27.3 Toxic epidermal necrolysis. (A) Bullae on dusky erythema. (B) Bullae rupture to leave large areas of denuded skin. (C) Haemorrhagic crusts on lips and eye involvement are frequent. (Note for Creative Commons: This figure appears as Fig. 5.21 in Khanna N. *Illustrated synopsis of dermatology and sexually transmitted diseases*, 4th ed. Philadelphia: Elsevier, 2012.)

27

with AKI, pleural effusions and LFT derangement being possible features. AGEP develops more quickly than other SCARs, with symptoms usually developing within 48 hours of ingestion of the causative agent (Table 27.1). The condition resolves within 15 days of withdrawal of the medication.

Generalized pustular psoriasis

Generalized pustular psoriasis (GPP) is a rare but severe form of psoriasis, presenting as acute, generalized, tender erythema covered by nonfollicular sterile pustules. These pustules often merge to form larger collections of pus

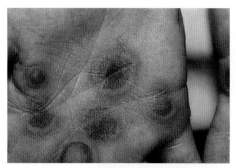

Fig. 27.4 Erythema multiforme-target lesions. (From Bolognia J, Jorizzo J, Rapini R. *Dermatology*, 1st ed. London: Mosby, 2003.)

(Fig. 27.6). Though pustules tend to resolve within days, resolution is often followed by further crops of pustules. The rash is accompanied by systemic upset, including fever. Complications associated with loss of skin integrity may develop. Though plaque psoriasis is associated with GPP, not all patients will have a prior history of psoriasis. Potential triggers include withdrawal of systemic corticosteroid treatment, drugs, infections and pregnancy.

Urticaria/angioedema

Urticaria (Fig. 27.7) is oedema within the dermis secondary to mast cell degranulation and is a common skin reaction. Angioedema (Fig. 27.8) results from oedema deeper within the dermis and subcutaneous tissues and may occur in up to 40% of cases of urticaria. Acute urticaria presents with well-circumscribed areas of itchy skin swelling with surrounding erythema (wheals). Angioedema causes swelling of the face, lips, genitals, or extremities. It can affect the structures of the upper airway, resulting in airway compromise that requires emergency intervention. Although commonly thought to be allergic, many cases of acute urticaria are not mediated by immunoglobulin E (IgE). Those that

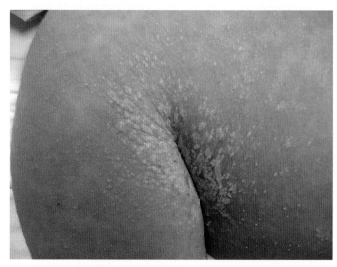

Fig. 27.5 Acute generalized exanthematous pustulosis. (Note for Creative Commons: This figure appears as Fig. 6.59 in Micheletti RG, James WD, Elston DM, McMahon PJ. *Andrews' diseases of the skin clinical atlas*, 2nd ed. Philadelphia: Elsevier, 2023.)

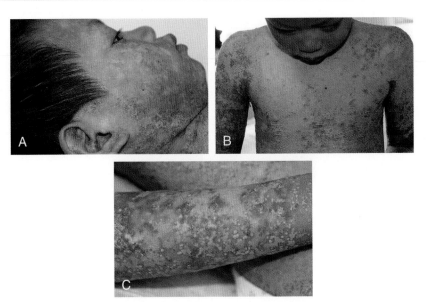

Fig. 27.6 Generalized pustular psoriasis in a child involving (A) the face, (B) trunk, and (C) extremities. (From Kelly M. Cordoro. Management of childhood psoriasis. *Advances in Dermatology* 24:125–169; 2008.)

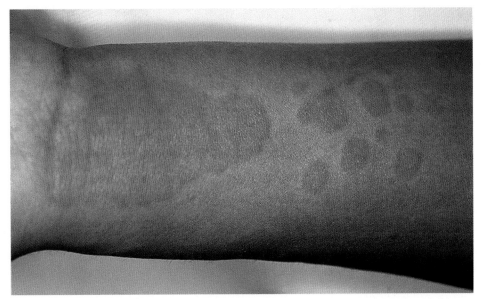

Fig. 27.7 Urticaria. (From Gawkrodger DJ. *Dermatology: an illustrated colour text*, 4th ed. Edinburgh: Churchill Livingstone, 2008.)

27

are arise in response to drugs (especially antibiotics), foods (peanuts, eggs, shellfish) and skin contact (latex, plants, bee/wasp stings) and may progress to anaphylaxis. Non-IgE causes include concurrent infection (especially upper respiratory tract infections), drugs that promote mast cell degranulation (opiates, aspirin, NSAIDs, ACE inhibitors) and foods that contain salicylates and additives.

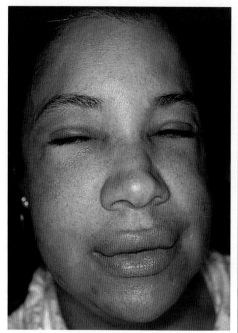

Fig. 27.8 Angioedema. (Note for Creative Commons: This figure appears as Fig. 232-3 in Goldman L, Cooney KA. *Goldman-Cecil medicine*, 27th ed. Philadelphia: Elsevier, 2024.)

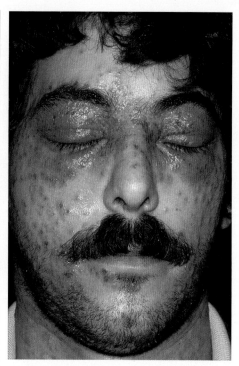

Fig 27.9 Eczema herpeticum. (Note for Creative Commons: This figure appears as Fig. 12.48 in Dinulos JG. *Habif's clinical dermatology: a color guide to diagnosis and therapy*, 7th ed. Philadelphia: Elsevier, 2021.)

Eczema Herpeticum

Eczema herpeticum (Fig. 27.9) is caused by cutaneous *Herpes simplex* infection in patients with atopic eczema. It presents with painful, itchy clusters of vesicles over inflamed skin, which over a period of 7 to 10 days can spread to healthy skin and in severe cases can become widespread. Once vesicles rupture, they leave punched-out erosions with overlying haemorrhagic crusts. Other clinical features may include fever and lymphadenopathy. Superadded bacterial infections (e.g., cellulitis, impetigo), ocular involvement (keratoconjunctivitis), and meningoencephalitis are potential complications.

Pemphigus/pemphigoid

Autoimmune diseases attacking structural components of the epidermis result in separation of keratinocytes from each other, or from the underlying dermis, resulting in the formation of bullae.

- Pemphigus vulgaris (Fig. 27.10) is the most serious of these diseases. It is characterized by flaccid cutaneous bullae which rupture, leaving erosions. Skin manifestations are usually preceded by painful oral erosions which interfere with eating and drinking.
- Bullous pemphigoid (Fig. 27.11) typically presents in older adults with itchy eruptions of tense bullae on either normal or erythematous-appearing skin on the flexor surfaces of the limbs, the trunk, and the abdomen. Oral lesions occur in less than one third of patients.

Both conditions are associated with an increased risk of sepsis due to breakdown of the normal skin barrier and the use of immunosuppressive medications to manage them.

Purpura (including vasculitis)

Purpura (Fig. 27.12) is fixed staining of the skin by leakage of blood from the intravascular

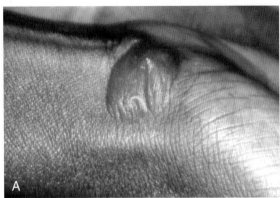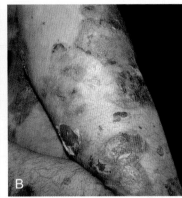

Fig. 27.10 Pemphigus vulgaris. (A) Flaccid blisters rupture easily to expose erosions (B). (Reeves JT, *Clinical Dermatology Illustrated: A regional approach*, 2nd edn. Elsevier, 1991.)

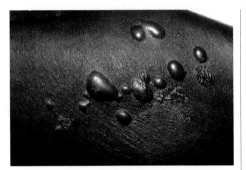

Fig. 27.11 Bullous pemphigoid. (Note for Creative Commons: This figure appears as Fig. 2.28 in Micheletti RG, James WD, Elston DM, McMahon PJ. *Andrews' diseases of the skin clinical atlas*, 2nd ed. Philadelphia: Elsevier, 2023.)

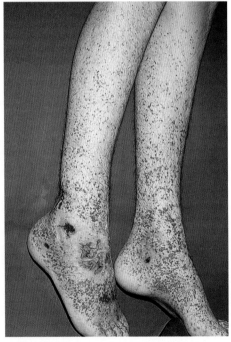

Fig. 27.12 Vasculitis/purpura. (From Gawkrodger DJ. *Dermatology ICT*, 4th ed. Edinburgh: Churchill Livingstone, 2008.)

space and needs to be distinguished from simple bruising. The appearance of purpura should prompt investigation for serious systemic disease. Causes include:

- Septic emboli from systemic infectious diseases
- Haematological disorders
- Thrombosis involving microcirculation
- Vasculitis (inflammation in vessel walls)

27

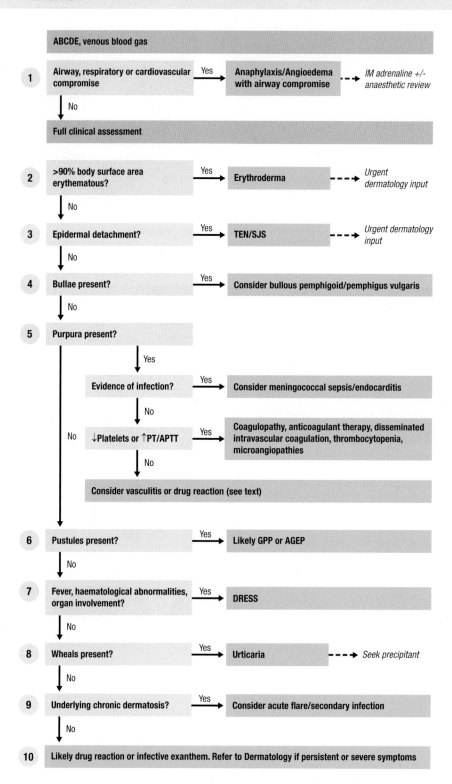

1 Airway, respiratory or cardiovascular compromise?

Skin and mucosal changes are present in 80% of patients with anaphylaxis and may be the first indication of anaphylactic reaction. If urticaria or angioedema are accompanied by life-threatening airway, respiratory, or cardiovascular compromise, urgent treatment with intramuscular adrenaline is required. Further treatment is described in the Advanced Life Support (ALS) anaphylaxis guidelines (https://www.resus.org.uk/library/additional-guidance/guidance-anaphylaxis). Diagnosis is supported by exposure to a known allergen.

Many cases of urticaria with angioedema are not IgE-mediated and therefore do not cause anaphylactic reactions. However, they can still be life-threatening if the angioedema causes airway swelling and obstruction. If there is concern about airway compromise, seek urgent Anaesthetic review.

2 >90% body surface area erythematous?

Estimate the proportion of skin that is erythematous using the guide in Box 27.2; >90% of BSA indicates erythroderma. Admit any patient with acute erythroderma to hospital, assess and stabilize as described in Box 27.3, and arrange urgent Dermatology review. Subsequent treatment is based on the exact diagnosis and guided by expert dermatological assessment.

Box 27.2 Calculating body surface area

Originally developed for calculating surface area for burn victims, in adults a simple way of calculating the BSA affected by a cutaneous disorder is the Wallace rule of nines. This system allocates to different body parts 9% (or half thereof) of the total BSA. In extensive skin disease it is sometimes easier to identify unaffected skin, and assessment is aided by remembering that the patient's hand is approximately 1% of BSA.

Wallace rule of nines.

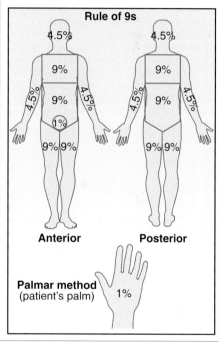

3 Epidermal detachment?

Suspect TEN/SJS if there is extensive blistering with epidermal detachment to reveal bright red oozing dermis (Fig. 27.3), along with mucous membrane involvement. Estimate BSA involvement (Box 27.2); diagnose TEN if epidermal detachment ≥30%, TEN/SJS overlap if epidermal detachment 10–30%, and SJS if epidermal detachment <10%. Stop any potentially causative medications, stabilize as described in Box 27.3, seek immediate Dermatology review, and manage in a Burns or CCU.

4 Bullae present?

If the patient has widespread bullae, consider an autoimmune bullous disease. Distinguishing between autoimmune bullous diseases can be challenging.

- In bullous pemphigoid (Fig. 27.11), lesions are tense, itchy, and may be preceded by erythematous or urticarial lesions. They are usually distributed over flexural surfaces of the limbs and the abdomen. Nikolsky sign (lateral pressure of the skin surrounding a bulla results in blistering of previously normal skin is negative). Bullous

27

Box 27.3 Assessment and immediate management of skin dysfunction

The mainstay of emergency dermatology treatment is to provide surrogate skin function until the underlying condition has resolved or is suppressed with suitable medication. Look for evidence of shock (Box 2.1) and dehydration, and monitor U+Es regularly.

Replenish fluid lost through defective skin barrier function with IV fluids and supplementary electrolytes. Optimize nutrition, ideally by supporting oral intake.

Take swabs of all areas of suspected infection and, if the patient is pyrexial, take blood cultures before commencing antibiotic therapy. Use strict aseptic technique for blood cultures, ideally through nonaffected skin, to try to avoid contaminants (more likely in dermatological patients due to ↑skin flora load).

Remember that many acute cutaneous eruptions are associated with pyrexia, due not to systemic infection but to loss of temperature homeostasis through vasodilatation.

Maintain body temperature with a warm room and regular antipyretics. Assess the extent of skin compromise as detailed above and restore its barrier function with regular application of thick emollients (liquid paraffin:white soft paraffin, 50:50) and dressings. Remove any potential exacerbates by discontinuing all unnecessary medication.

pemphigoid is uncommon in patients <70 years.

- In pemphigus vulgaris (Fig. 27.10), flaccid bullae tend to be distributed over the face, scalp, and torso. Rupture of bullae leaves painful cutaneous erosions. Nikolsky sign is positive. Unlike the situation in bullous pemphigoid, where oral lesions occur in the minority of cases, most patients with pemphigus vulgaris will have painful oral erosions which precede cutaneous manifestations, often by months. Pemphigus vulgaris often occurs in middle age.

More localized bullae may be associated with severe cellulitis, necrotizing fasciitis, fixed drug eruptions, or insect bites.

5   Purpura present?

Classify the rash as purpuric when there are dark red or purple macules/patches that do not blanch with pressure (Fig. 27.12).

Suspect meningococcal sepsis and treat as described in Chapter 13 if the patient has fever, shock, drowsiness or meningism.

Consider septic emboli from endocarditis if the patient is febrile and has a predisposing cardiac lesion or a new murmur.

Look for evidence of an underlying bleeding tendency—ask about and examine for ecchymoses, epistaxis, GI bleeding, menorrhagia, haemarthrosis, and mucosal haemorrhage, and check FBC, PT and APTT. Unless the cause is obvious (e.g., excessive anticoagulation, chronic liver disease), discuss with Haematology, particularly if there is coagulopathy or ↓platelets.

If ↓platelets are present with normal coagulation, look for associated features of thrombotic thrombocytopenic purpura:

- ↓Hb without an obvious alternative cause
- Red cell fragmentation on blood film
- ↑↑LDH and bilirubin (suggestive of haemolysis)
- Neurological abnormalities (↓GCS score, headache, seizures)
- Fever
- AKI (Chapter 29)

If any of these are present, seek immediate Haematology input, as urgent plasma exchange may be life-saving.

Suspect a systemic vasculitis (e.g., polyarteritis nodosa, Henoch–Schönlein purpura, cryoglobulinaemia, or ANCA-associated vasculitis) if there is palpable purpura accompanied by fever, ↑ESR/CRP, constitutional upset, joint disease and/or renal involvement (↓GFR, proteinuria, haematuria). Check ANA, ANCA, ENA, and dsDNA, and consider skin biopsy ± biopsy of other affected organs.

Many new cases of purpura are caused by a cutaneous vasculitis without any systemic involvement. This is frequently a hypersensitivity vasculitis caused by new medications (Table 27.1) or infection (e.g., hepatitis B, hepatitis C, HIV), though other causes include autoimmune disease and malignancy. Evaluate for sinister causes, systemic disease, and potential triggers. In patients with a clear infectious/drug-related trigger, the purpura should resolve spontaneously. Seek Dermatology input if the cause remains unclear.

6   Pustules present?

Generalized pustular eruptions should raise the possibility of GPP or AGEP. Features that suggest AGEP (Fig. 27.5) include recent exposure (typically within 48 hours) to a new medication; rash predominantly affecting skin folds; and pinhead-sized pustules. Facial oedema may be present. GPP (Fig. 27.6) is suggested by a history of plaque psoriasis, larger pustules that coalesce into lakes of pus, and a more generalized distribution. Admit the patient and seek an urgent dermatological opinion.

7 Fever, haematological abnormalities, organ involvement?

Suspect DRESS in any patient with a generalized morbilliform rash (Fig. 27.1) with associated fever, haematological abnormalities, lymphadenopathy, and organ involvement. Haematological abnormalities that are suggestive of DRESS include eosinophilia, leukocytosis, and atypical lymphocytes. Organ involvement may present as hepatitis, AKI, myocarditis, or interstitial pneumonitis. Review all prescribed and nonprescribed medications, stop any potential causative agents and discuss urgently with Dermatology.

8 Wheals present?

Classify the rash as urticaria if there are wheals: transient (<24 hours), erythematous, intensely pruritic raised skin lesions (Fig. 27.7). Look for swelling of the lips, face and throat, suggesting associated angioedema (Fig 27.8); patients may describe the skin sensation as burning rather than itchy. Take a careful food and drug history to identify possible precipitants, although in many cases, a cause cannot be identified (idiopathic urticaria). Other than avoidance of any identified precipitant, the mainstay of treatment is regular antihistamines; most cases subside quickly with avoidance of the precipitant and/or antihistamine treatment. Refer patients with persistent

(>24 hours) or chronic (>6 weeks) lesions for outpatient dermatological assessment.

9 Underlying chronic dermatosis?

Ask about previous skin disease, recent changes to dermatological or other medications, and specifically whether the present eruption resembles previous rashes. In patients with acute flares of atopic eczema, consider bacterial infection. If there is evidence of vesicles or punched-out erosions, start antiviral treatment for eczema herpeticum (Fig. 27.9).

It is very common for hospital patients to miss their dermatological medications due to lack of prescription or interruption of their regular topical application routine; if this is the case, suspect an acute flare-up and look for resolution of the rash after reinstating routine treatment.

10 Likely drug reaction or infective exanthem. Refer to Dermatology if persistent or severe symptoms

In the absence of any specific features detailed above, most acute generalized eruptions are likely to be either infective exanthems or drug eruptions.

Precise identification of infective exanthems is seldom required as most do not need specific treatment and will settle conservatively. Seek specialist advice if the patient is a returning traveler with fever or an unusual rash.

Review all recent medications, both prescribed and over-the-counter. There is significant variation in the morphology and exposure-to-onset time of cutaneous drug eruptions. If a drug reaction is suspected (e.g., a drug from Table 27.1 is involved or there is a clear temporal association) attempt to confirm by trialing discontinuation wherever feasible. Ensure the patient is using regular emollient. Consider Dermatology referral if symptoms are persistent or troublesome.

27

28 Poisoning

Poisoning can occur secondary to accidental exposure, medication errors, deliberate self-harm or drug misuse. While poisoning secondary to drug exposure is most common in the UK, patients may also present following exposure to chemicals, plants or fauna. Assessment of the poisoned patient can be challenging as patients may be unable or unwilling to provide an accurate history. It is important to utilize a poisons information resource such as TOXBASE® (www.toxbase.org) to ensure the best possible care is provided for the patient.

Acute poisoning

Acute poisoning accounts for most poisoning episodes presenting to hospital in the UK. Obtaining an accurate history of events is critical, and this should include information about both the patient and the agent(s) in question (Table 28.1). The escalation and treatment of many poisons (e.g., paracetamol) relies on an accurate timeline of events, including both the time of exposure and the time to presentation at hospital. Obtaining this information accurately may be challenging, and management should always err on the side of caution if there is any doubt about the circumstance.

In situations where there is little or no information about the agent of exposure, a thorough knowledge and understanding of the common toxidromes can help to elucidate the nature of the poison and in turn, help to determine appropriate management. The clinical features displayed can be mapped to the appropriate toxidrome as demonstrated in Table 28.2.

In the UK, the most common drugs to be taken in intentional overdose include analgesics (e.g., paracetamol, ibuprofen, codeine), hypnotics (e.g., diazepam, zopiclone), antidepressants (e.g., sertraline, amitriptyline) and antipsychotics (e.g., quetiapine). Drugs commonly used recreationally include heroin, cocaine, diazepam, amphetamines and novel psychoactive agents. It is almost impossible to have a detailed knowledge of the toxicity of every drug. Instead, the focus should be on general principles of the assessment of poisoned patients to identify the underlying toxidrome and risk-assess the patient, before organizing relevant investigations and appropriate management. Use of a poisons information database such as TOXBASE® to guide this process is essential. Despite the many drugs that may be involved, poisoned patients generally present in either a sedated or agitated state. These states will be used to frame the diagnostic process.

Chronic poisoning

Chronic poisoning is a rarer presentation to hospital and can often pose a diagnostic challenge. Patients may not be as acutely unwell and can report vague, nonspecific symptoms that have often been present for weeks or months. There are often clues in the history, although these may be subtle, with some patients having several contacts with health professionals before a diagnosis can be established. Carbon monoxide (CO) is a cause of both acute and chronic poisoning and most commonly occurs secondary to faulty boilers in domestic properties. While acute CO poisoning presents with a sudden deterioration in consciousness level, chronic CO poisoning has a much more insidious onset, which may go undetected. Patients experience nonspecific symptoms such as headaches, nausea, and reduced appetite which improve when the patient is not within the immediate environment, e.g., leaves home and goes to work. It is only through recognition of this temporal relationship that the diagnosis may be considered. Similarly,

Table 28.1 **History in the poisoned patient**	
Agent	
Type	Drug, chemical, plant, fauna
Time	Time of exposure, correlating to paramedic history if required
Duration	Length of time of exposure
Route	Ingestion, injection, inhalational, skin or eye contact
Nature	Deliberate versus accidental
Patient	
Symptoms	Detailed history of symptoms patient is experiencing
Medical history	Relevant medical history including previous poisoning episodes
Psychiatric history	Relevant psychiatric history
Medication history	Detailed medication history, including over-the-counter medicines, recreational drug use and allergies.
	It may also be important to establish what the patient has access to, such as other household members' medication.
Alcohol history	Detailed history of current and previous alcohol use
Collateral history	Depending on information provided by the patient, a collateral history of events leading up to the admission may be important.

lead poisoning is associated with nonspecific symptoms such as abdominal pain, nausea and vomiting, which may be present for weeks before the diagnosis is made. Common sources of lead include contaminated drinking water from lead pipes or inhaled dust from lead paint that is being removed during renovations.

Table 28.2 Toxidromes				
The stimulated patient toxidromes	Observations	Pupils	Other features	Example agents
Opioid	Temperature ↓/ normal Heart rate ↓ Blood pressure ↓ Respiratory rate ↓	Miosis	↓ GCS Coma Hyporeflexia	Heroin Morphine Methadone Oxycodone
Sedative/Hypnotic	Temperature ↓/ normal Heart rate ↓/normal Blood pressure ↓/ normal Respiratory rate ↓/ normal	Miosis, mydriasis, normal	↓ GCS Confusion Coma Hyporeflexia	Benzodiazepines Alcohol GHB/GBL Barbiturates
Cholinergic	Normal temperature Heart rate ↓ Blood pressure ↓ Respiratory rate ↓	Miosis	Salivation, lacrimation Incontinence Diarrhoea Diaphoresis Bronchoconstriction Muscle fasciculations Convulsions	Organophosphate and carbamate insecticides Nerve agents
Carbon monoxide	Temperature ↓/ normal Heart rate ↑/↓ Blood pressure ↓/ normal Respiratory rate ↑	Normal	Headache Nausea and vomiting Confusion Ataxia v GCS Seizures	Carbon monoxide

Table 28.2 Toxidromes—cont'd				
The stimulated patient toxidromes	**Observations**	**Pupils**	**Other features**	**Example agents**
Sympathomimetic	Temperature ↑ Heart rate ↑ Blood pressure ↑ Respiratory rate↑	Mydriasis	Diaphoresis Agitation Hyperreflexia Seizures Paranoia	Cocaine Amphetamine Ephedrine Cathinones
Anticholinergic	Temperature ↑ Heart rate ↑ Blood pressure ↑/ normal Respiratory rate ↑	Mydriasis	Dry, flushed skin Dry mucous membranes Urinary retention Agitation and delirium Visual hallucinations (picking at objects in air)	TCAs Antihistamines Phenothiazines Atropine
Serotonin toxicity	Temperature ↑ Heart rate ↑ Blood pressure ↑ Respiratory rate ↑	Mydriasis	Hyperreflexia Myoclonus Clonus (lower extremities) Diaphoresis Diarrhoea	SSRIs SNRIs TCAs MAOIs MDMA
Methaemoglobinaemia	Temperature ↑/ normal Heart rate ↑ Blood pressure ↓/↑ Respiratory rate ↑	Normal	Apparent cyanosis SpO_2 85–90% with normal PaO_2 Headache Myocardial ischaemia Convulsions ↓ GCS	Alkyl nitrites Dapsone Prilocaine Benzocaine

28

The sedated poisoned patient

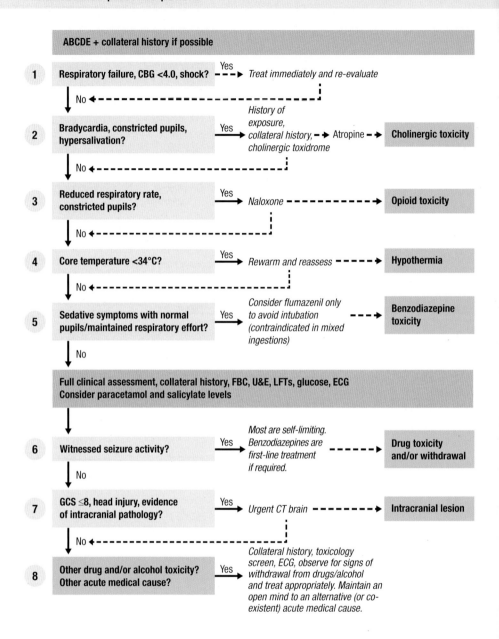

1 | Respiratory failure, CBG<4.0, shock?

Ensure a patent airway and provide cervical spine control if trauma is suspected. If the GCS score is ≤8, then definitive airway management may be required. Look for and treat rapidly reversible causes of reduced GCS score as per the ABCDE assessment:

- Assess oxygenation and ventilation by blood gas analysis. Treat hypoxia and hypercapnia urgently.
- Consider CO poisoning (Table 28.2) and check the carboxyhaemoglobin (COHb) concentration on the blood gas. Clinical features of CO poisoning are nonspecific; the diagnosis may be missed unless specifically considered. Nonsmokers typically have a COHb concentration of 1–2%, while in smokers this baseline may be 5–10%.
- Give a therapeutic/diagnostic dose of naloxone if there are features of opioid toxicity and evidence of respiratory depression (e.g., $PaCO_2$ ↑).
- Check capillary blood glucose (CBG) level; if <4.0 mmol/L, treat immediately with IV dextrose or IV/IM glucagon. Send blood for formal laboratory glucose measurement.
- Look for evidence of shock and, if present, treat appropriately (Box 2.1).

2 | Bradycardia, constricted pupils and hypersalivation?

Cholinergic toxidrome results in some clinical features which are similar to opioid toxicity. Some of the critical distinguishing clinical features of cholinergic toxicity are the presence of secretions (e.g., salivation, lacrimation, diarrhoea, diaphoresis), bronchoconstriction, fasciculations, and convulsions. Consider cholinergic toxicity if there is a history of exposure to a precipitating agent or supportive clinical features are present. A history of exposure particularly to agents which cause cholinergic poisoning may not always be apparent.

3 | Reduced respiratory rate and constricted pupils?

Consider opioid toxicity in any patient who has clinical features of opioid toxidrome (Table 28.2). Look for additional clues in the history (e.g., medication history, use of recreational drugs) and examination findings (e.g., presence of needle marks, fentanyl patch). Give a therapeutic/diagnostic dose of naloxone if opioid toxicity is suspected. A rapid improvement in consciousness level and oxygenation supports the diagnosis and indicates that opioids are, at least in part, contributing to the clinical state. The half-life of naloxone is shorter than that of most opioids, and so ongoing monitoring and repeated naloxone doses ± an infusion may be required. If the toxidrome is not fully reversed by naloxone, e.g., improved respiratory rate but GCS score remains low, then consider mixed overdose of sedative agents.

4 | Core temperature <34°C?

Poisoned patients are at risk of developing hypothermia, particularly after a prolonged period of immobility or exposure to cold or wet conditions. Diagnose hypothermia if there is a tympanic membrane reading <35°C. Rewarm and reassess whilst searching for additional causes.

28

5 **Sedative symptoms dominant with normal pupils/maintained respiratory effort?**

Benzodiazepines are a class of drug which is both commonly prescribed and misused recreationally. Benzodiazepine toxicity is therefore a common diagnosis in the poisoned patient population and should be considered in all patients displaying clinical features of the sedative toxidrome (Table 28.2). Flumazenil can reverse the effects of benzodiazepines and may be considered to avoid mechanical ventilation in patients with GCS score ≤8 where the cause is known to be solely due to benzodiazepines. However, it is not recommended as a diagnostic test (unlike naloxone, as described above) or in mixed ingestions where a proconvulsant drug may have been ingested, as its use has been associated with convulsions. Most other drugs associated with a sedative toxidrome have no specific management, and patients should be cared for supportively (see below).

6 **Witnessed seizure activity?**

Seizures are common in poisoned patients. They are not only associated with exposure to the drugs themselves, but may also occur because of hypoglycaemia, head injury and alcohol withdrawal, which frequently occur in the context of poisoning. Reduced GCS is common in the postictal period and, if possible, a corroborating history from an eye-witness is helpful to support the diagnosis. For further information on the assessment of seizures, see Chapter 24. Seizures in toxicology are often brief and self-limiting. Benzodiazepines are appropriate first-line treatment. However, it is important when considering pharmacological therapy not to worsen poisoning, e.g., avoid phenytoin in seizing poisoned patients due to its sodium channel–blocking effects.

7 **GCS ≤8, head injury, evidence of intracranial pathology?**

Once reversible causes of reduced GCS scores have been identified and treated, arrange an urgent CT head if any of the following are present:
- GCS score ≤8
- Evidence of focal neurological symptoms or lateralizing signs (e.g., unilateral pupillary abnormality) or signs of raised ICP (Box 15.1)
- Head injury

8 **Other drug or alcohol toxicity?**

For most poisonings, there is no diagnostic test or specific management, and best supportive care should be prioritized. Mixed ingestions are common, and patients may exhibit a range of clinical features. Check routine blood tests, CK and paracetamol level (if in UK) in all patients, and consider salicylate levels if there is any suggestion of metabolic disturbance. Capillary BG should be continuously monitored. Many drugs have the potential to cause cardiotoxicity, and so a 12-lead ECG should be performed with particular attention being paid to the QRS and QT intervals.

Alcohol misuse often coexists with poisoning. However, it is important never to assume that reduced GCS score is secondary to alcohol, even in patients with a known history of alcohol misuse. The correlation between breath or blood alcohol levels and consciousness level is poor, and so these values are helpful only in confirming alcohol is present. Patients with a history of alcohol excess should be treated with thiamine to prevent Wernicke's encephalopathy and monitored for signs of withdrawal. Urine or oral toxicology screens may be carried out and help to inform future practice, but they seldom are available in a sufficiently timely fashion to affect acute management.

The stimulated poisoned patient

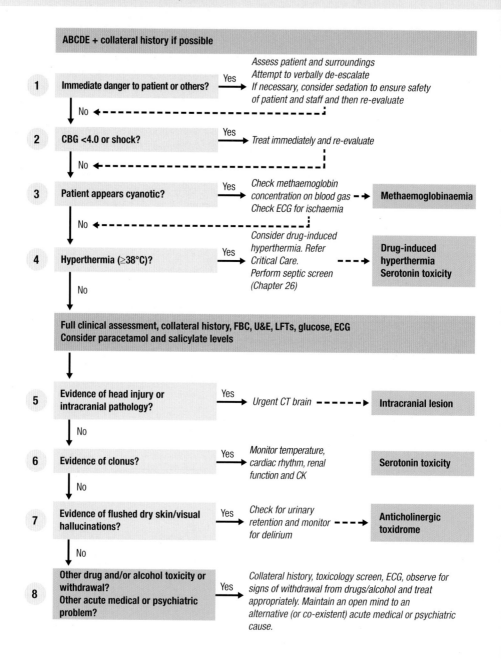

1 Immediate danger to patient or others?

Stimulated poisoned patients can pose a particular management challenge. It is important to call for senior help early and consider the safety of the patient, yourself, and anyone else in the immediate vicinity. While every effort should be made to diagnose the problem and instigate appropriate management, it may be necessary to administer sedation in the first instance to ensure the safety of the patient and others before other investigations can be carried out.

2 CBG <4.0 or shock?

Hypoglycaemia may present in a variety of ways, and patients can become confused and agitated as their blood glucose level falls. Check CBG and if <4.0 mmol/L, treat immediately with IV dextrose or IV/IM glucagon. Send blood for formal laboratory glucose measurement. Look for evidence of shock (Box 2.1); if present, treat appropriately.

3 Patient appears cyanotic?

Poisoned patients may appear cyanotic in the presence of methaemoglobinaemia. Methaemoglobinaemia (MetHb) is a condition of an elevated concentration of methaemoglobin in the blood. Methaemoglobin is an altered state of haemoglobin in which ferrous ions (Fe^{2+}) of haem are oxidized to ferric ions (Fe^{3+}) and unable to carry oxygen. Methaemoglobinaemia may occur following exposure to certain drugs (Table 28.2) and the patient may appear cyanotic with, if severe, signs of reduced oxygen delivery to vital organs (e.g., chest pain, ischaemic ECG). Oxygen saturations via finger probe measurements are unreliable and typically read 85–90%, while PaO_2 via blood gas measurement is normal. Check a MetHb level on blood gas measurement (normal level <1.5%). Mild effects are observed with levels of 10-30%, moderate effects occur when MetHb is 30-50% and severe effects occur with levels >50%.

4 Hyperthermia (≥38°C)?

Drug-induced hyperthermia in the poisoned patient is an important clinical sign which is associated with a poor prognosis without treatment. Hyperthermia can be a feature of several different stimulant toxidromes (Table 28.2), but it is a particularly important prognostic marker in the sympathomimetic and serotonin toxidromes, which are associated with high morbidity and mortality. Drug-induced hyperthermia can be associated with disseminated intravascular coagulation, rhabdomyolysis and multiorgan failure. Patients should be identified early and transferred to a critical care environment for active cooling and pharmacological intervention, e.g., benzodiazepines, cyproheptadine. Paracetamol is not effective as an antipyretic for drug-induced hyperthermia.

Hyperthermia may also signify sepsis, which may coexist in the poisoned patient. Perform a septic screen and commence antibiotics if appropriate. It is important in poisoned patients not to assume that pyrexia is the result of infection, as drug-induced hyperthermia is associated with significant morbidity and mortality if untreated.

5 Evidence of head injury or intracranial pathology?

Agitation may occur in the context of a head injury or other intracranial pathology. Arrange an urgent CT head if there is any evidence of a head injury, focal neurological symptoms or lateralizing signs (e.g., unilateral pupillary abnormality) or signs of raised ICP (Box 15.1).

6 Evidence of clonus?

Mild to moderate serotonin toxicity may occur in the absence of pyrexia. The presence of clonus in the context of poisoning is diagnostic of serotonin toxicity. Patients require careful monitoring for drug-induced pyrexia and the emergence of neurological excitation (seizures) and cardiovascular instability. Patients

28

with mild-moderate serotonin toxicity are at risk of rhabdomyolysis and require careful assessment of CK and renal function.

7 Evidence of flushed dry skin/visual hallucinations?

Anticholinergic toxidrome is underrecognized and underdiagnosed in clinical practice. Patients often have a florid delirium manifesting as visual hallucinations, restlessness and picking at objects. Patients with an anticholinergic toxidrome are at substantial risk from seizures and arrhythmias and require careful monitoring. Ensure urine output is monitored as urinary retention is a common clinical sign.

8 Other drug or alcohol toxicity or withdrawal? Other acute medical or psychiatric problem?

Agitation is a common clinical feature in poisoned patients as it can be associated with drug toxicity and/or withdrawal in regular drug users. It may also be associated with alcohol misuse and/or withdrawal which commonly coexist in poisoned patients. It is imperative to gather as much information about the history as possible, including a collateral from relatives or friends if available. As described above, patients with a history of alcohol excess should be treated with thiamine to prevent Wernicke's encephalopathy and monitored for signs of withdrawal. GHB/GBL are associated with profound sedation (toxicity) and agitation (withdrawal). If clinically suspected, seek senior support early.

Check routine blood tests to look for abnormalities in renal and liver function as well as raised inflammatory markers which may be associated with infection. Consider paracetamol and salicylate levels if there is any suggestion that these drugs may be involved. Monitor CBG and perform a 12-lead ECG. Stimulatory drugs are frequently associated with QRS and QT prolongation or ischaemia with ST/T wave changes. Urine or oral toxicology screens may be carried out and help to inform future practice, but they seldom are available in a sufficiently timely fashion to affect acute management.

Psychotic features may occur because of drug exposure but can also signify an underlying psychiatric illness. All patients displaying psychotic features should be referred to Psychiatry. It may be possible to confirm the diagnosis only after a period of time to allow the effects of the drug to wear off. If the psychosis persists beyond this time, this supports the presence of an underlying psychiatric condition.

Acute kidney injury 29

Acute kidney injury (AKI) is the acute impairment of kidney function, defined by either a rise in serum creatinine or a fall in urine output. The numerical thresholds for defining and determining the severity of AKI can be found in Table 29.1. It is not a diagnosis in itself but represents kidney dysfunction as a result of one or more underlying aetiologies. Many presentations can be complicated by AKI, to be identified during the assessment of those illnesses. AKI may also be the primary cause for a patient's presentation, or it may develop during a patient's hospital admission. Factors that increase susceptibility to developing AKI can be found in Box 29.1.

AKI is associated with increased risk of mortality and progression to CKD. Severity of AKI correlates to worse outcomes and, therefore, early identification and management is essential. Susceptible patients (Box 29.1) who are exposed to known precipitants such as infection, major surgery, and new medications that can impair renal function (Table 29.2) should be monitored for the development of AKI. Acute management should focus on the management of any complications (such as hyperkalaemia and fluid overload) and the treatment of contributing causes. These causes are typically classified as prerenal, renal, or postrenal.

Prerenal causes

Prerenal AKI is caused by reduced glomerular filtration due to impaired renal perfusion. Provided there is prompt restoration of renal perfusion, prerenal AKI is reversible. Impairment of renal perfusion can be due to:
- Shock (Chapter 2)
- Hypovolaemia e.g., reduced oral intake, haemorrhage, diarrhoeal illness, over-diuresis, third-space losses in pancreatitis and burns
- Reduced cardiac output, e.g., heart failure, massive PE, cardiac tamponade
- Decreased systemic vascular resistance e.g., sepsis, liver failure
- Renovascular disease e.g., renal artery stenosis or thrombosis, renal vein thrombosis
- Medications (Table 29.2)

Renal causes

Renal causes of AKI include intrinsic renal disease and damage to the renal parenchyma. Causes include:
- Acute tubular necrosis (ATN)—damage to the tubular epithelial cells as a result of either ischaemia or toxins. Ischaemia can develop in response to a prolonged or severe decrease in renal perfusion. Therefore, unrecognized or undertreated causes of prerenal AKI can result in ATN. Most causes of AKI are either prerenal or ATN after a persistent drop in renal perfusion. Toxins include medications (Table 29.2), myoglobin (in rhabdomyolysis), and serum-free light chains (in myeloma).
- Rapidly progressive glomerulonephritis (RPGN)—immune-mediated glomerular injury with an associated rapid loss of renal function. Causes to consider are ANCA-associated vasculitis, anti-GBM disease, and conditions associated with immune complex deposition in the glomerulus e.g., postinfectious glomerulonephritis, lupus nephritis and infectious endocarditis.
- Acute interstitial nephritis (AIN)—inflammation of the renal tubules and interstitium, typically due to a hypersensitivity reaction to medications (Table 29.2). Other causes include infections and some inflammatory conditions (e.g., sarcoidosis, Sjogren syndrome).

Table 29.1 Staging of AKI		
Stage	Serum creatinine	Urine output
1	1.5–1.9 times baseline[a] OR ≥ 26.5 µmol/L increase[b]	<0.5 ml/kg/hr for 6–12 hours
2	2.0–2.9 times baseline	<0.5 ml/kg/hr for ≥12 hours
3	3.0 times baseline OR Increase in serum creatinine to ≥353.6 µmol/L OR Initiation of renal replacement therapy (RRT)	<0.3 ml/kg/hr for ≥24 hours OR Anuria for ≥12 hours

[a]Known or presumed to have occurred in previous seven days.
[b]Within 48 hours.
Adapted from Kellum JA, Lameire N, Aspelin P, et al. Acute Kidney Injury Work Group. Kidney disease: improving global outcomes (KDIGO). Clinical practice guideline for acute kidney injury (AKI). Kidney International Supplements 2012:1(2):1–138.

Box 29.1 **Factors that increase susceptibility to developing AKI**

- Age > 65 years
- Female gender
- Black race
- Chronic Kidney Disease
- History of AKI
- Heart failure
- Atherosclerotic cardiovascular disease
- Liver disease
- Diabetes mellitus
- Use of medications that impair renal function (Table 29.2)
- Anaemia
- Frailty
- Cognitive impairment

- Microangiopathies—haemolytic uraemic syndrome, malignant hypertension, and thrombotic thrombocytopenic purpura all cause damage to the renal microvasculature.

Postrenal causes

Postrenal causes of AKI include any condition that obstruct the normal urinary outflow tract causing back-pressure of urine into the kidneys. The obstruction can be at the level of the lower urinary tract (urethra, bladder, prostate) or the upper urinary tract (kidneys and ureters). Unless there is a single functioning kidney, an obstruction will usually affect both kidneys to cause an AKI, as one kidney will compensate for a decrease in function of the other. Most postrenal AKI is therefore caused by lower urinary tract obstruction. Causes of lower urinary tract obstruction include benign prostatic hyperplasia (BPH), prostate cancer, bladder cancer, urethral strictures, neurogenic bladder and medications. Obstruction of the upper urinary tract can be caused by urinary calculi, external compression from pelvic cancer, and retroperitoneal fibrosis. Like prerenal AKI, permanent damage to the renal parenchyma can be avoided with prompt treatment.

Table 29.2 Medications associated with AKI/hyperkalaemia

Medication	Effect	Action in AKI
Diuretics	Exacerbate hypovolaemia	Withhold in AKI
ACE inhibitors/angiotensin receptor blockers	Inhibit constriction of glomerular efferent arteriole resulting in ↓glomerular transcapillary pressure and ↓GFR; exacerbate hyperkalaemia	Withhold in AKI
Other antihypertensives	Exacerbate renal hypoperfusion in hypotensive patients	Withhold if hypotensive
NSAIDs	Inhibit vasodilation of glomerular afferent arteriole resulting in ↓glomerular transcapillary pressure and ↓GFR. Rarely causes AIN. Can cause ATN	Withhold in AKI
Aminoglycoside antibiotics	Toxicity to tubular epithelial cells	Stop if felt to be cause of AKI. Avoid if possible in patients with established AKI. If used, reduce dose and monitor levels carefully
Amphotericin B	Toxicity to tubular epithelial cells	Stop if felt to be cause of AKI. Avoid if possible in patients with established AKI
Contrast media	Toxicity to tubular epithelial cells	Consider as cause for AKI. Use with caution in established AKI
Vancomycin	Toxicity to tubular epithelial cells at high levels	Careful dosing and drug monitoring
Cisplatin	Toxicity to tubular epithelial cells	Consider in patients with AKI who are receiving chemotherapy
β-lactam antibiotics Co-trimoxazole Vancomycin Phenytoin Allopurinol Ciprofloxacin Thiazide diuretics Furosemide Protein pump inhibitors H2 antagonists	Possible causes of AIN	Consider as precipitant for AKI if intrinsic renal disease suspected
Trimethoprim	May exacerbate hyperkalaemia	Use with care in AKI. Either avoid or reduce dose
Digoxin	May exacerbate hyperkalaemia	Monitor drug levels and consider reducing dose

Overview

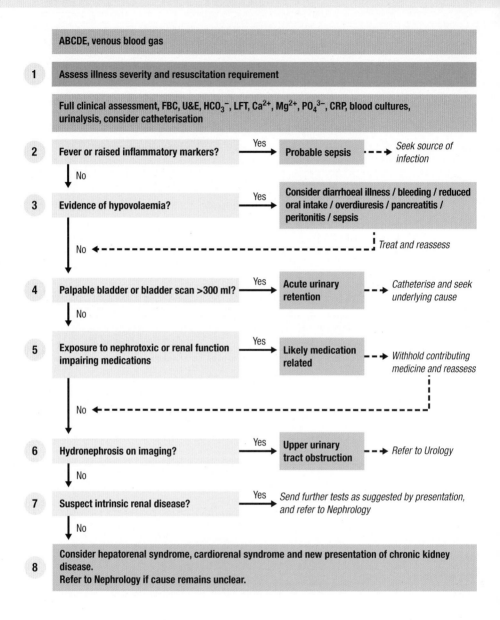

ABCDE, venous blood gas

1   **Assess illness severity and resuscitation requirement**

Full clinical assessment, FBC, U&E, HCO_3^-, LFT, Ca^{2+}, Mg^{2+}, PO_4^{3-}, CRP, blood cultures, urinalysis, consider catheterisation

2   Fever or raised inflammatory markers?   Yes → **Probable sepsis** - - → *Seek source of infection*

No ↓

3   Evidence of hypovolaemia?   Yes → **Consider diarrhoeal illness / bleeding / reduced oral intake / overdiuresis / pancreatitis / peritonitis / sepsis**

No ← - *Treat and reassess*

4   Palpable bladder or bladder scan >300 ml?   Yes → **Acute urinary retention** - - → *Catheterise and seek underlying cause*

No ↓

5   Exposure to nephrotoxic or renal function impairing medications   Yes → **Likely medication related** - - → *Withhold contributing medicine and reassess*

No ← -

6   Hydronephrosis on imaging?   Yes → **Upper urinary tract obstruction** - - → *Refer to Urology*

No ↓

7   Suspect intrinsic renal disease?   Yes → *Send further tests as suggested by presentation, and refer to Nephrology*

No ↓

8   Consider hepatorenal syndrome, cardiorenal syndrome and new presentation of chronic kidney disease.
Refer to Nephrology if cause remains unclear.

1 Assess illness severity and resuscitation requirement

Step 1 Are there features of shock?
Diagnosis of AKI requires either the availability of blood results or the close monitoring of urine output. Therefore, it is likely that a patient assessment has been carried out prior to AKI being identified, and appropriate treatment for the precipitant of AKI may have already been initiated, such as fluid resuscitation in hypovolaemic shock. In cases where treatment has not been started, identification of an AKI should trigger a reassessment and specific consideration of shock as a cause. Look for ↓BP or evidence of tissue hypoperfusion (Box 2.1). If shock is suspected, then assess and manage as per Chapter 2.

Step 2 Is there hyperkalaemia?
Hyperkalaemia is a serious complication of AKI. Early identification and treatment are critical as it is associated with arrhythmia and cardiac arrest. Moderate hyperkalaemia is a potassium concentration of 6–6.4 mmol/L, and severe hyperkalaemia is a potassium concentration ≥6.5 mmol/L. In all patients with moderate/severe hyperkalaemia, perform an urgent 12-lead ECG. If there are any ECG changes suggestive of hyperkalaemia (Figure 29.1), or when K^+ is ≥6.5 mmol/L, attach the patient to a cardiac monitor and give immediate intravenous calcium (30 mL 10% calcium gluconate or 10 mL 10% calcium chloride) to stabilize the myocardium. In any patient with moderate/severe hyperkalaemia, lower the serum potassium with an insulin/dextrose infusion (e.g., 10 units of insulin in 50 mL 50% dextrose followed by an infusion of 10% glucose at 50 mL/hour for 5 hours (25g) in patients with a pretreatment blood glucose >7 mmol/L) and a 10–20 mg salbutamol nebulizer. Sodium zirconium cyclosilicate and patiromer are potassium binders that can be used as additional options to lower potassium in severe hyperkalaemia. Patients should have their potassium repeated after 1, 2 and 4 hours to monitor the effect of treatment. Those with severe hyperkalaemia, which is refractory to medical management, should be referred to Nephrology and/or Critical Care for consideration of renal replacement therapy (RRT).

Step 3 Is there any indication for urgent renal replacement therapy?
Other acute complications of AKI include fluid overload ± pulmonary oedema, metabolic acidosis, and uraemic complications such as encephalopathy and pericarditis. Suspect pulmonary oedema in patients with classic clinical features such as ↑ RR, ↓ SpO_2, hypertension, peripheral oedema, ↑ JVP and bilateral crepitations. Arrange a CXR and give oxygen and diuretic. Metabolic acidosis will be identified on a venous blood gas. IV sodium bicarbonate can be given under expert supervision. Emergency RRT should be considered, and patients referred to Nephrology or Critical Care, if there is:

- Refractory metabolic acidosis (pH <7.15)
- Refractory fluid overload, including pulmonary oedema
- Uraemic complications of AKI — encephalopathy, pericarditis, myopathy, neuropathy, uraemic bleeding
- Refractory hyperkalaemia (K^+ ≥6.5)

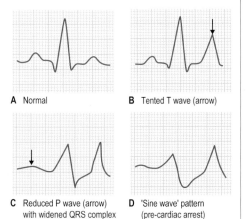

A Normal **B** Tented T wave (arrow)

C Reduced P wave (arrow) with widened QRS complex **D** 'Sine wave' pattern (pre-cardiac arrest)

Fig. 29.1 Progressive ECG changes with worsening hyperkalaemia. (Note for Creative Commons: This figure appears as Fig. 9.12 in Feather A, Randall D, Waterhouse M. Kumar and Clark's clinical medicine, 10th ed. Philadelphia: Elsevier, 2021.)

2 Fever or raised inflammatory markers?

In patients with an undifferentiated AKI, sepsis is the first cause to exclude. Sepsis can cause AKI, even in the absence of shock. Suspect sepsis in patients with fever, raised inflammatory markers, tachycardia, or hypotension. Perform a septic screen (Chapter 26). If a source of infection is identified, initiate targeted antibiotics and start IV fluids. If there is no clear source but a high index of suspicion for sepsis, start fluids and broad-spectrum antibiotics pending investigation results. If sepsis is deemed unlikely, antibiotics are not required. However, remain vigilant for developing signs of infection.

3 Evidence of hypovolaemia?

Assessment of a patient's volume status is key to the management of AKI. Factors in the history which suggest hypovolaemia include diarrhoea and vomiting, bleeding, reduced oral intake, thirst, postural dizziness and use of diuretic medications. On examination, look for cool peripheries, dry mucous membranes, prolonged capillary refill time, reduced skin turgor, ↑RR, ↑HR and ↓BP. Postural hypotension can be a useful early sign of hypovolaemia. Note that a patient can appear to be normotensive, but a low blood pressure compared to their normal suggests relative hypotension.

Be aware of hypovolaemia in conditions where fluid losses are less overt. Pancreatitis, burns, and peritonitis are all associated with third-space losses that will result in hypovolaemia. Hypovolaemia often coexists with sepsis due to increased insensible losses.

Give IV crystalloid to restore circulating volume. AKI secondary to hypovolaemia is confirmed by an improvement in creatinine/urine output following fluid resuscitation. Consider other causes if AKI does not improve.

4 Palpable bladder or bladder scan >300mL?

Consider urinary retention in all patients presenting with an AKI and perform a bedside bladder USS. Patients may be asymptomatic or have symptoms of anuria, lower abdominal pain and/or have a palpable bladder. A post-void residual volume of >300 mL is diagnostic of urinary retention, and a catheter should be inserted to relieve the obstruction. A new diagnosis of urinary retention should prompt investigation to determine the underlying cause.

Evaluate for UTI, constipation, and conditions that could cause a neurogenic bladder (e.g., multiple sclerosis). Review any medications that could contribute (Box 23.2). In men, ask about lower urinary tract symptoms, perform a digital rectal examination to assess the prostate, and refer to Urology for further evaluation if prostatic disease is suspected. In women, ask about previous pelvic surgery or radiation, perform a pelvic examination to check for prolapse or pelvic tumours, and refer to Urology.

5 Exposure to nephrotoxic or renal function impairing medications?

Medications cause AKI either by impacting glomerular perfusion (e.g., ACE inhibitors) or by toxicity to the renal parenchyma (e.g., aminoglycoside antibiotics). They can be a contributing factor to AKI in patients with sepsis, hypovolaemia, and urinary retention, or can be the primary cause of AKI. All patients with an AKI should have a detailed medication review to identify medications that may be contributing to AKI, and renally excreted medications that could accumulate in the presence of AKI. This review should include over-the-counter medications and recreational drugs. Medications that could contribute to AKI (Table 29.2) should be withheld and renally excreted medications may require a dose reduction or temporary cessation to prevent toxicity.

When no other precipitant for AKI has been identified, suspect medications as the primary cause if there has been a recent exposure to a nephrotoxic medication, or the introduction or change in dose of a medication that is known to impair glomerular perfusion (Table 29.2). Withhold the medication, ensure adequate hydration, and monitor kidney function.

6 Hydronephrosis on imaging?

In patients with AKI, fever, and flank pain, an infected upper urinary tract obstruction (i.e., pyonephrosis) should be suspected, and urgent imaging with renal tract US should be arranged within 6 hours, as infected obstructions of the upper urinary tract are associated with a high risk of septic shock. If US is unavailable urgently, then a CTKUB (kidneys, ureter, bladder) should be performed. Refer urgently to Urology if obstruction is identified.

Any other patient in whom obstruction is suspected, AKI is unexplained, or in whom AKI is not improving with treatment, should have renal tract US within 24 hours. All patients with evidence of upper urinary tract obstruction, suggested by hydronephrosis on imaging, should be referred to Urology for further management.

7   Suspect intrinsic renal disease?

Intrinsic renal disease is the least common cause of AKI. Most cases of AKI have one or more clear precipitants. Intrinsic renal disease should be suspected when no precipitants have been identified or when the patient has suggestive symptoms, signs, or investigation results.

Consider RPGN in patients with positive urinalysis for blood and protein. Diagnosis of RPGN is supported by a subacute presentation of fever and fatigue with evidence of multisystem disease. Suspect ANCA-associated vasculitis or anti-GBM disease in patients with haemoptysis or evidence of pulmonary haemorrhage. Vasculitis may also be suggested by involvement of the skin, upper airways, joints, or nerves. Consider lupus nephritis in patients with a history of joint pains, photosensitive rash, mouth and genital ulceration, dry eyes and dry mouth, alopecia, or Raynaud phenomenon. A recent history of infection may suggest postinfectious glomerulonephritis. If RPGN is suspected, send the investigations listed in Table 29.3.

Investigate for rhabdomyolysis by sending a CK if there is muscle pain, haematuria on dipstick, brown discolouration of the urine, or a history of a long lie. Consider multiple myeloma in patients with bone pain, anaemia, and hypercalcaemia. If suspected, send serum-free light chains and a urinary Bence Jones protein. Microangiopathies should be considered in patients with haemolysis (see Further Assessment of Anaemia, Chapter 25) and thrombocytopenia associated with AKI. Presentation of AIN is often nonspecific but may be associated with fever, maculopapular rash, and eosinophilia.

Table 29.3 Serological investigations in suspected glomerulonephritis

Test	Underlying diagnosis
ANA	Connective tissue disease, such as SLE
Anti-dsDNA	—
Extractable nuclear antigens	—
Anti-GBM antibodies	Goodpasture disease
ANCA	Vasculitis, for example, granulomatosis with polyangiitis
Anti-streptolysin O titre	Post-streptococcal glomerulonephritis
Cryoglobulins	Cryoglobulinaemia

If intrinsic renal disease is suspected, refer urgently to Nephrology for ongoing investigation and management.

8   Consider hepatorenal syndrome, cardiorenal syndrome and new presentation of chronic kidney disease. Refer to Nephrology if cause remains unclear

Hepatorenal syndrome should be considered as a cause of AKI in any patient with advanced liver disease and AKI when other causes have been excluded. Its management requires specialist input from the Hepatology team.

Cardiorenal syndrome (CRS) describes a condition in which a deterioration of heart function causes a deterioration of kidney function, and vice versa. AKI caused by acute heart failure is categorized as type 1 CRS. Suspect this in patients presenting with acute decompensated heart failure, MI, or cardiogenic shock with associated AKI, and refer to Cardiology for ongoing management.

In patients in whom there is no recent creatinine result available, a diagnosis of CKD can be considered. This would be supported by small kidneys on renal US, anaemia, secondary hyperparathyroidism, and symptoms of fatigue and pruritis. However, if there is any doubt, treat as AKI.

If the cause remains unclear, or the AKI is worsening despite intervention, refer to Nephrology for further assessment and consideration of kidney biopsy.

29

Appendix

	Reference range[a]	
Analyte	**SI units**	**Non-SI units**
Alanine aminotransferase (ALT)	10–50 U/L	–
Albumin	35–50 g/L	3.5–5.0 g/dL
Alkaline phosphatase (ALP)	40–125 U/L	–
Aspartate aminotransferase (AST)	10–45 U/L	–
Bilirubin (total)	2–21 µmol/L	0.18–1.23 mg/dL
Calcium (total)	2.1–2.6 mmol/L	4.2–5.2 mEq/L or 8.5–10.5 mg/dL
Chloride	95–107 mmol/L	95–107 mEq/L
Cholesterol (total)	3.5 – 6.5 mmol/L (ideal <5.2 mmol/L)	–
C-reactive protein (CRP)	<5 mg/L	–

Creatine kinase (CK) (total)
  Male
  Female
	
	55–170 U/L
	30–135 U/L
		
		–
		–

Creatinine
  Male
  Female
	
	64–111 µmol/L
	50 – 98 µmol/L
		
		0.72–1.26 mg/dL
		0.57–1.11 mg/dL

Gamma-glutamyl transferase (GGT)
  Male
  Female
	
	10–55 U/L
	5 – 35 U/L
		
		–
		–

Glucose (fasting)	3.6–5.8 mmol/L	65–104 mg/dL
Glycated haemoglobin (HbA_{1c})	4.0 – 6.0% 20 – 42 mmol/mol Hb	–
Lactate	0.6–2.4 mmol/L	5.40–21.6 mg/dL
Lactate dehydrogenase (LDH) (total)	125–220 U/L	–
Phosphate (fasting)	0.8–1.4 mmol/L	2.48–4.34 mg/dL
Potassium (serum)	3.6–5.1 mmol/L	3.6–5.1 mEq/L
Protein (total)	60–80 g/L	6–8 g/dL
Sodium	135–145 mmol/L	135–145 mEq/L

Triglycerides (fasting)
  Male
  Female
	
	0.7–2.1 mmol/L
	0.5–1.7 mmol/L
		
		–

Normal values for biochemical tests in venous blood

Normal values for biochemical tests in venous blood—cont'd

Analyte	Reference range[a] SI units	Non-SI units
Urate		
Male	120 –420 µmol/L	2.0–7.0 mg/dL
Female	120 – 360 µmol/L	2.0–6.0 mg/dL
Urea	2.5–6.6 mmol/L	15–40 mg/dL

[a]Note these values may vary according to local laboratory calibration.

Arterial blood analysis

Analysis	Reference range SI units	Non-SI units
Bicarbonate (HCO₃)	21–29 mmol/L	21–29 mEq/L
Hydrogen ion (H⁺)	37–45 nmol/L	pH 7.35–7.43
PaCO₂	4.5–6.0 kPa	34–45 mmHg
PaO₂	12–15 kPa	90–113 mmHg
Oxygen saturation (SpO₂)	>97%[a,b]	

[a]Breathing room air.
[b]Varies with age.

Haematological values

Analysis	Reference range SI units	Non-SI units
Bleeding time (Ivy)	<8 min	–
Blood volume		
Male	65–85 mL/kg	–
Female	60–80 mL/kg	
Coagulation screen		
Prothrombin time	10.5–13.5 secs	–
Activated partial thromboplastin time	26–36 secs	–
Erythrocyte sedimentation rate (ESR)	Higher values may be normal in older patients	
Adult male	0–10 mm/hr	
Adult female	3–15 mm/hr	–
Ferritin		
Male (and postmenopausal female)	20–300 µg/L	20–300 ng/mL
Premenopausal female	15–200 µg/L	15–200 ng/mL
Fibrinogen	1.5–4.0 g/L	0.15–0.4 g/dL
Folate		
Serum	2.8–20 µg/L	2.8–20 ng/mL
Red cell	120–500 µg/L	120–500 ng/mL
Haemoglobin		
Male	130–180 g/L	13–18 g/dL
Female	115–165 g/L	11.5–16.5 g/dL

Continued

Haematological values—cont'd	Reference range	
Analysis	SI units	Non-SI units
Haptoglobin	0.4–2.4 g/L	0.04–0.24 g/dL

Iron
  Male
  Female
	
	14–32 µmol/L
	10–28 µmol/L
		
		78–178 µg/dL
		56–157 µg/dL

Leukocytes (adults)	$4.0–11.0 \times 10^9$/L	$4.0–11.0 \times 10^3$/mm^3

Differential white cell count
  Neutrophil granulocytes
  Lymphocytes
  Monocytes
  Eosinophil granulocytes
  Basophil granulocytes
	
	$2.0–7.5 \times 10^9$/L
	$1.5–4.0 \times 10^9$/L
	$0.2–0.8 \times 10^9$/L
	$0.04–0.4 \times 10^9$/L
	$0.01–0.1 \times 10^9$/L
		
		$2.0–7.5 \times 10^3$/mm^3
		$1.5–4.0 \times 10^3$/mm^3
		$0.2–0.8 \times 10^3$/mm^3
		$0.04–0.4 \times 10^3$/mm^3
		$0.01–0.1 \times 10^3$/mm^3

Mean cell haemoglobin (MCH)	27–32 pg	–
Mean cell volume (MCV)	78–98 fL	–

Packed cell volume (PCV) or haematocrit
  Male
  Female
	
	0.40–0.54
	0.37–0.47
		
		–
		–

Platelets	$150–350 \times 10^9$/L	$150–350 \times 10^3$/mm^3

Red cell count
  Male
  Female
	
	$4.5–6.5 \times 10^{12}$/L
	$3.8–5.8 \times 10^{12}$/L
		
		$4.5–6.5 \times 10^6$/mm^3
		$3.8–5.8 \times 10^6$/mm^3

Red cell lifespan
  Mean
  Half-life (^{51}Cr)
	
	120 days
	25–35 days
		
		–
		–

Reticulocytes (adults)	$25–85 \times 10^9$/L	$25–85 \times 10^3$/mm^3
Transferrin	2.0–4.0 g/L	0.2–0.4 g/dL

Transferrin saturation
  Male
  Female
	
	25–50%
	14–50%
		
		–
		–

Vitamin B$_{12}$
  Normal
  Intermediate
  Low
	
	>210 pg/mL
	180–200 pg/mL
	<180 pg/mL
		
		–

Source: Reproduced with permission from Innes A. Davidson's Essentials of Medicine. Edinburgh: Churchill Livingstone, 3rd ed. 2020.

Index